DORLAND'S DERMATOLOGY WORD BOOK FOR MEDICAL TRANSCRIPTIONISTS

DORLAND'S DERMATOLOGY WORD BOOK FOR MEDICAL TRANSCRIPTIONISTS

Series Editor:
SHARON B. RHODES, CMT, RHIT

Edited & Reviewed by:
Susan M. Goeltzenleuchter, CMT

SAUNDERS

SAUNDERS
An Imprint of Elsevier Science

11830 Westline Industrial Drive
St. Louis, Missouri 63146

DORLAND'S DERMATOLOGY WORD BOOK FOR MEDICAL
TRANSCRIPTIONISTS   0-7216-9526-4

International Standard Book Number 0-7216-9526-4

Acquisitions Editor: Karen Fabiano
Developmental Editor: Ellen Wurm
Publishing Services Manager: Peggy Fagen
Designer: Ellen Zanolle

KI/MVY
Printed in the United States of America
Last digit is the print number: 9   8   7   6   5   4   3   2   1

PREFACE

I am proud to present the *Dorland's Dermatology Word Book for Medical Transcriptionists* – one of the ongoing series of word books being compiled for the professional medical transcriptionist. For one hundred years, W.B. Saunders has published the *Dorland's Illustrated Medical Dictionary*. With the advent of medical transcription, it became the dictionary of choice for medical transcriptionists.

When I was approached several years ago to help develop a series of Dorland's word books for medical transcriptionists, I have to admit the thought absolutely overwhelmed me. The *Dorland's Illustrated Medical Dictionary* was one of my first book purchases when I began my transcription career over thirty years ago. To participate in this project is an honor I could never have imagined for myself!

Transcriptionists need and will continue to need trusted up-to-date resources to help them research difficult terms quickly. In developing the *Dorland's Dermatology Word Book for Medical Transcriptionists*, I had access to the entire Dorland's terminology database for the book's foundation. In addition to this immense database, a context editor, Susan M. Goeltzenleuchter, CMT, a recognized leader in the field of medical transcription, was selected to review the material from the database, to contribute new and unique terms, and to remove outdated and obsolete ones. With Susan's extensive research and diligent work, I believe this to be the most up-to-date word book for the field of dermatology.

In developing the dermatology word book, I wanted the size to be manageable so the book would be easy to handle, provide a durable long-lasting binding, and use a type font large enough to read while providing extensive terminology not found in other resources available to medical transcriptionists.

Anatomical plates are included showing the structure of the skin, epidermis, and nails; cutaneous lesions; comedones; and staging for melanomas. I have also included a list of the most commonly used dermatologic pharmaceutical agents.

Although I have tried to produce the most thorough word book for dermatology available to medical transcriptionists, it is difficult to include every term as the field of medicine is constantly evolving. As you discover new terms, please feel free to share them with me for inclusion in the next edition of the *Dorland's Dermatology Word Book for Medical Transcriptionists*.

I may be reached at the following e-mail address: Sharon@TheRhodes.com.

SHARON B. RHODES, CMT, RHIT
Brentwood, Tennessee

A

A
   A and D ointment
   A and D medicated
      ointment

Å
   Ångström
   Å unit

a
   erythema a calore

A-200 Pyrinate

AA
   arachidonic acid
      AA amyloidosis

AAD
   American Academy of
      Dermatology

AAP
   American Academy of
      Pediatrics

AAV
   adeno-associated virus

Ab
   antibody

ab
   erythema ab igne

abacillary disease

ABC
   aspiration biopsy
      cytology

ABCDE
   asymmetry, irregular
      border, variegated color,
      larger than 5 mm
      diameter, elevation
         ABCDE criteria
         ABCDE of pigmented
            lesions

abdominal

abducens nerve paralysis

Abelcet

Abernethy sarcoma

aberrant
   a. basal cell carcinoma
   a. mongolian spots
   a. synthesis of
      glycosaminoglycans

aberration

abest saliva

ab igne
   erythema ab i.

abiotrophy

ablation
   argon laser a.
   CO_2 laser a.
   laser a.
   surgical a.
   ultrapulse laser a.

ablative treatment

abnormal
   a. DNA repair
   a. pigmentation

abnormality
   calcinosis cutis, osteoma
      cutis, poikiloderma, and
      skeletal a's (COPS)
   hematologic a.
   nail fold capillary loop a.
   pigmentary a.

abnutzung pigment

ABO

ABO antigens
   ABO incompatibility
   ABO system

abortive
   a. neurofibromatosis

abradant

abrade

1

abrasion
  brush burn a.
  mechanical a.

abrasive cleansers

abrasor

Abrikosov's (Abrikossoff's) tumor

abscedens

abscess
  acute a.
  cold a.
  dry a.
  follicular a.
  fungal a.
  metastatic tuberculous a.
  Munro a.
  Paget a.
  Paget a. syndrome
  Pautrier's a.
  perifollicular staphylococcal
    a.
  phlegmonous a.
  pulp a.
  pulpal a.
  sterile a.
  subcutaneous a.
  subepidermal a.
  subungual a.
  sudoriparous abscess

abscessus
  Mycobacterium a.

absent
  a. dermal component
  a. dermatoglyphic
  a. lacrimal puncta

Absidia

absolute
  a. anergy

absorbent gelling material
  (AGM)

Absorbine
  A. Jock Itch
  A. Jr. Antifungal

absorption
  cutaneous a.
  external a.
  percutaneous a.
  a. spectrum

abtropfung

abuse
  sexual a.

AC
  acanthosis nigricans

ACA
  acrodermatitis chronica
    atrophicans

acacia
  a. tree

ACADERM patch test

a calore
  erythema a c.

acanthamebiasis

Acanthamoeba
  A. astronyxis
  A. castellanii
  A. culbertsoni
  A. glebae
  A. hatchetti
  A. palestinensis
  A. polyphaga
  A. rhisodes

acanthoid

acantholysis
  a. bullosa
  incipient a.

acantholytic
  a. acanthoma
  a. cell
  a. dermatosis
  a. dyskeratoma
  a. dyskeratosis
  a. dyskeratotic
    keratinocytes
  a. squamous cell
    carcinoma

acanthoma *pl.* acanthomata,
  acanthomas
    a. adenoides cysticum
    basal cell a.
    clear cell a.
    Degos a.
    epidermolytic a.
    a. fissuratum
    a. inguinale
    intraepidermal a.
    pilar sheath a.
    a. tropicum
    a. verrucosa seborrheica

acanthome
    a. à cellules claires of
      Degos and Civatte

acanthorrhexis

acanthosis
    malignant a. nigricans
    a. nigricans (AN)
    a. palmaris
    a. papulosa nigra
    psoriasiform a.
    a. seborrheica
    a. verrucosa

acanthotic
    a. epidermal proliferation

acari (*plural of* acarus)

acarian

acariasis
    demodectic a.
    psoroptic a.
    sarcoptic a.

acaricide

acarid

acaridiasis

Acarina

acarine

acarinosis

acariosis

acarodermatitis
    a. urticarioides

acaroid

acarologist

acarology

acarophobia

acarotoxic

Acarus
    A. balatus
    A. folliculorum
    A. gallinae
    A. hordei
    *A. rhyizoglypticus
      hyacinthi*
    A. scabiei
    A. siro
    A. tritici

acatalasemia

acatalasia

acatastatic

accelerated
    a. actinic elastosis
    a. phase
    a. platelet destruction

accelerator

accentuation
    abdominal a.
    follicular a.
    perifollicular a.

accessory
    a. facial fissures
    a. spleen

Accolate

Accutane

ACD
    allergic contact
      dermatitis
    angiokeratoma corporis
      diffusum

ACE
  angiotensin-converting
    enzyme
    ACE inhibitors

Ace bandage

acetabulum *pl.* acetabula

acetamidine

acetaminophen
  chlorpheniramine and a.
  chlorpheniramine,
    phenylpropanolamine,
    and a.
  a., chlorpheniramine, and
    pseudoephedrine
  a. and diphenhydramine
  a. and isometheptene
    mucate
  a. and phenyltoloxamine
  phenyltoloxamine,
    phenylpropanolamine,
    and a.

acetate
  aluminum a.
  cortisone a.
  cyproterone a.
  dexamethasone a.
  Florinef A.
  fludrocortisone a.
  hydrocortisone a.
  Hydrocortone A.
  mafenide a.
  m-cresyl a.
  megestrol a.
  methylprednisolone a.
  paramethasone a.
  pirbuterol a.
  sermorelin a.

acetazolamide

acetic acid
  glacial a. a.

acetoacetic acid

acetone dermatitis

acetonide

acetonide (*continued*)
  fluocinolone a.
  triamcinolone a.

acetowhite lesions

acetowhitening

acetylator

acetylcholine
  a. depletion

acetylcysteine

achalasia

Achard-Thiers syndrome

Achenbach's syndrome

Achilles' tendon
  A. t. xanthoma tendinosum

achlorhydria

achloric algae

Achorion schoenleinii

achromasia

achromatosis

achromia
  congenital a.
  consecutive a.
  a. parasitica
  a. unguium

achromians
  incontinentia pigmenti a.

achromic
  a. lesion
  a. nevus

achromoderma

achromotrichia

Achromycin
  A. V Oral

acid
  acetic a.
  all-*trans*-retinoic a.
  alpha-hydroxy a.

acid (*continued*)
- amino a.
- ε-aminocaproic a.
- δ-aminolevulinic a.
- aminosalicylic a.
- antifibrinolytic tranexamic a.
- arachidonic a.
- argininosuccinic a.
- arsenious a.
- ascorbic a.
- aspartic a.
- azelaic a.
- benzoic a.
- boric a.
- carbolic a.
- a. ceramidase
- chenodeoxycholic a.
- chlorosulfonic a.
- cholic a.
- chromic a.
- citrulline a.
- a. deficiency
- delta-aminolevulinic a.
- dicarboxylic a.
- dichloroacetic a.
- epsilon-aminocaproic a.
- essential fatty a.
- fluoroboric a.
- folic a.
- free fatty a.
- a. fuchsin
- ginkgolic a.
- glutamic a.
- glycolic a.
- a. hemolysis test
- homogentisic a.
- hyaluronic a.
- hydriodic a.
- hydrobromic a.
- hydrochloric a.
- hydrofluoric a.
- iodic a.
- kojic a.
- linoleic a.
- *a*-linolenic a.
- a. mantle
- mefenamic a.
- a. mucopolysaccharides

acid (*continued*)
- muramic a.
- muriatic a.
- nalidixic a.
- nicotinic a.
- nitric a.
- okadaic a.
- oxalic a.
- para-aminobenzoic a.
- perchloric a.
- periodic a.–Schiff stain
- a. pH
- phenylpyruvic a.
- phosphoric a.
- phytanic a.
- picric a.
- polyunsaturated fatty acid
- salicylic a.
- silicofluoric a.
- sorbic a.
- sulfonic a.
- sulfuric a.
- sulfurous a.
- tannic a.
- thiosalicylic a.
- 13-*cis*-retinoic a.
- tranexamic a.
- trichloroacetic a.
- tungstic a.
- valproic a.
- a. violet 6B

acid-fast
- a.-f. bacillus (AFB)
- a.-f. mycobacteria
- a.-f. organism

acidophilic
- a. condensation
- a. hyaline
- a. inclusion body
- a. polygonal cell

acidosis
- lactic a.
- starvation a.

aciduria

aciduric

acinar
    a. cell carcinoma
    a. glandlike structure

acinous

acitretin

acladiosis

Acladium castellani

ACLE
    acute cutaneous lupus
      erythematosus

Aclovate
    A. topical

acne
    adolescent a.
    a. aestivalis
    a. albida
    apocrine a.
    a. artificialis
    atrophia a.
    a. atrophica
    axillary cystic a.
    a. bacillus
    bromide a.
    a. cachecticorum
    a. cheloidalis
    chlorine a.
    a. ciliaris
    colloid a.
    a. comedo
    comedo a.
    common a.
    a. conglobata
    conglobate a.
    contact a.
    a. cosmetica
    cystic a.
    a. cystica
    a. decalvans
    a. detergicans
    a. disseminata
    a. dorsalis
    drug-induced a.
    epidemic a.
    a. erythematosa

acne (*continued*)
    a. estivalis
    excoriated a.
    a. excoriée des filles
    a. excoriée des jeunes filles
    a. frontalis
    a. fulminans
    a. generalis
    halogen a.
    a. hypertrophica
    a. indurata
    infantile a.
    a. inversa
    iodide a.
    a. keloid
    keloid a.
    keloidal a.
    a. keloidalis
    a. keloidalis nuchae
    a. keratosa
    lupoid a.
    Mallorca a.
    a. mechanica
    mechanical a.
    a. medicamentosa
    menstrual a.
    a. mentagra
    a. miliaris
    a. miliaris necrotica
    miliary a.
    a. necrotica
    a. necroticans et exulcerans
      serpiginosa nasi
    a. necrotica miliaris
    neonatal a.
    a. neonatorum
    nodulocystic a.
    occupational a.
    oil a.
    papular a.
    a. papule
    a. papulosa
    a. pathogens
    petroleum a.
    picker's a.
    pomade a.
    preadolescent a.
    premenstrual a.

acne (*continued*)
 propionobacterium a.
 pubertal a.
 a. punctata
 pustular a.
 a. pustule
 a. pustulosa
 a. rosacea
 a. scorbutica
 a. scrofulosorum
 a. seborrheica
 severe inflammatory a.
 severe scarring a.
 simple a.
 a. simplex
 steroid a.
 summer a.
 a. surgery
 a. syphilitica
 systemic a.
 tar a.
 a. tarsi
 a. telangiectodes
 a. tetrad
 trade a.
 tropical a.
 a. tropicalis
 a. urticata
 a. varioliformis
 a. venenata
 a. vulgaris

acné
 a. chéloïdique
 a. excoriée des filles
 a. excoriée des jeunes filles

Acne-5

Acne-10

Acne Lotion

acneform, acneiform
 a. dermatitis
 a. eruption
 follicular a.
 a. lesion
 pitted a.
 a. pustules
 a. syphilid

acneforme, acneiforme
 erythema a.

acnegen

acnegenic
 a. cosmetics

acneic

acneiform eruption

acne-pustulosis-hyperostosis-
 osteitis

acnes
 Bacillus a.
 Corynebacterium a.
 Propionibacterium a.

acnitis

Acno
 A. cleanser

Acnomel

Acnotex

acomia

acquired
 a. acral fibrokeratoma
 a. angioedema I
 a. angioedema II
 a. benign vascular
  neoplasm
 a. chronic bullae
 a. clubbing
 a. cutis laxa
 a. dermatosis
 a. digital fibrokeratoma
 a. disorder
 a. dyskeratotic leukoplakia
 a. forms
 a. generalized lipodystrophy
 a. genital warts
 a. hair kinking
 a. hemangioma
 a. hemolytic anemia
 a. hyperostosis syndrome
 a. hypertrichosis lanuginosa
 a. hypogammaglobulinemia
 a. ichthyosis

acquired (*continued*)
  a. immunodeficiency
    syndrome (AIDS)
  a. intravascular hemolytic
    anemia
  a. isolated plaques
  a. leukoderma
  a. localized trichorrhexis
    nodosa
  a. longitudinal pigmented
    band
  a. lymphangiectasia
  a. lymphangioma
  a. melanoma
  a. nevus
  a. palmoplantar keratosis
  a. perforating dermatosis
  a. pigmented anomaly
  a. platelet function defect
  a. progressive kinking of the
    hair
  a. progressive
    lymphangioma
  a. reactive perforating
    collagenosis
  a. secondary process
  a. sensitivity
  a. syndromes
  a. systemic infiltrative
    process
  a. toxoplasmosis
  a. tufted angioma

acquisita
  epidermolysis a.
  epidermolysis bullosa a.
    (EBA)

acquisitum
  leukoderma a. centrifugum

acral
  a. area
  a. arteriolar ectasia
  a. blister
  a. bullus
  a. erythema
  a. fibrokeratoma
  a. gangrene

acral (*continued*)
  a. hyperkeratosis
  a. keratosis
  a. keratotic papule
  a. lentiginous melanoma
  a. lesion
  a. microlivedo
  a. mycoses fungoides
  a. nodule
  a. persistent papular
    mucinosis
  a. pseudolymphomatous
    angiokeratoma
  a. vitiligo

Acremonium
  A. falciforme
  A. kiliense
  A. pelletier
  A. recifei

acrid

acritochromacy

acrivastine/pseudoephedrine

acroangiodermatitis

acroasphyxia

acrocephalosyndactyly

acrochordon

acrocyanosis

acrodermatitis
  a. chronica atrophicans
  a. continua
  a. continua of Hallopeau
  a. enteropathica
  Hallopeau's a.
  a. hiemalis
  infantile a.
  papular a. of childhood
  a. papulosa infantum
  a. perstans
  pustular a.
  a. pustulosa
  a. vesiculosa tropica

acrodermatosis

acrodynia

acrodynic erythema

acrofacial vitiligo

acrogeria

acrohyperhidrosis

acrokeratoelastoidosis
  a. of Costa

acrokeratosis
  a. neoplastica
  paraneoplastic a.
  a. paraneoplastica
  a. verruciformis
  a. verruciformis of Hopf

acrokeratotic poikiloderma
  (Weary-Kindler)

acrolein

acroleukopathy

acromastitis

acromegalic
  a. arthropathy

acromegalogigantism

acromegaloidism

acromegaly

acromelalgia

acromelanosis progressiva

acrometagenesis

acromicria

acromikria

acromiodeltoideus
  nevus fuscoceruleus a.

acro-osteolysis

acropachy
  thyroid a.

acropachyderma
  a. with pachyperiostitis

acroparesthesia

acroparesthesia (*continued*)
  Nothnagel-type a.
  Schultze-type a.

acropigmentatio reticularis of
  Kitamura

acropigmentation
  a. of Dohi
  a. of Kitamura
  a. reticularis of Kitamura

acropolyneuritis

acropurpura

acropustulosis
  infantile a.
  a. of infancy

acroscleroderma

acrosclerosis

acrospiroma
  eccrine a.
  giant eccrine a.
  malignant clear cell a.

acrostealgia

acrosyringeal cell

acrosyringium *pl.* acrosyringia

acroteric

acroterica
  morphea a.

Acrotheca aquaspersa

acrotrophodynia

acrylate

acrylic
  a. acid therapy
  a. bone cement
  a. monomer
  a. monomer dermatitis
  a. plastics
  a. resin

Acsorex

Actagen

ACTH
    adrenocorticotropic
        hormone
    ACTH stimulation test

ACTH therapy

Acthar

Acticel wound dressing

Acticoat bandage

Actiderm

Actifed

actin

Actinex
    A. topical

actinic
    a. burn
    a. cheilitis
    a. damage
    a. dermatitis
    a. elastosis
    a. granuloma
    a. keratosis
    a. lichen nitidus
    a. lichen planus
    a. plaques
    a. porokeratosis
    a. prurigo
    a. purpura
    a. reticuloid
    a. reticuloid syndrome
    a. telangiectasis

actinica
    dermatitis a.

actinically damaged elastic
    tissue

actinicity

actiniform

actinism

actinobacillosis

Actinobacillus
    A. actinomycetemcomitans

Actinobacillus (*continued*)
    A. equuli
    A. hominis
    A. lignieresii
    A. suis
    A. ureae

actinodermatitis

actinodermatosis

actinolyte

Actinomadura
    A. madurae
    A. pelletieri

actinometer

actinometry

actinomycelial

Actinomyces
    A. bovis
    A. hominis
    A. israelii
    A. naeslundii
    A. viscosus

Actinomycetaceae (*genera*)
    Actinomyces
    Arachnia
    Bacterionema
    Bifidobacterium
    Rothia

Actinomycetales (*families*)
    Actinomycetaceae
    Actinoplanaceae
    Dermatophilaceae
    Frankiaceae
    Micromonosporaceae
    Mycobacteriaceae
    Nocardiaceae
    Streptomycetaceae

actinomycetemcomitans
    Actinobacillus a.

actinomycete
    nocardioform a.

actinomycetoma

actinomycin D

actinomycoma

actinomycosis
cervical a.

actinomycotic

actinomycotin

actinoneuritis

actinoquinol sodium

actinophage

actinophytosis

actinotherapeutics

actinotherapy

action
mechanism of a.
a. spectrum

activated
a. endothelial cell
a. keratinocytes
a. T cell

activation

activator
lipoprotein lipase a.
plasminogen a.

active
a. infectious disease

activity
tumoricidal a.

acuminata *pl.* acuminatae
verruca acuminata
verrucae acuminatae

acuminate
a. papular syphilid
a. warts

acuminatum *pl.* acuminata
condyloma acuminatum
condylomata acuminata
papilloma a.

acuminatus

acuminatus (*continued*)
lichen ruber a.

acupuncture

acupuncturist

acuta
parapsoriasis a.
parapsoriasis lichenoides et
varioliformis a.
pityriasis lichenoides et
varioliformis a. (PLEVA)
pustulosis vacciniformis a.
urticaria a.

acute
a. allergic urticaria
a. anaphylactic reaction
a. atrophic oral candidiasis
a. boric acid ingestion
a. cellulitis
a. cutaneous leishmaniasis
a. cutaneous lupus
erythematosus (ACLE)
a. decubitus ulcer
a. diffuse iridocyclitis
a. digital gangrene
a. disseminated lupus
erythematosus
a. febrile illness
a. febrile neutrophilic
dermatitis
a. febrile neutrophilic
dermatosis
a. folliculitis
a. generalized
exanthematous pustulosis
a. glomerulonephritis
a. graft-versus-host disease
a. guttate
a. guttate eruption
a. guttate psoriasis
a. hemolytic anemia
a. hemorrhagic edema of
infancy
a. herpes zoster
a. herpetic gingivostomatitis
a. immunosuppression
a. infectious mononucleosis

acute (*continued*)
 a. inflammation
 a. inflammatory stage
 a. intermittent porphyria
 a. lupus erythematosus
 a. lupus pneumonitis
 a. lymphoblastic leukemia
 a. lymphocytic leukemia
 a. meningitis
 a. migratory polyarthritis
 a. military tuberculosis
 a. myelogenous leukemia
 a. myeloid leukemia
 a. necrotizing ulcerative
  gingivitis
 a. necrotizing ulcerative
  gingivostomatitis
 a. pemphigus
 a. phototoxic event
 a. porphyrias
 a. respiratory distress
  syndrome
 a. retinal necrosis
 a. rheumatic disease
 a. rheumatic fever
 a. sarcoidosis
 a. scalp cellulitis
 a. seroconversion syndrome
 a. upper respiratory infection
 a. urticaria
 a. vascular purpura

acute-phase reactant

acutum
 ulcus vulvae a.

acutus
 pemphigus a.

acyclic

acyclovir
 a. sodium
 a. suppression
 a. therapy

adactyly

Adamantiades-Behçet
 syndrome

adamantinoma

Adams-Oliver syndrome

Adamson's "fringe"

adapalene gel

ADCC
 antibody-dependent
  cellular cytotoxicity
 antibody-dependent cell-
  mediated cytotoxicity

addicted scrotum syndrome

Addison
 A's disease
 A's keloid
 A's morphea
 A's pigmentation
 Addison-Gull disease

addisonian
 a. steroid dependency
 a. syndrome

addisonism

additive
 food a.

addressin

Aden
 A. fever
 A. ulcer

adenitis
 suppurative inguinal a.

adeno-associated virus (AAV)

adenocarcinoma
 aggressive digital papillary
  a. (ADPA)
 ceruminous a.
 colonic a.
 follicular a.
 mixed papillary/follicular a.
 ovarian a.
 sebaceous a.

adenocystic
 a. basal cell carcinoma

adenoepithelioma

adenoid
    a. cystic carcinoma
    a. proliferation
    a. tubular proliferation

adenoidal facies

adenoides
    epithelioma a. cysticum

adenolipoma

adenolipomatosis

adenoma
    adrenocortical a.
    aggressive digital papillary
      a. (ADPA)
    apocrine a.
    eosinophil a.
    a. of nipple
    papillary eccrine a.
    a. sebaceum
    sebaceous a.
    senile sebaceous a.

adenomatoid

adenomatosis
    erosive a.
    a. oris

adenomatous
    a. cystic proliferation

adenopathy
    hilar a.
    shotty a.

adenosine
    a. deaminase
    a. deaminase deficiency
    a. diphosphate (ADP)

adenovirus

adenylate cyclase toxin

adermal

adermatoglyphia

adermia
    a. congenita

adermic

adermogenesis

adherent

adhesion molecule

adhesiotherapy

adhesive
    a. dermatitis

adiaphoresis

adiaphoretic

adipocyte

adipofibroma

adipogenic

adipogenous

adipometer

adiponecrosis
    a. subcutanea neonatorum

adiposa
    blepharoptosis a.
    a. dolorosa
    seborrhea a.

adiposalgia

adipose tissue

adiposis
    a. cerebralis
    a. dolorosa
    a. orchica
    a. tuberosa simplex
    a. universalis

adipositis

adiposity
    painful a.

adiposus
    panniculus a.

adjunctive
    a. antibiotic therapy
    a. therapy

adjuvant

adjuvant (*continued*)
    Freund's complete a.
    Freund's
        incomplete a.
    mycobacterial a.

Adlone injection

admixture

adnata
    alopecia a.

adnexa (*plural of* adnexum)
    ocular a.
    a. oculi

adnexal
    a. carcinoma
    a. keratinocytes
    a. neoplasm
    a. tumor

adnexum

adolescent
    a. atopic dermatitis
    a. eczema

adontia

Adoxa

ADP
    adenosine diphosphate
    ALA dehydratase d
        eficiency porphyria

ADPA
    aggressive digital papillary
        adenocarcinoma
    aggressive digital papillary
        adenoma

adrenal
    a. adenoma
    a. cortical hyperplasia
    a. dysfunction
    a. insufficiency
    a. neoplasm
    a. tumor

adrenalectomy

adrenalitis

adrenergic
    a. urticaria

adrenocortical
    a. hypoplasia
    a. tissue

adrenocorticosteroid
    a. therapy

adrenocorticotropic
    a. hormone (ACTH)
    a. hormone therapy

adrenogenic

adrenogenital syndrome

adrenogenous

adrenoleukodystrophy (ALD)

adrenotrophic

adrenotropic

Adriamycin

Adrucil injection

Adson
    A's forceps
    A's toothed forceps

adult
    a. acquired reactive
        perforating collagenosis
    a. bullous dermatosis
    a. eczema
    a. form
    a. linear IgA bullous
        dermatosis
    a. Niemann-Pick disease
    a. phase
    a. progeria
    a. T-cell leukemia (ATL)
    a. T-cell lymphoma
    a. T-cell
        lymphoma/leukemia

adult-onset
    a.-o. colloid milium
    a.-o. GM_1 gangliosidosis
    a.-o. idiopathic
        erythromelalgia

advancing edge

adventitial
　a. dermis

adventitious matter

adverse
　a. drug reaction

Advil

AEC
　ankyloblepharon,
　　ectodermal defects, and
　　cleft lip and/or palate
　AEC syndrome

AECA
　antiendothelial cell
　　antibodies

Aedes
　A. aegypti
　A. albopictus
　A. aldrichi
　A. caballus
　A. communis
　A. excrucians
　A. leucocelaenus
　A. polynesiensis
　A. punctor
　A. scapularis
　A. sollicitans
　A. stimulans
　A. variegatus
　A. vexans

aerial
　a. mycelia
　a. mycelium

Aeroaid

aerobe

aerodermectasia

aerodigestive tract

Aeromonas
　A. caviae
　A. hydrophila
　A. infection

Aeromonas (*continued*)
　A. septicemia
　A. shigelloides
　A. sobria
　A. veronii

Aeroseb-Dex

Aeroseb-HC

aerosol

aerosolization

AeroZoin

aeruginosa

aesthetic

aestivale (*see* estivale)

aestivalis (*see* estivalis)

afferent

affinity *pl.* affinities

afibrinogenemia

African
　A. Burkitt's lymphoma
　A. cutaneous Kaposi's
　　sarcoma
　A. endemic relapsing fever
　A. histoplasmosis
　A. honeybee
　A. lymphadenopathic
　　Kaposi's sarcoma
　A. tick virus
　A. trypanosomiasis
　A. vector horsefly

Aftate

aftosa

AFX
　atypical fibroxanthoma

agammaglobulinemia
　acquired a.
　Bruton's a.
　common variable a.
　lymphopenic a.
　secondary a.

agammaglobulinemia
(*continued*)
 sex-linked a.
 Swiss type a.
 transient a.
 X-linked a.
 X-linked infantile a.

agar
 brain-heart infusion a.
 cystine glucose blood a.
 Mycosel a.
 a. precipitation
 Sabouraud's a.

agenesia

agenesis
 pilorum a.

agent
 alkylating a.
 blistering a.
 chemotherapeutic a.
 cytotoxic a.
 topical anticandidal a.
 TRIC a's

AGEP
 acute generalized
 exanthematous pustulosis

agerasia

agglomerated

agglomeration

agglutination
 a. test

agglutinin
 cold a.
 peanut a.

aggregate

aggregated
 a. IgA

aggregation

aggressive
 a. cutaneous squamous cell
 carcinoma

aggressive (*continued*)
 a. digital papillary
 adenocarcinoma (ADPA)
 a. digital papillary adenoma
 (ADPA)
 a. infantile fibromatosis

aging
 premature a. in Werner's
 syndrome

AGL
 acquired generalized
 lipodystrophy

agminata

agminate
 a. lesion

agminated
 a. follicle
 a. lentiginosis
 a. verrucous papule

AGN
 acute glomerulonephritis

agomphiasis

agomphious

agomphosis

agranulocytic state

agranulocytica
 a. cruris
 hypercyanotic a.
 a. lymphomatosa
 necrotic a.
 neutropenic a.
 a. pectoris vasomotoria

agranulocytosis
 feline a.

Agrimonia
 A. eupatoria

agrimony

AHLE
 angiolymphoid hyperplasia
 with eosinophilia

AHO
  Albright's hereditary
    osteodystrophy

AHS
  acquired hyperostosis
    syndrome

A-hydroCort

AHYS

acquired hyperostosis syndrome

AIDS
  acquired immune
    deficiency syndrome
  acquired
    immunodeficiency
    syndrome
      AIDS vaccine

AIL
  angioimmunoblastic
    lymphadenopathy

AILD
  angioimmunoblastic
    lymphadenopathy with
    dysproteinemia

ainhum

AIP
  acute intermittent porphyria

air
  liquid a.
  a. plethysonography

airborne
  a. material
  a. mold

akamushi
  Leptotrombidium a.
  Trombicula a.

akamushi disease

Akne-Mycin
  A. topical

ALA
  aminolevulinic acid

ALA (*continued*)
  ALA dehydratase deficiency
    porphyria (ADP)

ala nasi hypoplasia

Ala-Cort

Ala-Quin topical

Ala-Scalp

Alagille's syndrome

Alanko
  A. method
  method of A.

alastrim

alba
  linea a.
  miliaria a.
  morphea a.
  phlegmasia a.
  pityriasis a.
  stria a.

albae

albedo
  a. unguium

albendazole
  a. sulfoxide

albicans
  Candida a.
  Monilia a.
  stria a.

albinism
  a. I
  a. II
  acquired a.
  Amish a.
  autosomal dominant
    oculocutaneous a.
  autosomal recessive ocular
    a. (AROA)
  brown a.
  brown oculocutaneous a.
  circumscribed a.
  complete imperfect a.

albinism (*continued*)
    complete perfect a.
    cutaneous a.
    Forsius-Eriksson-type ocular
        a.
    localized a.
    Nettleship-Falls-type ocular
        a.
    ocular a.
    ocular a., autosomal
        recessive
    ocular a., Forsius-Eriksson
        type
    ocular a., Nettleship-Falls
        type
    ocular a., X-linked
        (Nettleship)
    oculocutaneous a.
    partial a.
    piebald a.
    red a.
    rufous a.
    rufous oculocutaneous a.
    temperature-sensitive
        oculocutaneous a.
    type IA oculocutaneous a.
    type IB oculocutaneous a.
    type II ocular a.
    type II oculocutaneous a.
    type I-MP oculocutaneous
        a.
    type I ocular a.
    type I oculocutaneous a.
    type I-TS oculocutaneous a.
    tyrosinase-negative (ty-neg)
        oculocutaneous a.
    tyrosinase-positive (ty-pos)
        oculocutaneous a.
    xanthous a.
    X-linked ocular a.
        (Nettleship) (XOAN)
    yellow a.
    yellow mutant (ym)
        oculocutaneous a.
    yellow oculocutaneous a.

albinismus
    a. circumscriptus

albinismus (*continued*)
    a. totalis
    a. universalis

albino

albinoidism
    oculocutaneous a.
    punctate oculocutaneous a.

albinotic

albopapuloid
    a. lesions
    a. type

Albright
    A's disease
    A's hereditary
        osteodystrophy
    A's dimpling sign
    A's osteodystrophy
    A's sign
    A's syndrome

albumin

albuminorrhea

albuminuria

Alcian blue
    A. b. staining

alclometasone dipropionate

alcohol
    benzyl a.
    cetyl a.
    cinnamic a.
    isopropyl a.
    medicated a.
    pantothenyl a.
    stearyl a.
    wool wax a.

alcoholic cirrhosis

alcoholism

Alcyonidrium
    A. hirsutum

ALD
    adrenoleukodystrophy

Aldactone

aldehyde

aldolase

aldosterone

aldosteronism

Aldrich-Mees lines

alefacept

Aleppo boil

alexandrite
    Q-switched a. laser

Alezzandrini's syndrome

alfa-2a
    interferon a.

alfa-2b
    interferon a.

alfalfa
    a. grass

Alferon N

algae
    achloric a.
    saprophytic a.

algoneurodystrophy

algorithm
    Dermatologic
     Diagnostic A.
    diagnostic a.
    problem-oriented a.

Alibert
    A's disease
    A's keloid
    A's mentagra

Alibour's solution

aliphatic
    a. alcohols
    stearyl a.

aliquot

alitretinoin

Alkaban-AQ

alkali *pl.* alkalis, alkalies
    a. patch test

alkaline
    a. irritant dermatitis
    a. permanent hair wave
     dermatitis
    a. phosphatase
    a. phosphatase and
     pyrophosphate
    a. sulfide dermatitis

alkalinization

alkalis

alkalization

alkaloid
    ergot a.
    Vinca a.

alkaptonuria

alkyl phenol

alkylating
    a. agent
    a. therapy

ALL
    acute lymphocytic
     leukemia

Alagille's syndrome

allantoin

allele
    HLA a.

allelic

allelomorph

allelomorphic

Aller-Chlor oral

allergen
    a. contact
    environmental a.
    epidermal a.
    a. exposure
    flux a.

allergen (*continued*)
    inhalant a.
    a. inhalation challenge test
    Lolium perenne a.
    occupational a.

allergenic principles

allergic
    a. cheilitis
    a. contact cheilitis
    a. contact dermatitis
        (ACD)
    a. eczema
    a. eczematous contact-type
        dermatitis
    a. eczematous dermatitis
    a. granuloma
    a. granulomatosis
    a. hypersensitivity
    a. manifestation
    a. mechanism
    a. nonthrombocytopenic
        purpura
    a. purpura
    a. rhinitis
    a. state
    a. stomatitis
    a. transformation
    a. urticaria
    a. vasculitis

allergologic

allergy
    atopic a.
    bacterial a.
    contact a.
    drug a.
    food a.
    hereditary a.
    immediate a.
    insulin a.
    latent a.
    nickel a.
    physical a.
    seafood a.
    a. unit (AU)

AllerMax oral

alliaceous

alligator
    a. boy
    a. skin

alloantigen

allochromasia

Allodermanyssus
    A. sanguineus

allodynia

allogenic, allogeneic
    a. bone marrow
        transplantation
    a. cultured keratinocytes
    a. graft
    a. human skin fibroblast

allograft
    epidermal a.
    a. rejection

allophore

allopurinol
    a. hypersensitivity
        syndrome

allotransplantation

alloy
    chrome a.

all-*trans*-retinoic acid

allylamines (*class of drugs*)

Aloe
    Cortaid with a.
    Dermtex HC with a.

aloe

aloetic

alogia

alopecia
    a. acquisita
    a. adnata
    adrenal-androgenic female
        pattern a.
    a. anagen effluvium

alopecia (*continued*)
    androgenic a.
    androgenetic a.
    a. androgenetica
    a. areata
    a. capitis totalis
    centrifugal scarring a.
    cicatricial a.
    a. cicatrisata
    a. circumscripta
    congenital a.
    a. congenitalis
    congenital sutural a.
    congenital triangular a.
    a. disseminata
    drug a.
    drug-induced a.
    endocrinologic a.
    favic a.
    favid a.
    female pattern a.
    follicular a.
    a. follicularis
    a. generalisata
    a. hereditaria
    hereditary a.
    hot comb a.
    a. leprotica
    a. liminaris
    a. liminaris frontalis
    lipedematous a.
    male pattern a.
    marginal a.
    a. marginalis
    mechanical a.
    a. medicamentosa
    moth-eaten a.
    a. mucinosa
    a. neoplastica
    a. neurotica
    ophiasic a. areata
    a. orbicularis
    patchy a.
    patchy cicatricial a.
    patterned a.
    physiologic a.
    pityriasic a.
    a. pityrodes

alopecia (*continued*)
    postoperative pressure a.
    postpartum a.
    premature a.
    a. prematura
    a. presenilis
    pressure a.
    pseudopelade-type a.
    psychogenic a.
    radiation a.
    radiation-induced a.
    roentgen a.
    a. sarcoid
    scarring a.
    a. seborrheica
    senile a.
    a. senilis
    stress a.
    a. symptomatica
    syphilitic a.
    a. syphilitica
    a. telogen effluvium
    a. totalis
    a. toxica
    traction a.
    traumatic a.
    traumatic marginal a.
    a. triangularis
    a. triangularis congenitalis
    a. universalis
    x-ray a.

alopecic

alpha
    a. adrenergic blocker
    a. adrenergic stimulation
    a. chain
    a. fetoprotein
    a. helical coiled pattern
    a. interferon
    a. nerve fibers

Alpha Keri
    A.K. Moisturizing Soap
    A.K. Spray
    A.K. Therapeutic Bath Oil

alpha-antitrypsin
    serum a.-a.

alpha-galactosidase A

alpha-hydroxy acids

alpha-interferon 3

alpha-L-fucosidase

alpha-L-iduronidase

alpha-lipoprotein deficiency

alpha-methyldopa

alpha-methylene

alpha-*N*-
acetylgalactosaminidase
deficiency

alpha-phytanic acid alpha
hydroxylase

Alphaherpesvirinae

Alphatrex

Alphavirus

Alström's syndrome

alteration
a. of flora
pigmentary a.
qualitative a.
quantitative a.
vacuolar a.

Alternaria
A. mold
A. tenuis

alternariatoxicosis

alternariosis

alum
ammonium a.
burnt a.
dried a.
potassium a.
exsiccated a.

aluminum
a. acetate
a. acetotartrate
a. acetylsalicylate

aluminum (*continued*)
a. ammonium sulfate
a. aspirin
a. bismuth oxide
a. chlorate nonahydrate
a. chlorhydroxide
a. chloride
a. chloride dermatitis
a. chloride hexahydrate
a. chloride hexahydrate in
anhydrous ethanol
a. chloride solution
a. chloride tincture
a. chlorohydrate
a. chlorohydrex
a. chlorhydroxy allantoinate
a. (Finn) chambers
a. hydrate
a. hydroxide gel
a. hydroxychloride
a. oleate
a. oxide
A. Paste
a. phenolsulfonate
a. potassium sulfate
a. subacetate
a. sulfate
a. sulfate octadecahydrate

Alu-Tab

Aluwets

alveolar
a. bone
a. proteinosis
a. ridges

alveoli (*plural of* alveolus)

amalgam
dental a.
a. tattoo

amantadine
a. HCl
a. hydrochloride

amastigote

amatol

Ambi 10

AmBisome

Amblyomma
    A. americanum
    A. cajennense
    A. hebraeum

amblyopia

ambustion

amcinonide

Amcort

amebiasis
    a. cutis
    pruritus ani a.

amebic
    a. ulcer

ameboid cell

amelanosis

amelanotic
    a. melanoma

ameliorate

amelioration

ameloblastoma
    melanotic a.
    peripheral a.
    pigmented a.

amenorrhea

American
    A. Academy of Dermatology
    A. Academy of Pediatrics
        (AAP)
    A. Celiac Society
    A. cockroach
    A. College of Rheumatology
        (ACR)
    A. cutaneous leishmaniasis
    A. elm
    A. elm tree
    A. Joint Committee on
        Cancer
    A. leishmaniasis

American (*continued*)
    A. mucocutaneous
        leishmaniasis
    A. Rheumatism Association
        (ARA)
    A. trypanosomiasis
    A. visceral leishmaniasis

A-methaPred injection

Amevive (alefacept)

amiantacea
    pityriasis a.
    tinea a.

amiantaceous
    a. crust

Amicar

amikacin
    a. sulfate

amiloxate

amine

amino
    a. acid
    a. acid metabolism
    a. acid peptide
    a. precursor uptake
    a. terminal end

aminoaciduria

aminobenzene

aminobenzoate
    a. potassium

p-aminobenzoic acid

aminocaproic acid

aminoglycoside

δ–aminolevulinic acid

Amino-Opti-E Oral

aminophylline
    a., amobarbital, and
        ephedrine

aminosalicylic acid

amiodarone
  a. photosensitivity
  a. pigmentation

amitriptyline
  a. hydrochloride

AML
  acute myelogenous
    leukemia

amlexanox

amlodipine

ammonia
  a. carbonate
  a. persulfate
  a. rash

ammoniated mercury
  a.m. dermatitis

ammonical ulcer

ammonium
  a. alum
  a. carbonate
  a. lactate lotion
  a. persulfate
  a. persulfate dermatitis
  quaternary a.
  a. thioglycolate
  a. thioglycolate dermatitis

amniocytes

amnion
  a. nodosum

amnionic

amniotic

Amoeba histolytica

amorphous
  a. eosinophilic material
  a. mass
  a. material
  a. matrix
  a. parenchymal
    opacification
  a. polysaccharide mass
  a. substance

amoxicillin
  a. and clavulanic acid

amoxicillin/clavulanate
  (AMX/CL)
  a. suspension

amphetamine

amphophilic

amphoteric

amphotericin
  a. B
  a. B cholesteryl
  a. B deoxycholate
  a. B liquid complex (ABLC)

ampicillin

amplification loop

amplitude

ampule, ampul

amputating ulcer

amputation
  spontaneous a.
  a. stump

AMX/CL
  amoxicillin/clavulanate
    AMX/CL suspension

amyloid
  a. bodies
  a. degeneration
  a. deposition
  a. disease
  a. fibers
  a. P component
  a. protein

amyloidosis
  bullous a.
  chronic a.
  cutaneous a.
  a. cutis
  dialysis-related a.
  familial a.
  focal a.
  frictional a.

amyloidosis (*continued*)
   hereditary a.
   heredofamilial a.
   lichen a.
   lichenoid a.
   macular a.
   nodular a.
   nodular cutaneous a.
   myeloma-associated a.
   a. of aging
   poikiloderma-like
    cutaneous a.
   primary a.
   primary cutaneous a.
   primary systemic a.
   secondary cutaneous a.
   secondary systemic a.
   senile a.
   systemic a.
   tumefactive cutaneous a.
   tumor-associated a.

amyloidosus
   lichen a.

amyopathic
   a. dermatomyositis

amyotrophia

amyotrophic lateral sclerosis
   (ALS)

amyotrophy
   diabetic a.
   a. hemiplegic
   neuralgic a.

AN
   acanthosis nigricans

ANA
   antinuclear antibody
   speckled-pattern ANA

Anacardium occidentale

Anacardiaceae

Anacin

anaerobe
   facultative a.

anaerobe (*continued*)
   obligate a.

anaerobic
   a. bacterial arthritis
   a. cellulitis
   a. organism
   a. rod

anaerobically

anaerobiosis

anaeroplasty

Anafranil

anagen
   a. effluvium
   a. hair
   a. phase
   a. release
   short a.

Ana-Kit

analgesia
   a. algera
   a. dolorosa
   narcotic a.

analgesic

analogous

anamnesis

anamnestic
   a. eruption
   a. reaction
   a. response

anaphylactic
   a. antibody
   a. crisis
   a. hypersensitivity reaction
   a. intoxication
   a. reaction
   a. shock
   a. state
   a. transfusion reactions

anaphylactogen

anaphylactoid

anaphylactoid (*continued*)
   a. crisis
   a. purpura
   a. reaction
   a. shock

anaphylatoxic

anaphylatoxin

anaphylaxis
   aggregate a.
   generalized a.
   local a.
   passive cutaneous a.
   penicillin-induced a.
   systemic a.

anaplasia

anaplastic

anasarca

anastomose

anastomosis *pl.* anastomoses

anatomic
   a. malformation
   a. nails
   a. tubercle
   a. wart

anatomical
   a. tubercle
   a. wart

anatomically predisposed
   blushing

anatoxic

anatoxin

ANCA
   antineutrophil cytoplasmic
      antibody

Ancef

anchoring fibrils

Ancobon

Ancylostoma
   A. braziliense

Ancylostoma (*continued*)
   A. caninum
   A. ceylanicum
   A. dermatitis
   A. duodenale

ancylostomiasis
   cutaneous a.
   a. cutis

Anders' disease

Anderson-Fabry disease

Andrews disease

androblastoma

androgen
   a. biosynthesis
   a.-blocking agent
   a. blood levels
   a.-dependent area
   a.-dependent hair growth
   a.-dependent syndrome
   a.-induced hair loss
   a. precursor
      androstenedione
   a. response
   a. stimulation
   synthetic a.
   a. testosterone

androgenetic
   a. alopecia
   a. change

androgenic
   a. alopecia

androstenedione

anecdotal observation

anemia
   acute hemolytic a.
   aplastic a.
   Coombs-positive hemolytic
      a.
   dermatopathic a.
   hemolytic a.
   hypochromic a.
   hypochromic normocytic a.

anemia (*continued*)
    Mediterranean a.
    megaloblastic a.
    microangiopathic a.
    microangiopathic hemolytic
      a.
    pernicious a.
    sickle cell a.

anemicus (*variant* anaemicus)
    nevus a.

anergic
    a. leishmaniasis

anergy

Anestacon

anesthesia

anesthetic
    intradermal a.
    a. leprosy
    preoperative a.
    topical a.

anetoderma
    congenital a.
    Jadassohn's a.
    Jadassohn-Pellizzari a.
    a. of prematurity
    perifollicular a.
    postinflammatory a.
    Schweninger-Buzzi a.
    a. scleroatrophy

anetodermatous

aneuploidy

aneurysm
    ascending aortic a.
    capillary a.
    cirsoid a.
    dissecting aortic a.

aneurysmal dilation

Angelica
    A. archangelica

angelica
    a. root

angiitis
    allergic a.
    choroidal a.
    Churg-Strauss a.
    consecutive a.
    cutaneous a.
    granulomatous a.
    hypersensitivity a.
    leukocytoclastic a.
    a. livedo reticularis
    necrotizing a.
    non-necrotizing a.
    systemic hypersensitivity a.

angina
    a. bullosa haemorrhagica
    herpetic a.
    Ludwig's a.
    a. pectoris
    Vincent's a.

anginal attack

angioblastic
    a. lymphadenopathy
    a. tumors

angioblastoma

angiocentric
    a. lymphoma

angioderm

angiodermatitis
    disseminated pruritic a.

angiodestructive

angiodysplasia
    papular a.

angioedema
    acquired a.
    allergic a.
    bullous a.
    cold urticaria and a.
    drug-induced a.
    episodic a.
    hereditary a.
    a. profile
    a. of urticaria
    vibratory a.

angioedema-urticaria-
  eosinophilia syndrome

angioedematous

angioelephantiasis

angioendothelioma
  endovascular papillary a.

angioendotheliomatosis
  malignant a.
  neoplastic a.
  a. proliferans
  proliferating systematized a.
  reactive a.
  systemic proliferating a.

angiofibrolipoma

angiofibroma
  a. contagiosum tropicum

angiofibromatous
  a. hamartoma

angiogenic

angiogranuloma

angiography

angiohistiocytoma

angioid streaks

angioimmunoblastic
  a. lymphadenopathy
    (AIL)

angiokeratoma
  a. circumscriptum
  a. corporis diffusum
  a. corporis diffusum
    universale
  diffuse a.
  localized a.
  a. of Fordyce
  a. of Mibelli
  a. of scrotum
  scrotal a.
  solitary a.
  verrucous a.
  vulvar a.
  a. of vulva

angiokeratosis

angioleiomyoma
  solitary a.

angiolipofibroma

angiolipoleiomyoma

angiolipoma

angiolupoid

angiolymphatic invasion

angiolymphoid
  a. hyperplasia
  a. hyperplasia with
    eosinophilia (AHLE)

angioma
  acquired tufted a.
  a. arteriale racemosum
  capillary a.
  a. cavernosum
  cavernous a.
  cherry a.
  hereditary hemorrhagic a.
  infectious a.
  keratotic a.
  a. lymphaticum
  a. pigmentosum
  plane a.
  plexiform a.
  sclerosing a.
  senile a.
  a. serpiginosum
  a. simplex
  spider a.
  stellate a.
  strawberry a.
  sudoriparous a.
  superficial a.
  telangiectatic a.
  tuberous a.
  tufted a.
  a. venosum racemosum
  venous a.

angiomatoid

angiomatosis
  bacillary a.

angiomatosis (*continued*)
    dermal a.
    encephalotrigeminal a.
    Sturge-Weber a.
    universal a.

angiomatous

angiomyolipoma

angioneurosis

angioneurotic
    a. edema

angioneurotica
    purpura a.

angio-osteohypertrophy
  syndrome

angiopathy

angioplasty

angiosarcoma

angiotensin-converting enzyme
  (ACE)

angle-closure glaucoma

angry
    a. back reaction
    a. back syndrome

angstrom, Ångström (Å)

Ångström unit (A unit)

angular
    a. cheilitis
    a. crease
    a. conjunctivitis
    a. macule
    a. stomatitis

anhidrosis
    thermal a.
    thermogenic a.

anhidrotic
    a. ectodermal dysplasia

anhydrous
    a. facial foundation
    a. theophylline

ani
    pruritus a.

anicteric

anidrosis

anidrotic

aniline
    a. dye dermatitis

animal
    a. dander
    a. dander sensitivity
    a. scabies

anionic
    a. detergents

anisakiasis

Anisakis
    A. marina
    A. simplex

anise oil

anisocoria

ankle-brachial index

ankyloblepharon
    congenital a.
    a. filiforme adnatum

ankyloglossia

ankylosing spondylitis (AS)

ankylosis spondylitis

Ankylostoma

annelid

Annelida

annual bluegrass

annular
    a. array
    a. atrophic connective
      tissue panniculitis
    a. borders
    a. configurations
    a. constriction
    a. elastolytic giant cell
      granuloma

annular (*continued*)
 a. erythema
 a. erythema of infancy
 a. erythematous plaque
 a. lesion
 a. lichen planus
 a. lipoatrophy
 a. patch
 a. patterns
 a. pustules
 a. sarcoidosis
 a. syphilid
 a. urticarial drug reaction

annulare
 erythema a.
 generalized granuloma a.
 granuloma a.
 a. lesions
 localized granuloma a.
 macular granuloma a.
 perforating granuloma a.
 subcutaneous granuloma a.

annularis
 leukotrichia a.
 lichen a.
 lichen planus a.
 lipoatrophia a.
 prurigo a.
 psoriasis a.
 purpura a. telangiectodes

annulati
 pili a.

annulus
 a. migrans

Anobium punctatum

anoderm

anodontia
 partial a.
 total a.
 true a.
 a. vera

anogenital
 a. herpes
 a. lichen sclerosus

anogenital (*continued*)
 a. wart

anomalous

anomaly *pl.* anomalies
 Jordan a.
 morning glory a.

anonychia

anonychosis

Anopheles
 A. albimanus
 A. freeborni
 A. funestus
 A. gambiae

Anoplura (*genera*)
 Haematopinus
 Linognathus
 Pediculus
 Phthirus
 Solenopotes

anorectal
 a. melanoma
 a. mucosa

anorexia nervosa

ANOTHER
 *a*lopecia, *n*ail dystrophy, *o*phthalmic complications, *t*hyroid dysfunction, *h*ypohidrosis, *e*phelides and *e*nteropathy, and *r*espiratory tract infections syndrome

anovulation

anovulatory agent

ansa lenticularis

ansate

anserina
 cutis a.

anserine

ansiform

ant
    a. bite
    black a.
    fire a.
    harvester a.
    red a.
    red imported fire a.
    a. sting
    velvet a.

antagonist
    serotonin a.

antecedent

antecubital
    a. area
    a. fossa
    a. space

anterior
    a. axillary fold
    a. cervical hypertrichosis
    a. faucial pillars
    a. hairline
    a. nares

anteverted pinnae

anthracis
    Bacillus a.

anthelix
    elastotic nodules of a.

anthracene

Anthra-Derm

anthralin
    a. paste
    a. therapy

anthranilate anthelminthics

anthrarobin

anthrax
    cutaneous a.
    intestinal a.
    a. spores
    a. toxin

Anthrenus
    A. scrophulariae

Anthrenus (*continued*)
    A. verbasci

anthropophaga
    Cordylobia a.

anthropophilic
    a. dermatophytes
    a. species

antiacetylcholine receptor
  antibody

antiandrogen

antiandrogenic
    a. substance

antiantibody

antibacterial
    a. soap
    a. therapy

anti–basement membrane
    anti–b. m. antibody

antibiotic
    a. anaphylaxis
    broad-spectrum a.
    a. candidiasis
    a. dermatitis
    a. prophylaxis

antibiotic-resistant

anti-BMZ specificity

antibody (Ab)
    antiacetylcholine receptor
      a.
    antiandrogen
    anti–basement membrane
      a.
    anti–basement membrane
      zone a.
    anti–basement zone a.
    anti-*Borrelia* a.
    anticardiolipin a. (ACA,
      ACLAb)
    anticentromere a.
    antidesmosomal a.
    antineutrophilic
      cytoplasmic a. (ANCA)

antibody (*continued*)
  antinuclear a. (ANA)
  antiphospholipid a. (APLA)
  anti-BP 180 a.
  anti-BP 230 a.
  anti-CD3 a.
  anti-DJ a.
  anti-ds DNA a.
  anti-EJ a.
  antierythrocyte a.
  anti-Jo-1 a.
  anti-Ku a.
  anti-La a.
  anti-Mi-2 a.
  anti-nRNP a.
  antinuclear circulating a.
  anti-PL-7 a.
  anti-PL-12 a.
  anti-PM/Scl a.
  anti-Ro a.
  anti-RNP a.
  anti-single stranded DNA a.
  anti-Sm a.
  anti-ss DNA a.
  antisynthetase a.
  antivaricella a.
  a. assay system
  complement-fixing specific
    a.
  a.-dependent cellular
    cytotoxicity
  drug-specific a.
  a. excess
  fluorescent a.
  heterophile a., heterophile
    a.
  IgA a.
  IgD a.
  IgE a.
  IgG anti–type II collagen a.
  IgM a.
  intracellular a.
  isohemagglutinin a.
  microsomal a.
  a. molecule
  monoclonal a.
  nuclear ribonucleoprotein
    a.

antibody (*continued*)
  passively infused a.
  pemphigus intracellular a.
  PM-Scl a.
  Ro a.
  a. synthesis
  thyroid a.
  thyroid-stimulating a.
  Treponema a.

antibody-complement
  interaction

antibody-dependent
  a.-d. cell-mediated
    cytotoxicity (ADCC)
  a.-d. cellular cytotoxicity

antibody-mediated
  a.-m. cellular cytotoxicity
  a.-m. disease

anti-*Borrelia* antibody

antibromics (*class of drugs*)

anticandidal
  a. agents
  a. imidazoles

anticardiolipin
  a. antibody (ACA, ACLAb)
  a. antibody syndrome

anticentromere
  a. antibody
  a. pattern

anticholinergic
  a. agent
  a. drug

anticoagulant
  circulating a.
  lupus a. (LA)
  a. therapy

anticonvulsant
  hydantoin a.
  a. hypersensitivity reaction
  a. hypersensitivity
    syndrome

anticorrosion solutions

anticytoplasmic

antidepressant
    heterocyclic a.
    tricyclic a.

antidesmosomal antibody

anti–double-stranded DNA

antieczematic

antiedematous

antiedemic

antielastase

antiendothelial cell antibody

antiepileptic
    a. medication

antiepiligrin cicatricial
    pemphigoid

antiepithelial serum

antifibrinolytic
    a. agents
    a. tranexamic acid

antifungal
    Absorbine Jr. A.
    a. agents
    Breezee Mist A.
    oral azole a.
    a. therapy

antigen (Ag)
    a. 5
    97-kD a.
    105-kD a.
    145-kD a.
    180-kD bullous pemphigoid
       a.
    180-kD a.
    200-kD a.
    230-kD a.
    230-kD bullous pemphigoid
       a.
    290-kD a.
    antineutrophilic
       cytoplasmic a.
    booster a.

antigen (*continued*)
    carcinoembryonic a. (CEA)
    cardiolipin-cholesterol-
       lecithin a.
    CD-7 a.
    complement-opsonized a.
    cryptococcal a.
    cutaneous lymphocyte a.
       (CLA)
    cytoplasmic a.
    exogenous a.
    Frei a.
    histocompatability a.
    HL-A a.
    HLA-D a.
    Intracellular a.
    Kveim a.
    LDA-1 a.
    leukocyte function a.
    lipoidal a.
    MHC class II a.
    Mitsuda a.
    a.-nonspecific helper
    nucleolar a.
    paracoccidioidin a.
    phagocytosed extracellular
       a.
    a.-presenting cells
    Ro/SSA a.
    SM a.
    soluble a.
    soluble protein a.
    a.-specific helper
    T cell-independent a.
    transplantation a.
    treponemal a.
    tumor a.
    unbound a.
    vaccine a.

antigen-antibody
    a.-a. complex
    a.-a. interaction
    a.-a. reaction

antigen-binding site

antigenemia

antigenic

antigenic (*continued*)
a. challenge
a. determinant
a. exposure
a. trigger

antigenicity

antigen-presenting cell (APC)

antiherpetic antibiotic

antihidrotic

Antihist-1

antihistamines (*class of drugs*)
H1 a.
H2 a.
nonsedating a.
oral a.

antihistaminic ointment

anti-HIV antiretroviral therapy

antihuman

antihidrotics (*class of drugs*)

anti-icteric

anti-idiotype
a.-i. antibody
a.-i. response

antiinfective

antiinflammatory
nonsteroidal a.
a. therapy

anti-influenza vaccine

antikeratin

antilaminin cicatricial
pemphigoid

antileprotic

antiluetic

antimalaria-induced
hyperpigmentation

antimalarial
a. agent

antimalarial (*continued*)
a. drug
a. therapy

antimetabolite

antimicrobial
a. contact dermatitis
a. preparation
a. spectrum

antimitochondrial antibody

antimonial drug therapy for
leishmaniasis

antimony
a. dermatitis
a. *n*-methyl glutamine
pentavalent a.
a. potassium tartrate
a. sodium tartrate
a. sodium thioglycollate
tartrated a.
a. thioglycollamide
a. trichloride

antinative DNA

antineoplastic

antineutrophilic
a. cytoplasmic antibody
(ANCA)

anti-nRNP
antinuclear ribonucleic acid
protein

antinuclear
a. antibody (ANA)
a. antibody immunodiffusion
a. antibody
immunofluorescence
a. antibody screening by
enzyme immunoassay
a. antibody screening test
a. factor (ANF)
a. ribonucleic acid protein

antioxidant
a. dermatitis
hydroquinone a.

antiparasitic

antiparastata

antiperspirant
   a. dermatitis

antiphospholipid
   a. antibody (APLA)
   a. antibody syndrome (APS)
   a. syndrome

antiplatelet

antipruritic
   a. agent
   a. therapy
   topical a.

antipseudomonal
   a. Cortisporin otic
      solution
   a. Cortisporin otic
      suspension
   a. penicillin

antipsoriatic

antipyogenic

antipyresis

antipyretic

antipyrotic

antiretroviral agents

anti-Ro antibody

antiscabietic

antiseborrheic

antiseptics (*class of drugs*)

antiserum *pl.* antisera

antispasmodic

antistaphylococcic

antistreptolysin
   a. O (ASLO)
   a. O titer

antisudoral

antisudorific

antisynthetase syndrome
   a. s. antibody

antisyphilitic

antithrombin
   a. III

antithrombotic

antithymocyte globulin

antithyroglobulin

antithyroid

antitoxin
   a. rash

antituberculous therapy

antivaricella antibody

antivenin
   black widow spider a.
   a. (Crotalidae) polyvalent

antivenom
   tiger snake a.

antivenomous serum

antiviral
   a. drug
   a. immunity
   a. therapy

antiwrinkle band

antiwrinkling chemicals

antlerlike projections

anucleate squames

ANUG
   acute necrotizing ulcerative
      gingivitis

anulus

anuric

Anusol
   A. HC-1
   A.-HC 2.5%
   A.-HC suppository

Anxanil

anxiety

aorta adventitia

aortic

aortitis

APACHE
  acute physiology and
    chronic health evaluation
      APACHE II score
      APACHE II system

apathy

APC
  antigen-presenting cell
    APC gene

APECED
  autoimmune
    polyendocrinopathy,
    candidiasis-ectodermal
    dystrophy
      APECED syndrome

Apert
  A's hirsutism
  A's syndrome

aphasia

aphtha *pl.* aphthae
  Bednar's aphthae
  herpetiform a.
  Mikulicz's aphthae
  recurrent scarring aphthae

aphthaelike lesions

Aphthasol

aphthoid

aphthosis

aphthous
  a. genital ulcer
  a. oral ulcer
  a. stomatitis
  a. ulcer

Aphthovirus

apical dental abscess

apices

aplasia
  a. cutis congenita
  a. cutis congenita areata
  a. cutis congenita
    circumscripta

aplastic anemia

Apligraf

apocrine
  a. adenoma
  a. carcinoma
  a. cell
  a. chromhidrosis
  a. cystadenoma
  a. epithelial antigen
  a. gland
  a. gland carcinoma
  a. epithelioma
  a. hidrocystoma
  a. metaplasia
  a. malaria
  a. miliaria
  a. retention cyst
  a. secretion
  a. sweat gland
  a. sweat fluoresce

apocrinitis

apolipoprotein (apo)

aponeurosis *pl.* aponeuroses
  bicipital a.
  a. bicipitalis
  epicranial a.
  a. epicranialis
  extensor a.
  a. linguae
  lingual a.
  a. musculi bicipitis brachii
  a. palatina
  palatine a.
  palmar a.
  a. palmaris
  pharyngeal a.
  a. pharyngis
  pharyngobasilar a.

aponeurosis (*continued*)
    a. pharyngobasilaris
    plantar a.
    a. plantaris
    temporal a.
    a. of vastus muscles

aponeurositis

aponeurotic fibroma

Apophysomyces
    A. elegans

apoprotein

apoptosis

apostematosa
    cheilitis glandularis a.

apparatus
    Golgi a.
    pilosebaceous a.

appearance
    clinical a.
    cluster-of-grapes a.
    cushingoid a.
    enamel paint spot a.
    "figure-eight" a.
    finger-in-glove a.
    granulomatous a.
    ground-glass a.
    hair-on-end a.
    hair-standing-on-end a.
    "hourglass" a.
    monomorphous a.
    slapped-cheek a.
    slapped-face a.
    stuck-on a.

appendage
    epidermal a.
    a. of the skin

appendageal
    a. structures

appetite suppressant

apple
    Indian a.
    a. jelly nodule

apple (*continued*)
    a. jelly papule of lupus
        vulgaris
    May a.

application sparganosis

apposing folds

APUD
    amino precursor uptake
        and decarboxylation

apurpuric

Aqua Tar

Aquacare

Aquacare topical

aquadynia

aquagenic
    a. pruritus
    a. urticaria

aquagenous urticaria

Aquanil

Aquaphor
    A. antibiotic topical

Aquasol E

aqueous
    a. epinephrine
    a. extract
    penicillin a.
    a. solution
    a. vaccine

arachidonic
    a. acid (AA)

Arachnia
    A. propionica

Arachnida

arachnidism
    necrotic a.

arachnodactylia

arachnodactyly
    congenital contractural a.

arachnoideus
    nevus a.

Aralen
    A. Phosphate
    A. Phosphate with
        Primaquine Phosphate

araneidism

araneus
    nevus a.

aranodactylia

arbor *pl.* arbores
    a. vitae
    a. vitae tree

arborescens
    lipoma a.

arborescent

arborization

arbovirus *(formerly arborvirus)*
    a. group

ARC
    AIDS-related complex

arc

*Arcanobacterium
    haemolyticum*

arcate

archipelago
    Indonesian a.

arciform

arcuate
    a. lesion

area
    butterfly a.
    dermatomic a.
    flush a.
    hairless atrophic a.
    intertriginous a.
    periocular a.
    perioral a.
    periorbital a.

areata
    alopecia a.
    keratolysis exfoliativa a.
        manuum
    pseudoalopecia a.

areate

areatus

Areca palm

Arenaviridae

Arenavirus

areola *pl.* areolae
    Chaussier a.
    a. mammae
    nevoid hyperkeratosis of
        nipple and a.
    a. of mammary gland
    a. of nipple
    a. papillaris
    primary a.
    umbilical a.
    vaccinal a.

areolar

areolate

Argas
    A. americanus
    A. brumpti
    A. miniatus
    A. persicus
    A. reflexus

Argasidae (*genera*)
    Antricola
    Argas
    Ornithodoros
    Otobius

argemone
    oil of a.

argentaffin

argentaffinoma

arginine codon

argininosuccinate synthase
    deficiency

argininosuccinic acid synthetase
  deficiency

argininosuccinicaciduria

argon
  a. laser
  a. laser ablation
  a. pumped tunable dye
    laser

Argyll Robertson pupil

argyria

argyriasis

argyric

argyrism

argyrosis

argyrophil, argyrophile

Aristocort
  A. Forte
  A. intralesional suspension

Aristospan

Arizona
  A. hinshawii

Arizona/Fremont
  A. cottonwood
  A. cottonwood tree

armamentarium
  dermatologist's surgical a.

armorlike plates

Arndt
  A.-Gottron disease
  A.-Gottron syndrome

AROA
  autosomal recessive ocular
    albinism

Arolla index

aromatherapy

aromatic

array

array (*continued*)
  linear a.
  reticulate a.

arrector *pl.* arrectores
  a. pili muscle
  a. pilus

arrhenoblastoma

arrhythmia

arrhythmogenic

arsenic
  a.-contaminated water
  a. dermatosis
  a. exposure
  a. fumes
  a. hyperpigmentation
  inorganic a.
  a. pesticides
  a. pigmentation
  a. squamous carcinomata
  a. trioxide
  white a.

arsenical
  a. cancer
  a. compounds
  a. dermatitis
  a. hyperpigmentation
  a. keratosis
  a. melanosis
  a. squamous carcinomata

arsenious

artegraft

arterial
  a. anomaly
  a. graft
  a. hypoxemia
  a. obliteration
  a. peripheral vascular
    disease
  a. thrombosis

arteriography

arteriohepatic dysplasia

arteriolar

arteriole
    ascending central a.
    terminal a.

arteriosclerosis
    a. obliterans

arteriosclerotic
    a. gangrene
    a. ulcer

arteriovenous (AV, A-V)
    a. aneurysm
    a. anomaly
    a. fistula
    a. malformation (AVM)
    a. shunt

arteritis
    brachiocephalic a.
    cranial a.
    equine viral a.
    extracranial a.
    giant cell a.
    granulomatous a.
    Horton's a.
    Takayasu a.
    temporal a.

arthralgia
    a. saturnina

arthralgic

arthrites pseudoseptiques et
    bacterides d'Andrews

arthritide

arthritis *pl.* arthritides
    asymmetrical a.
    gonococcal a.
    gonorrheal a.
    gouty a.
    hemophilic a.
    Jaccoud's a.
    juvenile a.
    juvenile chronic a.
    juvenile rheumatoid a.
    Lyme a.
    a. mutilans
    a. nodosa

arthritis (*continued*)
    polyarticular a.
    psoriatic a.
    pyogenic a.
    rheumatoid a. (RA)
    seronegative a.
    suppurative a.

Arthritis Foundation Pain
    Reliever

arthrochalasis multiplex
    congenita

arthroclasia

Arthroderma

arthrodynia

arthrogryposis
    congenital multiple a.
    a. multiplex congenita

arthrop bite

arthropathia
    a. psoriatica

arthropathy
    Jaccoud's a.
    myxedematous a.
    psoriatic a.

arthrophyma

arthropod
    a. bite
    a. sting

Arthropoda

arthropodic

arthropodous

arthrospore

arthrosteitis

Arthus
    A. phenomenon
    A.-type reaction

Articulose
    A. LA
    A.-50 injection

artifact

artificial
  a. fingernails
  a. ultraviolet light

arylsulfatase C

AS
  ankylosing spondylitis

ASA
  acetylsalicylic acid

Asacol Oral

asbestos
  a. corn
  a. wart

asbestosis

Asboe-Hansen disease

ascariasis

ascaricide

ascarid

ascaris

Ascaris lumbricoides

ascending
  a. aortic aneurysm
  a. central arteriole
  a. paralysis

Ascher's syndrome

ascitic fluid

ascospore

Ascriptin

ascus *pl.* asci

asepsis

aseptic
  a. necrosis
  a. technique

asepticism

ash
  Arizona a.

ash (*continued*)
  green a.
  Oregon a.
  a. tree
  white a.

ash-leaf
  a.-l. hypomelanotic macule
  a.-l. macule

ashy dermatosis

asiaticoside

ASO
  ASO test
  ASO titer

aspartic acid

aspartylglycosamine

aspartylglycosaminidase

aspartylglycosaminuria

aspen
  a. tree

aspergillin

aspergilloma

aspergillomycosis

aspergillosis

Aspergillus
  A. flavus
  A. fumigatus
  A. nidulans
  A. niger
  A. terreus

asphyxia
  birth a.
  blue a.
  a. cyanotica
  fetal a.
  a. livida
  local a.
  a. neonatorum
  a. pallida
  perinatal a.
  secondary a.

asphyxia (*continued*)
    traumatic a.
    white a.

asphyxiation

aspiration
    a. biopsy
    fine needle a. (FNA)
    recurrent a.

aspirin
    Bayer A.
    Bayer Buffered A.
    enteric-coated a.
    Extra Strength Bayer Enteric
      500 A.
    A. Free Anacin Maximum
      Strength
    a. sensitivity
    St. Joseph Adult Chewable
      A.
    a. triad

asplenic

Asprimox

assassin
    a. bug
    a. bug bite

assay
    hemolytic a.
    indirect a.

associated systemic disease

asteatodes

asteatosis
    a. cutis

asteatotic
    a. eczema

astemizole

asteroid body

asthenia
    cutaneous a.
    tropical a.
    tropical anhidrotic a.

asthma

astigmatism

astringents (*class of drugs*)

astrocytoma

asymmetric
    a. distribution
    a. periflexural exanthem of
      childhood

asymmetrical
    a. annular plaque
    a. clubbing
    a. distal interphalangeal
      joint
    a. sacroiliitis

asymptomatic
    a. carrier
    a. shedding

Atabrine

Atarax

ataxia
    a. cerebellar
    a. telangiectasia
    a. telangiectasia syndrome

ataxia-telangiectasia

atenolol

atheroma
    a. cutis

atheromata

atheromatosis
    a. cutis

atheromatous
    a. embolus

atherosclerosis

atherosclerotic disease

atherosis

athetoid

athetosis

athlete
  a's foot
  a's nodule

atlantoaxial
  a. joint

ATL
  adult T-cell leukemia

ATLL
  adult T-cell
    leukemia/lymphoma

atloaxoid

ATN
  tyrosinase-negative (ty-neg)
    oculocutaneous albinism

atonicity

atonia

atonic ulcer

atony

atopic
  a. dermatitis
  a. dermatitis rash
  a. diathesis
  a. disease
  a. eczema
  a. hand dermatitis
  a. sensitivity

atopy

Atozine

ATP
  adenosine triphosphate

ATPase activity

atresia

atrial
  a. myxoma
  a. septal defect

atrichia

atrichosis

atrichous

atrioventricular (AV, A-V)
  a. fistula

Atriplex

atriplicism

Atrisone

atrophedema

atrophia
  a. cutis
  a. cutis senilis
  a. maculosa

atrophic
  a. candidiasis
  a. erythematous
  a. filiform papillae
  a. glossitis
  a. lichen planus
  a. linear lesions
  a. macule
  a. papulosis
  a. pits
  a. plaque
  a. scar
  a. striae
  a. white scar
  a. wrinkling

atrophica *pl.* atrophicae
  acne a.
  hyperkeratosis figurata
    centrifuga a.
  macula a.
  stria a.

atrophicae (*plural of* atrophica)
  lineae a.
  lineae striae a.

atrophicans
  acrodermatitis chronica a.
  dermatitis a.
  epidermolysis bullosa a.
  keratosis pilaris a.
  lichen planus et
    acuminatus a.
  lichen sclerosus et a.
  pityriasis alba a.
  poikiloderma vasculare a.

atrophicus
    lichen sclerosis et a.
       (LS&A)

atrophie
    a. blanche
    a. cutis
    a. maculosa varioliformis
       cutis
    a. noire
    a. pilorum propria

atrophied

atropine

atrophoderma
    a. albidum
    a. biotripticum
    a. diffusum
    follicular a.
    idiopathic a. of Pasini and
       Pierini
    macular a.
    a. maculatum
    neuritic a.
    a. neuriticum
    a. of Pasini and Pierini
    Pasini-Pierini idiopathic a.
    progressive idiopathic a.
    a. reticulatum
       symmetricum faciei
    a. scleroatrophy
    senile a.
    a. senile
    a. striatum
    a. striatum et maculatum
    a. ulerythematosa
    a. vermicularis
    vermiculate a. of cheeks
    a. vermiculatum

atrophodermatosis

atrophodermia (variant of
    atrophoderma)
    a. reticulata
    a. ulerythematosa
    a. vermiculata

atrophy

atrophy (continued)
    black a.
    blue a.
    Buchwald's a.
    cutaneous a.
    cyanotic a.
    disuse a.
    epidermal a.
    fatty a.
    a. of fat
    fat-replacement a.
    idiopathic muscular a.
    linear a.
    macular a.
    optic a.
    pressure a.
    primary a.
    primary diffuse a.
    primary idiopathic macular
       a.
    red a.
    senile a.
    senile a. of skin
    skin a.
    smooth a.
    striate a. of skin
    traction a.
    villous a.
    wucher a.

atrophying papulosquamous
    dermatitis

atropine
    a. ointment
    a. sulfate

Atropine-Care Ophthalmic

A/T/S
    A. lotion
    A. topical

attenuated

atypia
    cellular a.
    cytologic a.

atypical
    a. cell

atypical (*continued*)
- a. cellulitis
- a. clinical course
- a. clone
- a. clostridial
- a. erythema multiforme
- a. fibroxanthoma
- a. histiocytosis
- a. ichthyosiform erythroderma
- a. Kawasaki disease (AKD)
- a. lesion
- a. lipoma
- a. lymphocytosis
- a. measles
- a. megakaryocyte
- a. melanocyte
- a. mitotic figure
- a. mole
- a. mole syndrome
- a. mononuclear cell
- a. morphology
- a. mycobacterial colonization
- a. mycobacterial infection
- a. mycobacteriosis
- a. nevus syndrome
- a. pityriasis rosea
- a. pneumonia
- a. purpuric targetoid lesion
- a. retinitis pigmentosa
- a. Sweet's syndrome
- a. target
- a. tumor cells

atypism

auditory

Audouin microsporon

audouinii
- *Microsporum a.*

augment

augmentation
- a. mammoplasty
- a. therapy

Augmentin

aura

aural fistula

Auralate

auranofin

aurantiasis

Aureobasidium pullulans

Aureomycin

auricle
- accessory a.
- cervical a.

auricular
- a. atresia
- a. fold
- a. nerve

auriculotemporal syndrome

aurid

aurotherapy

aurochromoderma

aurothioglucose

Auspitz's sign

Australian
- A. pine
- A. pine tree
- A. sea wasp
- A. sea wasp sting

autoallergy

autoamputation

autoantibody

autoantigen

autocytotoxicity

autocytotoxin

autoeczematization

autoerythrocyte
- a. sensitivity
- a. sensitization
- a. sensitization syndrome

autogeneic graft

autograft
   epidermal a.

autogram

autoimmune
   a. blistering disease
   a. bullous disease
   a. disease
   a. estrogen dermatitis
   a. hemolysis
   a. mechanism
   a. phenomenon
   a. polyendocrinopathy,
      candidiasis, ectodermal
      dystrophy syndrome
   a. progesterone dermatitis
   a. purpura
   a. thrombocytopenia
      (ATTP)

autoimmunity

autoimmunization

autoinoculable

autoinoculation

autologous
   a. bone marrow
      transplantation
   a. epidermal cell
   a. graft
   a. heat shock protein
   a. meshed split-thickness
      skin grafts
   a. minigraft
   a. mixed leukocyte reaction
   a. serum

Automeris
   A. io

autoplast

autoplastic
   a. graft

autosensitization
   a. dermatitis
   erythrocyte a.

autosomal
   a. dominant
   a. dominant characteristic
   a. dominant familial
      inheritance
   a. dominant fashion
   a. dominant
      genodermatosis
   a. dominant hypohidrotic
      ectodermal dysplasia
   a. dominant inheritance
   a. dominant inheritance
      pattern
   a. dominant inherited
      disorder
   a. dominant lamellar
      ichthyosis
   a. dominant manner
   a. dominant mode of
      transmission
   a. dominant syndrome
   a. dominant mode of
      transmission
   a. dominantly inherited
      condition
   a. dominantly inherited
      neuroectodermal
      syndrome
   a. recessive
   a. recessive disease
   a. recessive disorder
   a. recessive ichthyosis
   a. recessive inherited
      disease
   a. recessive mode of
      inheritance
   a. recessive severe
      combined
      immunodeficiency
      disorder (SCID)
   a. recessive trait
   a. recessive type of
      inheritance
   a. X-linked hereditary
      disorder

autotransplant

autotransplantation

AV, A-V
  atrioventricular
    AV block

avascular

Aveeno
  A. Anti-Itch cream
  A. Cleansing bar
  A. Cleansing for acne-prone
    skin
  A. lotion
  A. moisturizing cream
  A. Oilated Bath
  A. Regular Bath
  A. shave gel
  A. shower & bath oil

avian

avidin-biotin-peroxidase stain

avidity antibody

avitaminosis

Avlosulfon

avobenzone

Avon Skin-So-Soft

avulsion

axial lesions

axilla *pl.* axillae

axillary
  a. antiperspirant
  a. apocrine myoepithelial
    cells
  a. deodorant
  a. dermatitis

axillary (*continued*)
  a. freckles
  a. freckling
  a. hyperhidrosis
  a. malodor
  a. vault

axon sheath myxoma

azatadine maleate

azathioprine (AZA)

azelaic acid

azelastine

Azelex

azithromycin

azo
  a. compounds
  a. dye
  a. itch

azobenzene dye

azoles (*class of drugs*)

azotemia
  progressive a.

Azulfidine

azure lunula of nail

azurophil
  a. granule
  a. granule protein

azurophilia

azurophilic
  a. leukocytic inclusions

B

B
B cell
B lymphocyte
B virus

BA
betamethasone acetate

B&A
before and after

Babesia
B. bigemina
B. bovis
B. canis
B. divergens
B. equi
B. felis
B. major
B. microti
B. rodhaini

babesiosis

baboon syndrome

baby
blueberry muffin b.
collodion b.

Baby Magic soap

bacampicillin hydrochloride

bacciform

Baciguent topical

bacillary
b. angiomatosis (BA)
b.-barren tuberculid
b. fragment
b. index (BI)

bacille
bacille bilié de Calmette-
Guérin (BCG)
b. Calmette-Guérin (BCG)
b. Calmette-Guérin live
b. Calmette-Guérin
vaccine

bacilliformis
Bartonella b.

bacillosis

Bacillus
B. acnes
B. anthracis
B. anthracis toxin
B. cereus
B. licheniformis
B. stearothermophilus
B. subtilis
B. tularense

bacillus pl. bacilli
acid-fast b. (AFB)
acne b.
Battey b.
Boas-Oppler b.
Bordet-Gengou b.
Doderlein b.
Ducrey b.
enteric b.
Escherich b.
Flexner b.
Friedlander b.
Frisch b.
fusiform b.
Gartner b.
Ghon-Sachs b.
glanders b.
glanderslike b.
gram-negative b.
gram-positive b.
Hansen b.
hay b.
Hofmann b.
influenza b.
Klebs-Loeffler b.
Koch b.
Koch-Weeks b.
Lepra b.
leprosy b.
Morgan b.
Newcastle-Manchester b.
paracolon b.

bacillus (*continued*)
 Pfeiffer b.
 plague b.
 Preisz-Nocard b.
 rhinoscleroma b.
 Schmitz b.
 Shiga b.
 smegma b.
 Sonne-Duval b.
 Strong b.
 swine rotlauf b.
 tubercle b.
 typhoid b.
 Vincent b.
 Weeks b.
 Welch b.
 Whitmore b.

bacitracin
 b. zinc
 b. zinc and neomycin
  sulfate and polymyxin B
  sulfate
 b. zinc and polymyxin B
  sulfate
 b. zinc complex

baclofen

bacoti
 Liponyssus b.

bacteremia
 gram-negative b.
 gram-positive b.
 polymicrobial b.
 Pseudomonas aeruginosa
  b.

bacteria (*plural of*
 bacterium)
 pathogenic b.

bacterial
 b. agglutination assay
 b. agglutination test
 b. cell wall
 b. culture
 b. decomposition
 b. endocarditis
 b. exotoxins

bacterial (*continued*)
 b. folliculitis
 b. infection
 b. invasion
 b. lipase
 b. resistance
 b. septicemia
 b. sycosis
 b. tissue
 b. toxin

bactericide
 specific b.

bacterid
 pustular b.

bacteriocide

bacteriocidin

bacteriostatic

bacterium *pl.* bacteria
 gram-negative bacteria
 gram-positive bacteria
 lactic acid b.

Bacteroides
 B. fragilis
 B. fusiformis

Bactine

Bactocill
 B. injection
 B. Oral

BactoShield topical

Bactrim
 B. DS

Bactroban
 B. ointment
 B. cream

Baelz
 B. disease

Bäfverstedt's syndrome

Bagdad
 bouton de B.

baggy nevi

Baghdad boil

Bain de Soleil

Bairnsdale ulcer

Baker cyst

baker
  b's dermatitis
  b's eczema
  b's itch

baking soda paste

balanitic thrush

balanitis *pl.* balanitides
  Candida b.
  b. candidomycetica
  b. circinata
  circinate b.
  b. circumscripta
    plasmacellularis
  erosive *Candida* b.
  b. erosive circinata
  Follmann b.
  gangrenous b.
  perimeatal b.
  plasma cell b.
  b. plasmacellularis
  b. plasmacellularis zoon
  b. xerotica obliterans
  b. of Zoon
  Zoon's balanitis

balanoposthitis
  chronic circumscribed
    plasmocytic b.
  b. chronica circumscripta
    plasmacellularis
  b. erosive circinata

bald
  b. cypress
  b. cypress tree

Baldex

balding
  temporal b.

baldness
  common b.

baldness (*continued*)
  congenital b.
  male pattern b.
  moth-eaten b.
  pubic b.

Ballingall
  B. disease

balloon
  b. angioplasty
  b. cells
  b. cell melanoma
  b. cell nevus
  b. degeneration
  b. viral cells

ballooning degeneration

balm
  b. of Gilead

Balmex
  B. Baby
  B. Emollient

balnea
  pruritus b.

Balneol

balneotherapy

Balnetar

balsam
  b. of Gilead
  b. of Peru
  b. of tolu
  peruvian b.
  tolu b.
  Turlington's b.
  Wade's b.

balsamics

bamboo
  b. hair
  b. spine

banal
  b. condition
  b. perivascular infiltrate
  b. pyogens

banana-shaped body

band
    b. immunoglobulin
      deposition

bandage
    Ace b.
    Hollister medial adhesive b.
    b. sign
    TubiFast b.

Band-Aid
    B. dressing

bandlike
    b. inflammatory infiltrate
    b. pattern

Banker type

bankokcrend

Bannayan
    Bannayan-Riley-Ruvalcaba
      syndrome
    Bannayan-Zonana
      syndrome

Bannwarth's syndrome

Banophen Oral

Banthine

bantiana
    Cladophialophora b.
    Xylohypha

bar
    Aveeno Cleansing b.
    HI-CAL VM b.
    ZNP B.

barba *gen. and pl.* barbae
    eczema barbae
    folliculitis barbae
    pseudofolliculitis barbae
    sycosis barbae
    tinea barbae
    trichophytosis barbae

Barber
    B. psoriasis

barber
    b's itch
    b's pilonidal sinus

barb

barbula
    b. hirci

Barcoo
    B. disease
    B. rot

Bard-Parker scalpel blade

Bardet-Biedl syndrome

bare lymphocyte syndrome

barium sulfide

barley itch

Barraquer-Simons syndrome

barrier
    b. layer
    b. methods
    b. zone

basilar pigmentation

Bart
    B's syndrome
    B.-Pumphrey syndrome

Bartholin abscess

Bartonella
    B. bacilliformis
    B. clarridgeiae
    B. henselae
    B. henselae detection
    B. quintana

bartonellae

bartonellas

bartonellosis

basal
    b. ganglia
    b. hemidesmosome
    b. keratinocyte
    b. lamina
    b. layer

basal (*continued*)
    b. layer damage
    b. layer spongiosis

basal cell
    b. c. carcinoma
    b. c. carcinoma syndrome
    b. c. damage
    b. c. epithelioma
    b. c. layer
    b. c. nevus syndrome
    b. c. papilloma
    b. c. proliferation

basal cell carcinoma
    metatypic b. c. c.
    morpheiform b. c. c.
    pigmented b. c. c.
    solid-cystic b. c. c.
    superficial b. c. c.
    ulcerating b. c. c.

basalar

basalioma
    b. terebrans

basaloid
    b. cell
    b. hamartomatous
    b. nest

basaloma

base
    clean b.
    gummy b.
    b. of nail
    sessile b.

Basedow
    B. disease

baseline
    b. dermatologic
      photography
    b. liver biopsy
    b. metabolism

basement membrane
    b. m. zone (BMZ)
    b. m. zone collagen

basidiobolomycosis

Basidiobolus ranarum

basilar
    b. hyperpigmentation
    b. melanocytic
      hyperplasia
    b. pigmentation

basiloma terebrans

Basis soap

basket-weave
    b.-w. pattern
    b.-w. vacuolization

basocellular sheet

basophil
    b. degranulation test
    b. mediator

basophilic
    b. cell
    b. cytoplasm
    b. degeneration
    b. keratohyalin
      granules
    b. nuclear remnant
    b. nucleus

basosquamous
    b. carcinoma

Bateman
    B's disease
    B's purpura
    B's syndrome

bath
    alkaline b.
    Aveeno b.
    colloid b.
    emollient b.
    infrared b.
    b. itch
    oatmeal b.
    b. pruritus
    b.-PUVA

bathing-suit distribution

bathing-trunk nevus

battery acid

Battey strain

bavachi

bay sore

bayberry

Bayer
  B. aspirin
  B. buffered aspirin

bayonet hair

Bazex
  B's follicular atrophoderma
    syndrome
  B's syndrome

Bazin
  B's disease
  B's ulcer

BB
  borderline borderline

Bb
  Borrelia burgdorferi

BCC
  basal cell carcinoma

B-cell
  B-c. deficiency
  B-c. phenotype
  B-c. immunodeficiencies
  B-c. lymphocytoma cutis
  B-c. lymphoma
  B-c. lymphoma of follicular
    center cell origin
  B-c. lymphoid hyperplasia
  B-c. markers
  B-c. proliferation
  B-c. pseudolymphoma
  B-c. surface
  B-c. surface markers

BCE
  basal cell epithelioma

BCG

BCG (*continued*)
  bacille bilié de Calmette-
    Guérin
  bacille Calmette-Guérin
    BCG immunization
    TICE BCG
    TICE BCG Live
    BCG lupus
    BCG vaccine

BCH
  benign cephalic
    histiocytosis

BCNU therapy

beaded
  b. hair
  b. lizard

beaklike nose

beam

"bean bag" cell

beard
  ringworm of b.

bearded region

Beare-Stevenson cutis gyrata
  syndrome

Beau's lines

beautician

beauty mark

becaplermin

Beck (*see* Boeck)

Becker
  B's antigen
  B's hairy hamartoma
  B's nevus

Beckwith-Wiedemann
  syndrome

bed
  nail b.
  b. sore

bedbug
    b. bite
    b. disease transmission

Bednar
    B. aphtha
    B. tumor

Bedouin

bedsore

bee
    bumblebee
    honeybee
    b. sting
    sweat b.
    b. venom

beech
    b. tree

beefy red

Beepen-VK Oral

beeswax

beetle
    ash-gray blister b.
    blister b.
    carpet b.
    furniture b.
    rove b.
    striped blister b.

before and after (B&A)

behavioral therapy

Behçet
    B's disease
    B's oral and genital ulcers
    B's syndrome

Beigel
    B. disease

bejel

Belix Oral

belladonna alkaloids

Bell's palsy

Benadryl
    B. injection
    B. Oral
    B. topical

Ben-Aqua

Bence Jones
    B. J. cryoglobulin
    B. J. protein
    B. J. proteinuria

benign
    b. cephalic histiocytosis
    (BCH)
    b. dyskeratosis
    b. epidermal melanocytic
    neoplasm
    b. familial chronic
    pemphigus
    b. familial pemphigus
    b. giant cell synovioma
    b. hamartomatous
    dysplasia
    b. hemangiopericytoma
    b.
    hypergammaglobulinemic
    purpura
    b. inoculation
    lymphoreticulosis
    b. inoculation reticulosis
    b. juvenile melanoma
    b. leucoplakia
    b. lichenoid keratosis
    b. lipoblastomatosis
    b.
    lymphangioendothelioma
    b. migratory glossitis
    b. mucosal pemphigoid
    b. neonatal
    hemangiomatosis
    b. neoplasia
    b. neoplasm
    b. papular acantholytic
    dermatosis
    b. pigmented idiopathic
    hemorrhagic sarcoma
    b. plasma cell erythroplasia
    b. symmetric lipomatosis

benign (*continued*)
    transitory b., migrating
      plaques
    b. tumor

benigna
    lymphadenosis cutis b.
    lymphogranulomatosis b.
    variola b.

Benoquin cream

benoxaprofen

Benoxyl

bentonite
    b. flocculation test
    b. gel

Benzac
    B. AC Gel
    B. AC Wash
    B. W

benzalkonium chloride

Benzamycin

Benzashave

benzathine
    b. benzylpenicillin
    b. penicillin
    b. penicillin G

benzene

benzeneamine

benzethonium chloride

benzimidazole

benzin

benzoate and phenylacetate

benzocaine
    antipyrine and b.
    b. butyl aminobenzoate,
      tetracaine, and
      benzalkonium chloride
    b. gelatin, pectin, and
      sodium
      carboxymethylcellulose

benzocaine (*continued*)
    Orabase with b.
    b. and salicylic acid

benzodiazepine
    b. midazolam

benzoic acid
    b. a. and salicylic acid

benzoin
    tincture of b.

benzophenone
    b. dermatitis

benzoporphyrin derivative

benzoyl
    hydrous b. peroxide
    b. peroxide
    b. peroxide and
      hydrocortisone

p-benzyloxyphenol

benzpyrene
    3,4-b.

benzyl benzoate

benzylamines (*class of drugs*)

benzylhydrochlorothiazide

Beradinelli-Seip syndrome

beraprost sodium

bergapten

bergamot

beriberi

berlock, berloque
    b. dermatitis

Bermuda
    B. fire sponge
    B. dermatitis

berylliosis

beryllium
    b. disease
    b. granuloma

beryllium (*continued*)
  b. salts

Besnier
  B's disease
  B's lupus pernio
  prurigo of B.
  B's prurigo
  B.-Boeck disease
  B.-Boeck-Schaumann
    disease

beta (ß)
  b. blocker
  b. carotene
  b. carotene therapy
  b. catenin
  b. chain
  b. hemolytic streptococci
    infection
  b. lipoprotein

beta 2

beta 4 integrin genes

betacarotene

Betadine
  B. First Aid antibiotics +
    moisturizer

beta-glucocerebrosidase

beta-mannosidase deficiency

betamethasone
  b. and clotrimazole
  b. benzoate
  b. dipropionate
  b. group
  b. sodium phosphate and
    acetate suspension
  b. valerate

Betapen-VK Oral

beta-sitosterol

Betatrex

Beta-Val

betel pepper

Betula

BFP
  biologic false-positive

BHD
  Birt-Hogg-Dube syndrome

BI
  bacillary index

bicarbonate
  b. of soda

bichloracetic acid

Bicillin
  B. L-A injection

Bicitra

bidirectional

BIDS
  brittle hair, intellectual
    impairment, decreased
    fertility, short stature
      ichthyosis plus BIDS
      (IBIDS)
  BIDS syndrome

Bier's spots

Biet
  collarette of B.

bifid
  b. ribs
  b. scrotum
  b. uvula

bifonazole

bifunctional

bifurcated

bifurcation

bilaminate

bilateral
  b. adrenalectomy
  b. clavicular osteomyelitis
  b. dermatosis
  b. hilar adenopathy

bilateral (*continued*)
   b. index finger disease
   b. infraorbital nerve block
   b. pheochromocytomas
   b. port wine stains

bilayer

bilharzial
   b. granuloma
   b. ova

bilharziasis

bilharzioma

biliary
   b. cirrhosis
   b. colic
   b. disease
   b. pruritus

bilirubin
   b. level

Biltricide

bimodal

binder

binding
   b. activity
   b. elements

bindweed

bioavailability

Biobrane
   B. adhesive
   B. glove
   B. synthetic skin substitute

biochemical
   b. basis
   b. disturbance
   b. hyperandrogenism
   b. phenotypes
   b. studies

biocide

BioComplex 500 Revitalizing
   Conditioner

biogenesis

biologic
   b. false-positive (BFP)
   b. response modifier

Bioplastique

biopsy (Bx)
   aspiration b.
   biochemical b.
   elliptical b.
   excisional b.
   b. fixed erosive lesions
   b. in parte
   b. in toto
   incisional b.
   needle b.
   punch b.
   shave b.
   synovial b.
   total b.
   wedge b.

biosynthesis

biosynthetic pathway of
   melanin synthesis

Bio-Tab Oral

biotin
   b. deficiency

biotinidase
   b. deficiency

Biozyme-C

biparietal recession

biphasic tumor cell

biphosphonate

bipolar
   b. aphthosis
   b. current
   b. disorders
   b. electrical instrument
   b. electrosurgery

Bipolaris
   B. genera

Bipolaris (*continued*)
    B. spicifera

Birbeck
    B. granule
    B. granuloma

birch
    red b.
    river b.
    b. tree

birefringence
    apple-green b.

birefringent
    b. material

Birt-Hoff-Dubé syndrome (BHD)

birthmark
    port wine stain b.
    strawberry b.

BIS-GMA
    bisphenol A. and glycidyl
      methacrylate

Biskra
    bouton de B.
    B. button

bismuth
    basic b. carbonate
    b. aluminate
    b. line
    b. subcarbonate
    b. subgallate

bismuthia

bisphenol A

bisphosphonate

bite
    ant b.
    arthropod b.
    assassin bug b.
    bedbug b.
    black fly g.
    black widow spider b.
    brown recluse spider b.
    cat flea b.

bite (*continued*)
    centipede b.
    chigger b.
    conenose bug b.
    Congo floor maggot b.
    copperhead snake b.
    coral snake b.
    cottonmouth snake b.
    Ctenocephalides canis b.
    Ctenocephalides felis b.
    deer fly b.
    dog flea b.
    Eastern coral snake b.
    fiddle-back spider b.
    fly b.
    giant desert centipede b.
    Gila monster b.
    Glossina b.
    gnat b.
    harvest mite b.
    Heloderma suspectum b.
    horsefly b.
    insect b.
    kissing bug b.
    Latrodectus mactans b.
    Loxosceles reclusa b.
    midge b.
    mite b.
    moccasin snake b.
    mosquito b.
    northern rate flea b.
    Nosopsyllus fasciatus b.
    oriental rat flea b.
    b. pathology
    pit viper b.
    rat flea b.
    rattlesnake b.
    red bug b.
    sand flea b.
    sandfly b.
    Scolopendra heres b.
    sea snake b.
    snake b.
    spider b.
    stable fly b.
    Stomoxys b.
    Texas coral snake b.
    tick b.

bite (*continued*)
  Triatoma gerstaeckeri b.
  Triatoma sanguisuga b.
  tsetse fly b.
  Tunga penetrans b.
  violin-back spider b.
  Xenopsylla cheopis b.
  Yersinia pestis b.

bithionol

biting
  b. gnats
  b. insect
  b. midges
  nail b.
  b. reef worm

Bitot's spot

bitter dock

Bizzozero's nodes

Bjornstad's syndrome

B-K mole syndrome

blab

black
  b. ant
  b. central dot
  b. blowfly
  b. currant rash
  b. dermatographia
  b. dermatographism
  b. dots
  b. eschar
  b. eye
  b. fever
  b. fly
  b. fly bite
  b. hairy tongue
  b. heel
  b. ink
  b. jaundice
  b. jumping spider
  b. lacquer deposit
  b. locust
  b. measles
  b. toe

black (*continued*)
  b. piedra
  b. walnut
  b. widow spider
  b. widow spider bite

black and blue marks

black-dot
  b.-d. follicle
  b.-d. ringworm
  b.-d. tinea capitis

blackhead

blade
  copper and Teflon-coated
    standard scalpel b.
  No. 11 Bard-Parker scalpel
    b.

blain

blanchable red lesion

blanche
  atrophie b.

blanched
  b. cutaneous elevation
  b. halo

blanching
  delayed b.

Blancophor

bland
  b. emollients
  b. lubricants
  b. occlusive disorder

blankophore

Blaschko's line

blaschkoian

blast transformation

blastoconidia
  Candida b.

blastogenesis

blastogenetic

blastogenic
    T-cell b.

Blastomyces
    B. brasiliensis
    B. dermatitidis

blastomycete
    pathogenic b's

blastomycetic dermatitis

blastomycetica
    erosio interdigitalis b.

blastomycin

blastomycosis
    cutaneous b.
    European b.
    b.-like pyoderma
    North American b.
    South American b.
    systemic b.

blastomycotica
    dermatitis b.

blastospore

bleaching
    b. cream dermatitis
    b. creams
    b. hair dermatitis

bleb
    b. stapling

bleeding
    b. crater
    punctate b.

blemish

Blenderm patch technique

blennorrhagia

blennorrhagic

blennorrhagica
    keratoderma b.
    keratosis b.

blennorrhagicum
    keratoderma b.

blennorrhea
    acute b.

Blenoxane

bleomycin
    b. sulfate

blepharitis
    b. angularis
    marginal b.
    mixed seborrheic-
        staphylococcal b.
    staphylococcal b.

blepharochalasia

blepharochalasis

blepharochromidrosis

blepharocoloboma

blepharoconjunctivitis

blepharophimosis

blepharoplast

blepharoptosis adiposa

bleuâtre
    tache b.

blindness
    river b.

blister
    b. beetle
    b. beetle dermatitis
    b. beetle sting
    blood b.
    burn b.
    central b.
    diabetic b.
    fever b.
    b. fluid
    fly b.
    b. formation
    friction b.
    intraepidermal b.
    pressure b.
    b. rupture
    serosanguineous b.
    subcorneal b.

blister (*continued*)
    suprabasal acantholytic b.
    water b.

blistering
    b. collodion
    b. dermatitis
    b. distal dactylitis
    b. process
    b. skin
    b. skin lesion
    b. sunburn

Blis-To-Sol

Bloch
    B.-Siemens-Sulzberger
      syndrome
    B.-Sulzberger disease
    B.-Sulzberger incontinentia
      pigmenti
    B.-Sulzberger syndrome

block
    atrioventricular b.

blocker
    alpha-adrenergic b.
    calcium channel b.

blood
    b. blister
    b. coagulation
    b. dyscrasia
    b. fluke
    b. group incompatibility
    b.-tinged fluid
    b. transfusion
    b. worm

blood-borne

bloody diarrhea

Bloom
    B. syndrome
    B.-Torre-Machacek
      syndrome

blotch
    palpebral b.

blotchy

blowfly myiasis

blub

blubber

blue
    Alcian b.
    b. blade razor
    b. formazan
    methylene b.
    b. nails
    b. nevus
    b. nevus of Jadassohn-
      Tièche
    b. rubber-bleb nevus
    b. rubber-bleb nevus
      syndrome
    b. sclerae
    b. scleral dominant
    Selsun B.
    b. spot

blueberry
    b. muffin baby
    b. muffin child
    b. muffin lesion

bluebottle

Bluefarb-Stewart syndrome

blue-gray lesion

blunt
    b. dissection

blush

blushing

BMZ
    basement membrane
      zone
    BMZ antibody

boardlike

Bockenheimer's syndrome

Bockhart's
    B's folliculitis
    B's impetigo

Bodian stain

body
    banana-shaped b.
    b. cavity–based B-cell
        lymphoma
    Bollinger b's
    Civatte b.
    colloid b.
    cytoid b.
    b. dysmorphic disorder
    Farber b.
    Henderson-Paterson b.
    HX b.
    inclusion b.
    intracytoplasmic b.
    lamellar b.
    Leishman-Donovan b.
    b. lice
    Lipschütz b.
    b. louse
    Michaelis-Gutmann b.
    b. moisturizer
    molluscum b.
    Odland b.
    b. of nail
    b. of sweat gland
    pearly b.
    psittacosis inclusion b's
    residual b.
    ringworm of b.
    Schaumann b.
    sclerotic b.
    stellate b.
    Verocay b.
    stellate b.

Boeck
    B's disease
    B's itch
    B's sarcoid
    B's sarcoidosis
    B's scabies

Boerhaave
    B's sweat glands
    B's syndrome

boggy
    b. granuloma
    b. swelling

boil
    Aleppo b.
    Baghdad b.
    blind b.
    botfly b.
    date b.
    Delhi b.
    Madura b.
    Oriental b.
    salt water b., sea water b.
    tropical b.

Bollinger
    B. bodies
    B. granules

bone
    b. culture
    b. decay
    b. erosion
    b. formation
    b. marrow
    b. marrow aspiration
    b. marrow biopsy
    b. marrow failure
    b. marrow
        transplantation
    b. necrosis

bony
    b. ankylosis
    b. prominence

Böök's syndrome

boot
    Unna's b.
    Unna's paste b.

booster
    b. dose
    b. response

borax

border
    granulomatous b.
    indurated b.
    irregular b.
    raised b.
    scaly border
    vermilion b.

borderline
  b. borderline (BB)
  b. cases
  b. keorinatiys leprosy
  b. lepromatous (BL)
  b. lepromatous leprosy
  b. malignant
    hemangiopericytoma
  b. tuberculoid (BT)
  b. tuberculoid leprosy

boric acid

boring
  b. manner
  b. ulceration

boron

Borrelia
  B.-associated arthritis
  B. afzelii
  B. burgdorferi (*Bb*)
  B. burgdorferi sensu lato
  *B. burgdorferi sensu
    stricto*
  B. DNA
  B. duttonii
  B. garinii
  B.-induced cutaneous
    lymphoid hyperplasia
  B.-induced
    lymphocytoma
  B. lymphocytoma
  B. recurrentis
  B. vincentii

borrelial
  b. DNA
  b. lymphocytoma
  b. pseudolymphoma

borreliosis
  Lyme b.

Borst
  B.-Jadassohn epithelioma
  B.-Jadassohn type
    intraepidermal
    epithelioma

Boston exanthema

botfly
  b. boil
  b. facultative myiasis
  b. obligate myiasis

Botox

Botryomyces

botryomycoma

botryomycosis

botryosum
  Stemphylium b.

bottle brush dermatitis

botulin

botulinum antitoxin

botulism
  b. antitoxin
  wound b.

botulismotoxin

boubas

Bouchard's nodes

Bourneville
  B's disease
  B's syndrome
  B.-Brissaud disease
  B.- Pringle disease
  B.- Pringle syndrome

boutonneuse fever

bovine
  b. collagen dermal
    implant
  b. heparin
  b. papular stomatitis
  b. papular stomatitis virus

bovis
  Actinomyces b.

bowel
  b. bypass syndrome

Bowen's
  B. carcinoma
  B. disease

Bowen's (*continued*)
    B. precancerous dermatosis

bowenoid
    B. cell
    B. changes
    B. papulosis

box
    b. elder maple
    b. elder maple tree
    b. jellyfish
    b. jellyfish sting

BP
    bullous pemphigoid

bracelet

brachial plexus
    b. p. neuropathy

brachioradialis
    b. pruritus

brachycephaly

brachycheilia

brachychily

bradykinin

bradymetaphalangism

branched-chain amino acids

branchial
    b. cleft cyst
    b. cyst

branching tubules

branny
    b. desquamation

brassy taste

brawny induration

Brazilian
    B. pemphigus
    B. pepper tree
    B. rubber

breakbone fever

breaking out

breast
    b. carcinoma
    b. eczema

breastfeeding

Breezee Mist Antifungal

Breslow
    B. classification
    B. measurement technique
    B. thickness

Brethine
    B. injection
    B. Oral

Bretonneau
    B. angina
    B. disease

Brevoxyl

bridged sella

bridou

Brill
    B. disease
    B.-Symmers disease
    B.-Zinsser disease

Briska button

bristles

bristleworm

brittle
    b. bones
    b. hair, intellectual
      impairment, decreased
      fertility, short stature
      (BIDS)
    b. nail
    b. nail syndrome

brittleness

broad
    b. beta disease
    b. clinical spectrum
    b.-faced sack spider
    b. nasal root

broadband UVB

broad-spectrum
  b.-s. antibiotic

Brocq
  B's disease
  B's érythrose péribuccale
    pigmentaire
  B's lupoid sycosis
  B's pseudopelade

Broders calcification

broken veins

broken-off hairs

Bromarest

bromhidrosis

bromide
  b. acne

bromidrosiphobia

bromidrosis

bromine acne

bromism

bromocriptine

bromoderma

Bromphen
  B. elixir
  B. tablet

brompheniramine
  b. maleate
  b. and phenylephrine
  b. and
    phenylpropanolamine
  b. and pseudoephedrine

Bromsulphalein

bronchial
  b. adenoma
  b. carcinoid

bronchiectasis
  proximal b.

bronchiolitis

bronchiolitis (*continued*)
  b. obliterans with
    organizing pneumonia
    (BOOP)

bronchogenic
  b. carcinoma
  b. carcinoma–associated
    pachydermoperiostosis
  b. cyst

bronchospasm

bronopol dermatitis

bronze
  b. diabetes
  b. discoloration
  b. powder

bronzed skin

Brooke
  B's disease
  B's tumor

brow

brown
  b. albinism
  b.-black lesion
  b. hairy tongue
  b. moth larvae sting
  b. mucocutaneous
    hyperpigmentation
  b. oculocutaneous
    albinism
  b. recluse spider
  b. recluse spider bite
  b.-spot syndrome
  b.-to-black
    hyperpigmentation of
    flexures
  b. tumor

Brown's syndrome

brownish tint

brown-tail
  b.-t. moth caterpillar
  b.-t. moth larva

brown-tail (*continued*)
  b.-t. moth sting
  b.-t. rash

Brucella
  B. canis

brucellosis
  chronic b.
  contact b.

Bruch's membrane

Brugia
  B. malayi
  B. timori

bruise

bruiselike lesions

bruising
  easy b.

Brunsting
  B. type dermatomyositis
  B.-Perry cicatricial
    pemphigoid
  B.-Perry pemphigoid

brush fractures

Bruton
  B's disease
  B's syndrome

BT
  borderline tuberculoid

bubble
  b. gum dermatitis
  b. hair
  b. hair deformity

bubblelike defect

bubo *pl.* buboes
  Frei b.
  gonorrheal b.
  indolent b.
  nonvenereal b.
  pestilential b.
  b. pus
  strumous b.

bubo (*continued*)
  venereal b.

bubon
  b. d'emblée

bubonic plague

bubonulus

buccal
  b. commissures
  b. mucosa

Budd-Chiari syndrome

budding fungus

budesonide

budlike extensions

Buerger's disease

buffalo
  b. gnat
  b. hump

Bufferin

bulb
  b. of hair

bulbar

bulbous
  b. proliferation
  b. rete ridges

bulbus
  b. pili

bulging fontanelles

bulimia

bulla *pl.* bullae
  friction b.
  hemorrhagic b.
  intraepidermal b.
  pressure b.
  b.-spread
    phenomenon

bullate

bullation

bullectomy
transaxillary apical b.

Bullfrog

bullosa
Cockayne-Touraine
epidermolysis b.
Dowling-Meara
epidermolysis b.
Dystrophic
epidermolysis b.
epidermolysis b. (EB)
Hallopeau-Siemens
epidermolysis b.
Herlitz epidermolysis b.
impetigo b.
impetigo contagiosa b.
inherited
epidermolysis b.
junctional epidermolysis b.
(JEB)
Köbner epidermolysis b.
Pasini epidermolysis b.
urticaria b.

bullosis
diabetic b.

bullosum
erythema b.
erythema multiforme b.

bullosus
herpes circinatus b.

bullous
b. amyloidosis
b. congenital ichthyosiform
erythroderma
b. conjunctivitis
b. dermatosis
b. disease
b. drug eruption
b. edema
b. eruption
b. erythema multiforme
b. form

bullous (*continued*)
b. hemorrhagic pyoderma
gangrenosum
b. ichthyosiform
erythroderma
b. impetigo
b. impetigo of newborn
b. lesion
b. lichen planus
b. pemphigoid (BP)
b. pemphigoid antigen
(BPA)
b. pemphigoid-like eruption
b. pyoderma gangrenosum
b. skin lesion
b. syphilid

bull's eye lesion

bumblebee
b. sting

Bump Fighter razor

bump
goose b's

bundle
collagen b.

bunion

buphthalmos

bupivacaine
b. hydrochloride

Burkholderia
B. cepacia
B. pseudomallei

Burkitt's lymphoma

burn
actinic b.
brush b.
chemical b.
contact b.
electric b.
electrical b.
first-degree b.
flash b.

burn (*continued*)
    friction b.
    full-thickness b.
    mat b.
    millipede b.
    mokihana b.
    partial-thickness b.
    radiation b.
    road b.
    rope b.
    b. scars
    second-degree b.
    sun b.
    superficial b.
    thermal b.
    third-degree b.
    x-ray b.

burning
    b. lip syndrome
    b. mouth
    b. mouth syndrome
    b. paroxysm
    b. sensation
    b. tongue
    b. vulva syndrome

Burow solution

burrobrush
    white b.

burrow

burrowing

Buruli ulcer

burst
    spider b.

burweed

Buschke
    B's disease
    B's heat melanosis
    B's scleredema
    B.-Löwenstein giant
       condyloma
    B.-Löwenstein tumor
    B.-Ollendorff disease
    B.-Ollendorff sign

Buschke (*continued*)
    B.-Ollendorff syndrome

BuSpar

buspirone

busulfan

butamben
    b. picrate

butcher
    b's pemphigus
    b's tubercle

butenafine

Butesin

butethamine

buthionine sulfoximine

butter
    cacao b.
    cocoa b.

buttercup

butterfly
    b. area
    b. eruption
    b. facial erythema
    b. patch
    b. rash
    b. sign
    b.-wing pattern

button
    b. of Aleppo
    b. of Amboyna
    b. of Cairo
    b. of Delhi
    b. of Galsa
    b. hole sign
    b. of the Nile
    b. of the Orient
    b. of Yemen

buttonholing

butyl
    b. aminobenzoate

butylcatechol

butyric

butyrophenones

Bx
    biopsy

byproduct

Bywaters lesion

C

C
  complement component
  C group virus
  C syndrome
  C-terminal proline

C1 (*complement component*)
  C1 esterase
  C1 esterase inhibitor
  C1 inhibitor

C3 (*complement component*)
  C3 deposition

C3/C4 receptor

C9 (*complement component*)
  C9 deficiency

cable rash

cachecticorum
  acne c.
  melanoderma c.

cachexia

Cachexon

cactus needles

CAD
  chronic airway disease
  coronary artery disease

cadaverous

cadmium sulfide

cadre

CAE
  cefuroxime axetil
    suspension

caecutiens
  Onchocerca c.

caesiellus
  Aspergillus c.

café
  c. au lait macules
  c. au lait spots

cajennense
  Amblyomma c.

Cajuput oil

Calabar swelling

calamine

calcaneal
  c. petechia
  c. spur

calcar

Calciferol
  C. injection
  C. Oral

calcific
  c. periarthritis
  c. tenonitis

calcification
  soft tissue c.
  subcutaneous c.

calcified
  c. multinodular ovarian
    fibromas
  c. phleboliths

calcifying
  c. epithelioma
  c. epithelioma of Malherbe
  c. fibroma
  c. panniculitis

calcinosis
  c. circumscripta
  c. cutis
  c. cutis, osteoma cutis,
    poikiloderma, and skeletal
    abnormalities (COPS)
  c. cutis, Raynaud
    phenomenon, esophageal
    motility disorder,
    sclerodactyly,
    telangiectasia (CREST)
  c. cutis, Raynaud
    phenomenon, esophageal

calcinosis (*continued*)
  motility disorder,
    sclerodactyly,
    telangiectasia syndrome
  dystrophic c.
  idiopathic scrotal c.
  c. of the dermis
  primary
    hyperphosphatemic
    tumoral c.
  subcutaneous c.
  tumoral c.
  c. universalis

calciphylaxis

calcipotriene
  c. therapy

calcipotriol

calcitonin
  c. gene–related peptide
  c.-origin amyloid deposit

calcitriol

calcium
  c. ATPase
  c. carbonate crystal
  c. channel blocker
  c. chloride infusion
  c. citrate
  c. gluconate
  c. heparinate
  c. hydroxide
  c. hydroxide dermatitis
  c. oxide
  c. propionate
  c. salts
  c. thioglycolate
    dermatitis
  c. undecylenate

calcoaceticus
  Acinetobacter c.

Calcort

Caldecort
  C. Anti-Itch Spray

Caldesene topical

Caldwell's syndrome

California
  C. black-legged tick

Calliphora

Calliphoridae

Callitroga
  C. americana
  C. macellaria

callositas

callosities

callosity

callous

callus
  c. eczema

Calmette
  C. test
  bacille bilié de C.-Guérin
    (BCG)
  bacille C.-Guérin (BCG)
  C.-Guérin bacillus
  C.-Guérin vaccine

calomel disease

calor
  c. mordax
  c. mordicans

caloric
  c. hyperpigmentation
  c. intake

calorica
  dermatitis c.

caloricum
  erythema c.

calvarium

calvities

Calycophora dermatitis

Calymmatobacterium
  C. granulomatis

cAMP

cAMP (*continued*)
    cyclic adenosine
        monophosphate

camp pathway

Campbell-De Morgan spot

Campho-Phenique

camphor
    c., menthol, and phenol
    c. and phenol

camphoraceous

camphorated menthol

camptodactyly
    congenital c.

Campylobacter
    C. septicemia

Canada-Cronkhite syndrome

canal
    hair c.

canalicular obstruction

canaliculitis

cANCA
    cytoplasmic antineutrophil
        cytoplasmic autoantibody

cancer
    breast c.
    chimney-sweeps' c.
    c. en cuirasse
    epidermal c.
    epidermoid c.
    kang c.
    kangri c.
    melanotic c.
    mule-spinners' c.
    paraffin c.
    pitch workers' c.
    skin c.
    soot c.
    tar c.

cancericidal, cancerocidal

cancerophobia, cancerphobia

cancerous

cancrum
    c. nasi
    c. oris

Candida
    C. albicans
    C. albicans IgG
    C. balanitis
    C. colonization
    C. folliculitis
    C. granuloma
    C. infection
    C. intertrigo
    C. krusei
    C. leukoplakia
    C. paronychia
    C. pseudotropicalis
    C. quilliermondii
    C. skin test
    C. stellatoidea
    C. therapy
    C. tropicalis

candidal
    c. angular cheilitis
    c. infection
    c. intertrigo
    c. leukoplakia
    c. paronychia
    c. vulvovaginitis

candidemia

candidiasis
    acute atrophic oral c.
    antibiotic c.
    atrophic c.
    chronic c.
    chronic atrophic c.
    chronic hyperplastic c.
    chronic mucocutaneous c.
        (CMC)
    congenital c.
    cutaneous c.
    disseminated c.
    iatrogenic c.
    intertriginous c.
    invasive c.

candidiasis (*continued*)
  localized mucocutaneous c.
  mucocutaneous c.
  neonatal c.
  neonatal systemic c.
  oral c.
  oropharyngeal c.
  osteoarticular c.
  perianal c.
  systemic c.
  vulvovaginal c. (VVC)

candidid

candidosis

candiduria

candidus
  strophulus c.

canestick deformity

canimorsus
  Capnocytophaga c.

canine
  c. herpesvirus
  c. herpetovirus
  c. oral papilloma

caninum
  Ancylostoma c.
  Dipylidium c.

canis
  Demodex c.
  Microsporum c.
  Toxocara c.

canities
  rapid c.
  c. segmentata sideropenica
  c. unguium

canium
  Neospora c.

canker
  c. sore

Cann-Ease moisturizing nasal gel

cannonball pattern

cantharic acid

cantharidal solution

cantharidin

cantharis *pl.* cantharides

canthus *pl.* canthi
  inner c.
  nasal c.
  outer c.
  temporal c.

cap
  cradle c.

capacitor

Capastat sulfate

capillarectasia

capillariasis

capillaritis
  c. alba

capillaropathy

capillaroscopy
  nail fold c.

capillary *pl.* capillaries
  c. angioma
  c. bed
  c. hemangioma
  c. hemangioma of infancy
  c. loops
  c. nevus

capilli

capillitii
  dermatitis papillaris c.

capillitium

capillorum
  defluvium c.

capillus *pl.* capilli

capitate

capitis
  black dot tinea c.
  gray patch tinea c.

capitis (*continued*)
    inflammatory tinea c.
    pediculosis c.
    Pediculus c.
    Pediculus humanus c.
    pityriasis c.
    pthiriasis c.
    seborrhea c.
    tinea c.
    trichophytosis c.
    vitiligo c.

Capitrol

Capnocytophaga
    C. canimorsus

Capoten

Capozucca syndrome

capping

capreomycin
    c. sulfate

caprine
    c. herpes virus
    c. herpetovirus

Capripoxvirus

caprylic

capsaicin

capsid

Capsin

capsomer

capsulatum
    Histoplasma c.

capsulitis
    adhesive c.

Captia
    C. test
    C. test for syphilis

captopril

caput medusae

Capzasin-P

carate

carbamate

carbamazepine

carbamide

carbamoylphosphate synthase

carbenicillin indanyl sodium

Carbocaine injection

carbohydrate
    c. metabolism
    c. moieties

carbolfuchsin
    c. solution

carbolic acid
    c.a. burn

carbon
    c. baby
    c. dioxide
    c. dioxide arteriography
    c. dioxide laser
    c. dioxide laser ablation
    c. dioxide laser burn
    c. disulfide
    c. monoxide
    c. stain

carbonate

carbonization

carbovir

carbowax

carboxamide
    imidazole c.

carboxylase

multiple c. deficiency

carbuncle
    staphylococcal c.

carbuncular

carbunculoid
    c. eruption

carbunculosis

carcinoembryonic antigen (CEA)

carcinogen

carcinogenesis
cutaneous c.

carcinogenic
c. factor
c. rays

carcinogenicity

carcinogenesis

carcinoid
c. syndrome
c. tumor

carcinoma *pl.* carcinomata, carcinomas
adnexal c.
apocrine c.
basal cell c. (BCC)
basal cell c., alveolar
basal cell c., comedo
basal cell c., cystic
basal cell c., morphea-like
basal cell c., multicentric
basal cell c., nodulo-ulcerative
basal cell c., pigmented
basal cell c., sclerosing
basal cell c., superficial
basaloid c.
basosquamous c.
chimney sweep c.
c. cuniculatum
cutaneous squamous cell c.
eccrine c.
c. en cuirasse
epidermoid c.
c. erysipelatoides
fibroepithelioma basal cell c.
fungating c.
genital squamous cell c.
hair-matrix c.
infiltrative basal cell c.

carcinoma (*continued*)
c. in situ
in situ squamous cell c.
intermediate c.
intraepidermal c.
invasive squamous cell c.
melanotic c.
Merkel cell c.
metatypical cell c.
morbilliform basal cell c.
morpheaform basal cell c.
neuroendocrine c. of the skin
nevoid basal cell c.
nodular basal cell c.
pilomatrixoma c.
prickle cell c.
sebaceous c.
squamous cell c. (SCC)
superficial basal cell c.
c. telangiectaticum
trabecular c.
trabecular c. of the skin
sweat gland c.
verrucous c.
visceral c.

carcinomata
c. cuniculatum
c. en cuirasse
c. telangiectaticum

carcinomatosis

carcinomatous degeneration

cardiac
c. anomalies
c. catheterization
c. conduction defects
c. decompensation
c. disease
c. myxoma
c. sclerosis
c. valves

cardinal
c. features

cardiocutaneous
c. myxoma

cardiocutaneous (*continued*)
    c. syndrome

cardiofaciocutaneous syndrome

cardiolipin

cardiomegaly

cardiomyopathy
    restrictive c.

cardiopathy

cardiotoxic

cardiovascular system

carditis
    Lyme c.

carindacillin

Caripito itch

carmine

Carmol
    C. HC topical
    C. topical

carmustine (BCNU)

Carney
    C's complex
    C's syndrome

carnitine palmitoyltransferase
    deficiency

carotene
    beta c.

carotenemia

carotenoderma

carotenoid

carotenosis
    c. cutis

carotinemia

carotinosis
    c. cutis

carpal tunnel syndrome (CTS)

carpet beetle dermatitis

carpet-tack scale

Carpoglyphus passularum

carprofen

carrageenan

carrier *pl.* carriers
    c. female
    c. focus
    heterozygous c.
    plasma c.
    c. protein

Carrión's disease

carrionii
    Cladosporium c.

Carter black mycetoma

cartilage
    swollen c.

cartilaginous portion

caruncle

carunculae
    trichosis c.

Carybdea marsupialis

Casal
    C's collar
    C's necklace

cascade
    complex c.

caseating
    c. granuloma

caseation necrosis

casei
    Lactobacillus c.

casein

caseous
    c. necrosis

cashew
    c. nutshell oil dermatitis
    c. nut tree
    c. tree dermatitis

Casoni
  C. intradermal test
  C. reaction
  C. skin test

cassia oil dermatitis

cast
  hair c.

Castellani Paint Modified

castellani
  C. paint

Castleman
  C's disease
  C's tumor

castor bean dermatitis

cat
  c. dander
  c. flea
  c. flea bite

catabolism

catabolize

catagen
  c. hairs
  c. phase

catalase-positive bacteria

cataract
  corticosteroid-induced c.
  poikiloderma atrophicans
    and c.
  posterior subcapsular c.

cataracta dermatogenes

catarrhal jaundice

catarrhalis
  Branhamella c.
  herpes c.
  Moraxella c.

catastrophic illness

catatrichy

cat-back shape

catecholamine

catechols

caterpillar
  c. dermatitis
  puss c.
  c. rash
  saddleback c.
  c. sting
  stinging c.

catfish
  saltwater c.
  c. sting

Cath-Secure tape

catheter

cati
  Toxocara c.

cationic

cat-scratch disease (CSD)

cat-scratch fever

cat's tongue

cattle
  c. grub myiasis
  c. wart

caudal regions

cauliflower
  c.-like masses

causalgia

causative
  c. factor
  c. focus
  c. organism

caustic
  Churchill's iodine c.
  Filhos' c.
  Landolfi's c.
  Lugol's c.
  lunar c.
  mitigated c.
  Plunket's c.
  Rousselot's c.

caustic (*continued*)
Vienna c.
zinc c.

caustics (*class of drugs*)

cauterants (*class of drugs*)

cauterization

cauterize

cautery
chemical c.
gas c.

cavernosum
angioma c.

cavernosus
nevus c.

cavernous
c. angioma
c. hemangioma
c. lymphangioma
c. sinusoid

caviae
Aeromonas c.
Nocardia c.

cavitary

cavitation

cavity

cayenne
c. pepper spots

Cazenave
C's disease
C's lupus
C's vitiligo

CBC
complete blood count

CBDC
chronic bullous disease of
childhood

CD
cluster designation
CD system
CD molecules

CD4
CD4 cell
CD4 count
CD4 cell subset
CD4 T lymphocyte

CD4+
CD4+ helper/inducer cell
CD4+ measures
CD4+ T cell subset
CD4+ T lymphocyte

CD5
CD5 cell

CD8
CD8 cell
CD8 T cell subset

CD4/CD8 ratio

CDC
Center for Communicable
Diseases
Centers for Disease Control
Centers for Disease Control
and Prevention
CDC Drug Service

CDM
childhood dermatomyositis

CEA
carcinoembryonic antigen

Ceclor

cedar
c. poisoning

CeeNU Oral

cefaclor

cefadroxil monohydrate

Cefadyl

cephalexin

cefamandole
c. nafate

Cefanex

cefazolin
c. sodium

cefepime

Cefizox

cefixime

cefmenoxine

cefmetazole
    c. sodium

Cefobid

cefodizime

cefonicid
    c. sodium

cefoperazone
    c. sodium

ceforanide

cefotaxime
    c. sodium

cefotetan

cefoxitin sodium

cefpiramide

cefpodoxime
    c. proxetil

cefprozil

ceftazidime

Ceftin
    C. Oral

ceftizoxime sodium

ceftriaxone
    c. sodium

cefuroxime
    c. axetil suspension (CAE)

Cefzil

Celestone
    C. Soluspan

celiac
    c. disease
    C. Society

cell

cell (*continued*)
    activated endothelial c.
    antigen-presenting c. (APC)
    antigen-specific cytotoxic c.
    anti–red blood c. A
    anti–red blood c. B
    B c.
    balloon c.
    basal c.
    bowenoid c.
    cuboidal c.
    cytotoxic c.
    c. death
    dendritic c.
    effector c.
    endothelial c.
    epidermal Langerhans c.
    epidermic c.
    foam c.
    follicular dendritic c.
    foot c.
    granular c.
    heckle c.
    helper/inducer c.
    horny c.
    hybrid c.
    inflammatory c.
    interdigitating follicular c.
    interdigitating reticular c.
    interdigitating reticulum c.
    keratinized c.
    K c.
    killer c.
    Kupffer c.
    Langerhans' c.
    c. layer
    lepra c.
    Lipschütz c.
    long-lived memory c.
    c. lysis
    malpighian c.
    mast c.
    matrix c.
    c. membrane
    c. membrane antigen
    memory c.
    Merkel-Ranvier c.
    mesangial c.

cell (*continued*)
    microglial c.
    mononuclear c.
    multinucleated giant c.
    muriform c.
    mycosis c.
    natural killer c.
    neoplastic c.
    nests of nevus c's
    nevus c.
    c. nucleus
    c. organelles
    c. periphery
    phagocytic c.
    plasma c.
    polyhedral-shaped c.
    precursor B c.
    precursor stem c.
    prickle c.
    prototype antigen-
      presenting c.
    c. receptors
    regulator c.
    retained c.
    reticular c.
    reticuloendothelial c.
    Schwann c.
    sclerotic c.
    sentinel cells
    Sézary c.
    short-lived effector c.
    spindle c.
    squamous c.
    suppressor c.
    c.-surface IgE antibody
    c. surface glycoproteins
    T c.
    T Gamma/Delta c.
    Touton giant c.
    c. turnover process
    Tzanck c.
    veiled c.
    Virchow c.
    virus-infected c.
    c. wall
    xanthoma c.
cell-bound antibody

cell-mediated
    c.-m. drug reaction
    c.-m. hypersensitivity
    c.-m. immunity (CMI)
    c.-m. immunity response
    c.-m. immunologic drug
      reaction
    c.-m. reaction
Cellufresh
cellular
    c. arrangement
    c. atypia
    c. blue nevus
    c. casts
    c. disruption
    c. hypersensitivity reaction
    c. immune response
    c. immunodeficiency
    c. islands
    c. matrix
    c. nevus
    c. phospholipids
    c. proliferation
cellularis
    balanitis circumscripta
      plasma c.
Cellule claire
cellulite
cellulitis
    acute scalp c.
    anaerobic c.
    clostridial c.
    clostridial anaerobic c.
    demarcated c.
    dissecting c.
    dissecting c. of scalp
    eosinophilic c.
    epizootic c.
    facial c.
    finger c.
    gangrenous c.
    indurated c.
    necrotizing c.
    nonclostridial anaerobic c.
    orbital c.

cellulitis (*continued*)
  perianal streptococcal c.
  phlegmonous c.
  pneumococcal c.
  streptococcal c.

cellulose
  hydroxypropyl c.
  oxidized c.

cellulosic/cuprophan

Celluvisc

celonychia

Celsus
  C. alopecia
  C. area
  C. kerion
  C. papule
  C. vitiligo

Cel-U-Jec

cement eczema

cementoma

center
  necrotic c.

Centers for Disease Control
  (CDC)

Centers for Disease Control and
  Prevention (CDC)

centipede
  c. bite
  giant desert c.
  c. sting

central
  c. black keratin plug
  c. blister
  c. centrifugal scarring
    alopecia
  c. clearing
  c. cones
  c. depression
  c. dusky purpura
  c. fibrinoid necrosis
  c. hemorrhagic punctum

central (*continued*)
  c. hyalinized cores
  c. involution
  c. karyosome
  c. keratotic core
  c. lesion
  c. necrosis
  c. nervous system
    metastasis
  c. nonnucleated center
  c. papillary atrophy
  c. plug of horn
  c. pore
  c. pruritus
  c. punctum
  c. pyknotic nucleus
  c. red punctum
  c. rupture
  c. scaling
  c. suppuration
  c. thermoregulatory defect
  c. trunk
  c. type neurofibromatosis
  c. umbilication

centrifugal
  c. lipoatrophy
  c. pattern

centrifugum
  erythema annulare c. (EAC)
  leukoderma acquisitum c.
  c. marginatum

centripetal

centroblast

centroblastic-centrocytic
  lymphoma

centrofacial lentiginosis

Centruroides
  C. exilicauda
  C. exilicauda sting
  C. sculpturatus
  C. sculpturatus sting
  C. sting
  C. vittatus
  C. vittatus sting

CEP
   congenital erythropoietic
      porphyria

cephalad distribution

cephalalgia

cephalexin
   c. monohydrate

cephalic
   c. brainlike heterotopia
   c. skin

cephalo-oculocutaneous
   telangiectasia

cephalocele
   rudimentary c.

cephalosporin
   first-generation c.
   fourth-generation c.
   second-generation c.
   third-generation c.

Cephalosporium

cephalothin
   c. sodium

cephapirin sodium

cephradine

Ceptaz

ceramidase deficiency

ceramide trihexosidase

Ceratophyllus gallinae

Ceratopogonidae

cercaria *pl.* cercariae
   c.-infested water

cercarial
   c. dermatitis

cerea
   seborrhea c.

cerebellar
   c. ataxia
   c. dysfunction

cerebral
   c. calcification
   c. cortex
   c. palsy

cérébrale
   tache c.

cerebri
   pseudotumor c.

cerebriform
   c. appearance
   c. intradermal nevus
   c. nucleus
   c. surface

cerebrospinal
   c. meningitis

cerebrotendinous
   xanthomatosis

cerebrovascular
   c. accident
   c. disease

ceruminous
   c. adenocarcinoma
   c. glands

cerulea *pl.* caerulea
   macula c.
   maculae c.

ceruleus

ceruloplasmin

cerumen

ceruminal

ceruminous
   c. gland

cervical
   c. lymphadenitis
   c. lymphadenopathy
   c. lymph nodes
   c. lymph node swelling
   c. patagium
   c. rib
   c. shedding

cervicitis

cervicofacial area

cestodes

Cetacaine

Cetamide Ophthalmic

Cetaphil cream

Cetapred Ophthalmic

cetirizine

cetyl

CF
    carbolfuchsin

CFIDS
    chronic fatigue and
      immune dysfunction
      syndrome

CGD
    chronic granulomatous
      disease
        CGD phagocytes

CH50 assay

chafe

chaffeensis
    Ehrlichia c.

chafing

Chagas
    C's disease
    C's myocarditis

chagasic

chagoma

Chagres virus

chagrin
    peau de c.

chain
    alpha c.
    amino acid c.
    beta c.
    heavy c.
    J c.
    light c.

chain (*continued*)
    peptide c.
    polypeptide c.
    V c.

chalazion *pl.* chalazia
    c. knife

chalazodermia

chalk
    French c.

Chanarin-Dorfman
    syndrome

chancre
    erosive c.
    fungating c.
    hard c.
    hunterian c.
    indurated c.
    mixed c.
    monorecidive c.
    phagedenic c.
    c. recidive
    c. redux
    Ricord c.
    Rollet c.
    soft c.
    sporotrichositic c.
    sulcus c.
    syphyilis c.
    syphilitic c.
    tuberculous c.
    tularemic c.

chancriform
    c. lesion
    c. pyoderma
    c. syndrome

chancroid

chancroidal
    c. ulceration

chancrous
    c. bubo

change
    clinical c's
    environmental c.

change (*continued*)
    mitral valve prolapse, aortic
      anomalies, skeletal
      changes, and skin c's
      (MASS)
    nail c.
    pigment c.
    polyneuropathy,
      organomegaly,
      endocrinopathy,
      monoclonal gammopathy,
      and skin c's (POEMS)
    symmetric reticulonodular
      x-ray c.
    synovial fluid c's
    tinctorial c.

channel
    communicating c.
    lymphatic c.

channeling

Chaoul
    C. tube

chappa

chapped

chapping

characteristic
    c. appearance
    c. facies
    lesion surface c.
    morphologic c.

Charcot joint

Charlouis
    C. disease

Chédiak
    C.-Higashi disease
    C.-Higashi gene production
    C.-Higashi syndrome

cheek
    c. cosmetic

cheilitis (*variant* chilitis)
    c. abrasiva praecancerosa
      manganotti

cheilitis (*continued*)
    actinic c.
    c. actinica
    allergic c.
    angular c.
    apostematous c.
    candidal angular c.
    commissural c.
    contact c.
    c. exfoliativa
    exfoliativa c.
    c. glandularis
    c. glandularis simplex
    c. glandularis apostematosa
    glandularis apostematosa c.
    c. granulomatosa
    c. granulomatosa of
      Miescher
    granulomatous c.
    impetiginous c.
    Miescher's granulomatous
      c.
    migrating c.
    mycotic c.
    solar c.
    c. venenata
    Volkmann c.

cheilosis

cheiropompholyx

chelating agent

chelicera *pl.* chelicerae

cheloid

cheloidalis
    acne c.
    acné chéloïdique

cheloma

chelonae
    Mycobacterium c.

chemabrasion

chemes

chemexfoliation

chemical

chemical (*continued*)
    acnegenic c.
    c. agent
    c. burn
    c. carcinogenesis
    c. cocarcinogens
    c. contactants
    c. depilatory
    c. dermatitis
    c. leukoderma
    nonimmunogenic c.
    c. peel
    c. peeling
    c. phlebitis
    c. stimulus
    c. sunscreen

chemicocautery

chemocautery
    c. surgery
    c. therapy

chemoprophylaxis

chemoresistance

chemosis

chemosurgery
    Mohs c.

chemotactic
    c. factors
    c. peptide
    c. substances

chemotaxis

chemotherapeutic index

chemotherapy
    c. agent
    extracorporeal c.

chemotherapy-induced
    c.-i. acral erythema
    c.-i. hyperpigmentation

Cheney syndrome

chenodeoxycholic acid

cheopis
    Xenopsylla c.

cherry
    c. angioma
    c.-red spots
    c. spot

chest
    fissured c.

chevron nail

Cheyletiella
    C. blakei
    C. dermatitis
    C. infestation
    C. parasitovorax
    C. yasguri

cheyletiellosis

chicken
    c. flea bite
    c. pox

chickenpox
    c. immune globulin
      (human)
    c. immunoglobulin
    c. vaccine
    c. virus

chiclero ulcer

chigga

chigger
    c. bite
    c. flea

chigoe

chikungunya virus

chilblain
    c. lupus
    c. lupus erythematosus
    necrotized c.

chilblain-like erythema

CHILD
    congenital hemidysplasia
      with ichthyosiform
      erythroderma and limb
      defects
        CHILD syndrome

child
  blueberry muffin c.

childhood
  c. atopic dermatitis
  c. bullous dermatosis
  chronic bullous dermatosis
    of c.
  c. dermatomyositis (CDM)
  c. eczema
  c. erythromelalgia
  c. form
  c. hyperuricemia
  c. mastocytosis
  c. myositis
  papular acrodermatitis of c.
  polyarteritis in c.
  c. type tuberculosis

children
  chronic granulomatous
    disease of c.

Children's Advil

Children's Motrin suspension

Children's Silfedrine

Children's Vaccine Initiative
  (CVI)

chilitis (*variant of* cheilitis)

Chilopoda

CHIME
  colobomas of the eye, heart
    defects, ichthyosiform
    dermatosis, mental
    retardation, and ear
    defects
      CHIME syndrome

chimney sweep's cancer

Chinese
  C. herb

Chironex
  C. fleckeri
  C. fleckeri sting

chiropompholyx,
  cheiropompholyx

chitin

Chlamydia
  C. disease
  C. pneumoniae
  C. psittaci
  C. trachomatis

Chlamydiae

chlamydial
  c. conjunctivitis
  c. infection
  c. urethritis

chlamydospore

Chlo-Amine Oral

chloasma
  c. bronzinum
  c. faciei
  c. gravidarum
  c. hepaticum
  c. medicamentosum
  melanoderma c.
  c. periorale virginium
  c. phthisicorum
  c. traumaticum

chloracne

chlorambucil

chloramphenicol
  c., polymyxin B, and
    hydrocortisone

Chlorate Oral

chlordane

Chloresium

chlorhexidine
  c. gluconate
  c. HCl

chlorhydroxide dermatitis

chloride
  aluminum c.
  benzocaine, butyl
    aminobenzoate,
    tetracaine, and
    benzalkonium c.

chloride (*continued*)
    sweat c.
    c. sweat est

chlorine acne

chlorodeoxyadenosine
    2-c.

chloroform

chloroguanide hydrochloride

chloroma

Chloromycetin

chloronaphthalene
    c. chloracne

chlorophyllin
    c. copper complex

chloroprocaine hydrochloride

Chloroptic Ophthalmic

Chloroptic-P Ophthalmic

6-chloropurine

chloroquine
    c. phosphate
    c. and primaquine
    c. therapy

chloroquine-resistant
    c.-r. *Plasmodium*
       falciparum (CRPF)

chlorosis

chlorothiazide

chloroxine

Chlorphed

Chlorphed-LA Nasal Solution

chlorpheniramine
    c. maleate

chlorpromazine
    c. hydrochloride

chlorprothixene

chlortetracycline

chlortetracycline (*continued*)
    c. bisulfate
    c. calcium
    c. HCl

Chlor-Trimeton (CTM)
    C.-T. 4 Hour Relief Tablets
    C.-T. injection
    C.-T. Oral

cholecalciferol

choledochal disease

cholelithiasis

cholera-red reaction

cholestanol

cholestasia

cholestasis

cholestatic
    c. liver disease

cholesteroderma

cholesterol
    c. cleft
    c. embolus
    c.-rich particles
    c. sulfate

cholesterolized petrolatum

cholesterolosis
    c. cutis
    extracellular c.

cholesterosis
    extracellular c.

cholestyramine

cholic acid

choline
    c. magnesium trisalicylate
    c. salicylate

cholinergic
    c. urticaria

cholinesterase activity

chondritis

chondrodermatitis
    c. helicis nodularis
    c. nodularis chronica helicis

chondrodysplasia
    c. punctata
    c. punctata syndrome

chondrodystrophia
    c. calcificans congenitalis
    c. congenita punctata

chondroid syringoma

chondroitin
    c. sulfate

chondrolysis

chondroma

chondromatosis

chondrosarcoma

CHOP regimen

chord compression

chorda tympani syndrome

chordae tendineae

Chordata

chordoma

choreic movements

choreoathetoid

choreoathetosis

chorionic villous biopsy

chorioretinitis

choristoma

choroid plexus

choroiditis

choriocarcinoma

CHP
        cytophagic histiocytic
            panniculitis

Christ-Siemens-Touraine
    syndrome

Christian
        C's disease
        C's syndrome
        C.-Weber disease

Christmas tree pattern

chromaffin

chromate
    c. sensitivity

chromatica
    trichomycosis c.

chromatin

chromatism

chromatoblast

chromatogenous

chromatophore
    c. nevus of Naegeli

chromatosis

chrome
    c. dermatitis
    c. green
    c. patch test
    c.-tanned leather
    c. ulcer

chromhidrosis, chromidrosis
    apocrine c.
    eccrine c.

chromidrose
    c. pattern
    c. plantaire

chromidrosis

chromobacteriosis

Chromobacterium
    C. violaceum

chromoblastomycosis

chromogens

chromomycosis

chromonychia

chromophage

chromophobe

chromophobic

chromophore

chromophototherapy

chromophytosis

chromosomal
  c. aneuploidy condition
  c. mosaicism

chromosome
  c. arrangement
  c. 6, class III MHC
  c. number
  X c.

chromotherapy

chromotrichia

chromotrichial

chronic
  c. acral dermatitis
  c. actinic damage
  c. actinic degenerative
    change
  c. actinic dermatitis
  c. actinic cheilitis
  c. actinic exposure
  c. active hepatitis
  c. acyclovir suppression
  c. allograft rejection
  c. anaphylaxis
  c. arsenism
  c. atrophic candidiasis
  c. atrophic dermatitis
  c. atrophic vulvitis
  c. blistering disorder of the
    hand
  c. bullous dermatitis of
    childhood
  c. bullous dermatosis of
    childhood
  c. bullous disease of
    childhood
  c. candidiasis
  c. consumptive
    coagulopathy

chronic (*continued*)
  c. contact dermatitis
  c. cumulative irritant
    contact eczema
  c. cutaneous graft-versus-
    host reaction
  c. cutaneous leishmaniasis
  c. cutaneous lupus
    erythematosus
  c. discoid lupus
    erythematosus
  c. draining osteomyelitis
  c. eczema
  c. erythema multiforme
  c. erythema nodosum
  c. familial giant urticaria
  c. fatigue and immune
    dysfunction syndrome
    (CFIDS)
  c. graft-versus-host disease
  c. granulomatous disease
  c. granulomatous disease of
    children
  c. guttate parapsoriasis
  c. hereditary lymphedema
  c. hyperplastic candidiasis
  c. idiopathic
    thrombocytopenic
    purpura
  c. idiopathic urticaria
  c. immunosuppression
  c. inflammation (CI)
  c. inflammatory disease
  c. inflammatory pilonidal
    disease
  c. irritant dermatitis
  c. lichenified dermatitis
  c. lichenoid dermatitis
  c. low-grade anoxemia
  c. lymphangitis
  c. lymphedema
  c. lymphocytic leukemia
  c. mucocutaneous
  c. mucocutaneous
    candidiasis (CMC)
  c. mucocutaneous
    candidiasis syndrome
  c. multifocal osteomyelitis

chronic (*continued*)
    c. mycotic infection
    c. myelogenous leukemia
    c. papular dermatitis
    c. paronychia
    c. periapical infection
    c. photosensitivity
      dermatitis
    c. polyarthritis
    c. pulmonary disease
    c. pustular disease
    c. radiodermatitis
    c. recurrent aphthae
    c. recurrent erysipelas
    c. recurrent multifocal
      osteomyelitis
    c. redness
    c. relapsing eruption
    c. renal failure
    c. sinopulmonary disease
    c. skin disease
    c. solar radiation exposure
    c. suppurative folliculitis
    c. tophaceous gout
    c. ulcer
    c. undermining ulcer of
      Meleney
    c. urticaria
    c. venous insufficiency,
      grade I
    c. venous insufficiency,
      grade II
    c. venous insufficiency,
      grade III

chronica
    acrodermatitis c.
      atrophicans
    keratosis lichenoides c.
    mycosis cutis c.
    c. parapsoriasis lichenoid
    pityriasis lichenoides c.
    urticaria c.

chronicum
    erythema c.

chronicus
    genital lichen simplex c.

chronicus (*continued*)
    lichen c. simplex
    lichen simple c. (LSC)

chrotoplast

chrysanthemum dermatitis

chrysarobin

chrysiasis

chrysoderma

Chrysomyia

Chrysops
    C. caecutiens
    C. dimidiata
    C. discalis
    C. silacea

chrysorrhoea
    Euproctis c.

Chrysosporium pruinosum

Churg
    C.-Strauss granuloma
    C.-Strauss granulomatosis
    C.-Strauss syndrome (CSS)

chylidrosis

chyloderma

chylomicron band

chylomicronemia

chylous
    c. discharge
    c. lymphedema

CI
    chronic inflammation

Ciarrocchi
    C. disease

Ciba

cicatrices (*plural of* cicatrix)

cicatrice
    c's stellaires

cicatricial

cicatricial (*continued*)
    c. alopecia
    c. basal cell carcinoma
    c. bullous pemphigoid
    c. horn
    c. junctional epidermolysis
      bullosa
    c. patch
    c. pemphigoid
    c. pemphigoid antigen
    c. stenosis

cicatrisata
    alopecia c.

cicatrix *pl.* cicatrices
    hypertrophic c.
    c. hypertrophica
    c. process
    vicious c.

cicatrization
    exuberant c.

ciclopirox
    c. olamine

CID
    combined
      immunodeficiency
      disease

cidofovir

CIE
    congenital ichthyosiform
      erythroderma
    counter
      immunoelectrophoresis

cigarette burn
    self-inflicted c. b.

cigarette-paper wrinkling

ciguatera poisoning

cilia

ciliaris
    acne c.
    tylosis c.

ciliary
    c. body

Ciliata

Ciloxan Ophthalmic

cimetidine

Cimex lectularius

cimicosis

cinchona bark

cinnabar *(mercuric sulfate)*
    c. red spots

cinnamate
    c. dermatitis

cinnamic
    c. alcohol
    c. aldehyde

Cinnamomum zeylanicum

cinnamon
    c. oil
    c. oil dermatitis

Cipro
    C. injection
    C. Oral

ciprofloxacin
    c. hydrochloride

circinata
    balanitis c.
    impetigo c.
    pityriasis c.
    psoriasis c.
    tinea c.

circinate
    c. balanitis
    c. lesions
    c. patches
    c. pattern

circinatum
    erythema c.

circle of Hebra

circular macules

circulating
    c. anticoagulant
    c. testosterone

circumileostomy eczema

circumcised

circumcision

circumflexa
    ichthyosis linearis c.

circumoral tissue

circumscribed
    c. albinism
    c. area
    c. elevated lesion
    c. erythematous patch
    c. linear scleroderma
    c. myxedema
    c. neurodermatitis
    c. patch
    c. precancerous melanosis
        of Dubreuilh
    c. precancerous of
        Dubreuilh
    c. scleroderma
    c. telangiectasia

circumscripta
    allotrichia c.
    alopecia c.
    balanitis c. plasma
        cellularis
    calcinosis c.
    osteoporosis c.
    poliosis c.

circumscriptum
    c. angiokeratoma
    lymphangioma c.

circumvallate papilla

cirrhosis

cirsoid aneurysm

cisplatin

13-*cis*-retinoic acid

Citanest
    C. Forte
    C. Plain

citric acid

citronella oil

citrullinemia

Civatte
    C's bodies
    C's disease
    poikiloderma of C.
    C's poikiloderma

CLA
    cutaneous lymphocyte
        antigen

cladiosis

Cladophialophora bantiana

cladosporioides
    Cladosporium c.

cladosporiosis
    c. epidermica

Cladosporium
    C. carrionii
    C. cladosporioides
    C. mansonii
    C. werneckii

cladribine

clamdigger's itch

Clarinex

clarithromycin

Claritin

Claritin-D

Clark
    C. classification of
        malignant melanoma
        (levels I–V)
    C. levels (I–V)

class
    c. II storage molecule
    c. Mastigophora
    c. sporozoa

classic
    c. allergy symptom
    c. complement pathway
    c. Kaposi's sarcoma

classic (*continued*)
  c. lesion
  c. neurofibromatosis
  c. systemic periarteritis
  c. Woringer-Kolopp

classification
  Breslow c.
  Clark c. of malignant
    melanoma *(levels I–V)*
  Lund-Browder c.
  Ridley-Jopling c.

clastothrix

clausura

clavate microconidia

Claviceps purpurea

clavus *pl.* clavi
  c. durus
  c. mollis
  c. syphiliticus

claw
  c. hand
  c. nail

clawing
  c. deformity
  rheumatoid c.

clawlike
  c. nails
  c. prolongations

clean
  c. border
  Dey-Wash skin wound c.
  c. fracture

cleanser
  lipid-free c.
  Saf-Clens wound c.

cleansing cream

Clear
  C. Away Disc
  C. By design

clear cell
  c.c. acanthoma

clear cell (*continued*)
  c.c. hidradenoma
  c.c. papulosis
  c.c. myoepithelioma
  c.c. syringoma

Clearasil

clearing
  central c.

cleavage
  lines of c.

cleft
  intergluteal c.
  c. lip
  lucent c.
  c. palate

cleidocranial dysostosis

clemastine
  c. fumarate
  c. and
    phenylpropanolamine

clenched fist syndrome

Cleocin
  C. HCl
  C. Pediatric
  C. Phosphate

Cleocin T

climacteric flushing

climacterica
  keratoderma c.

climactericum
  keratoderma c.
  keratosis c.

climatotherapy

clindamycin

clinical
  c. changes
  c. hallmark
  c. hallmark of Woringer-
    Kolopp
  c. lepromatous process

clinical (*continued*)
    c. manifestation
    c. mark
    c. variant

clinician

clinicohistologic type

clinicopathologic
    c. features
    c. process

Clinique
    C. Daily Wash
    C. Extra Benefits
        Conditioner
    C. Shave Cream

clioquinol
    c. and hydrocortisone

clitoral
    c. dimension
    c. hood
    c. hypertrophy
    c. lesions

clitorimegaly

CLL
    chronic lymphocytic
        leukemia

cloacogenic carcinoma

clobetasol
    c. dipropionate
    c. propionate ointment
    c. solution

Clocort Maximum Strength

clocortolone pivalate

Cloderm
    C. topical

clofazimine
    c. palmitate

clomipramine

Clomycin

clonal
    c. B-cell proliferation

clonal (*continued*)
    c. deletion theory
    c. expansion
    c. immunoglobulin gene
        rearrangement
    c. proliferation
    c. rearrangement
    c. T-cell proliferation
    c. TCR rearrangement

clonality studies

clone

clonidine hydrochloride

clonorchiasis

Clorox

Clorpactin WCS-90

closed
    c. comedo
    c. curette
    c. patch test

"closed space" infection

clostridia

clostridial
    c. infection
    c. myonecrosis

Clostridium
    C. hemolyticum
    C. oedematiens
    C. perfringens
    C. septicum

closure
    Velcro c.

clothes louse

clothing
    c. dermatitis

clotrimazole
    betamethasone and c.
    c. cream
    c. suppository
    c. troche

clotted blood

clotting
  c. cascade
  c. disorders

Cloudman melanoma

cloudy cornea

Clouston's syndrome

clove oil

clover
  sweet c.

cloxacillin
  c. sodium

club
  c. foot
  c. hair
  c.-shaped

clubbed
  c. fingers
  c. nail

clubbing
  idiopathic c.
  nail c.
  c. of nail
  c. of the papillary bodies

cluster
  c. in a dermatome
  c.-of-jewels configuration
  c. of vesicles

cluster-of-grapes appearance

clustered papules

Clutton's joints

CMC
  chronic mucocutaneous
    candidiasis

CMM
  cutaneous malignant
    melanoma

CMV
  cytomegalovirus

Cnidaria

cnidarian
  c. envenomations
  c. larvae

cnidoblast

cnidosis

CNS
  central nervous system
    CNS lesions

CO_2 laser vaporization

Coactinon

coagulation
  blood c.
  c. factor deficiency
  c. factor disorder
  c. factor V
  c. necrosis
  c. phenomena

coagulopathy
  consumption c.

coal
  c. briquette
  c. tar
  c. tar bath
  c. tar, lanolin, and mineral
    oil
  c. tar and salicylic acid

coalescence

coalescing

coarctation of the aorta

coarse
  c. facies
  c. hair
  c. texture

coat
  proper c. of corium

coated tongue

Coats
  C's disease
  C's retinitis

cobalt

cobalt (*continued*)
 c. blue
 c. chloride
 c. dermatitis
 c. radiotherapy

cobblestone nevus

cobblestoned

cobblestoning

Cobb's syndrome

cobra
 c. hemotoxin
 c. itch
 c. venom cofactor
 c. venom factor

cocaine
 c. bug

cocardiform

cocci
 gram-negative c.
 gram-positive c.

Coccidia

coccidioidal
 c. granuloma
 c. osteomyelitis

Coccidioides immitis

coccidioidin
 c. skin test

coccidioidomycosis
 cutaneous c.
 disseminated c.
 primary c.
 primary pulmonary c.

coccidiosis

coccygeal sinus

Cochliomyia hominivorax

cockade

Cockayne
 C's syndrome

Cockayne (*continued*)
 C.-Touraine epidermolysis
 bullosa
 C.-Touraine type

cockscomb ulcer

cock-up deformity

co-climasone

coelenterate sting

coelom

coexistent
 c. disease
 c. infection

coffee fly

Cogan's syndrome

Cogentin

cohesion

coil
 c. gland

coiled
 c. ducts
 c. hairs

coincidental symptom

Cokeromyces

colchicine
 c. and probenecid

cold
 c. abscess
 c. agglutinin
 c. cream
 c. gangrene
 c. hemolysin
 c. injury
 c. panniculitis
 c. sore
 c. sore remedies
 c. ulcer
 c. urticaria

cold-dependent dermographism

cold-induced

cold-induced (*continued*)
   c.-i. urticaria
   c.-i. vasospasm

cold sore

colectomy

Coleoptera

coli
   Balantidium c.
   Escherichia c.
   c. granuloma

coliform

colistin, neomycin, and
   hydrocortisone

colitis
   ulcerative c.
   c. ulcerosa

collacin

collagen
   c. bundles
   c. disease
   c. fibers
   c. formation
   c. production
   c. remodeling
   type VII c.
   c. vascular disease

collagenase
   polymorphonuclear
      leukocyte c.
   type IV c.
   type V c.

collagenolysis

collagenoma

collagenosis
   reactive perforating c.

collagenous
   c. fibroma
   c. matrix
   c. plaques

collar
   Biett c.

collar (*continued*)
   Casal's c.
   keratotic c.
   c. of pearls
   venereal c.
   c. of Venus

collarette
   Biett's c.
   c. of Biett
   c. of scales
   c. scaling

collastin

colli
   leukoderma c.
   melanoleukoderma c.
   pterygium c.

colliquativa
   tuberculosis cutis c.

colliquative
   c. necrosis
   c. sweat

collodion
   c. baby
   blistering c.
   cantharidal c.
   hemostatic c.
   iodized c.
   c. membrane
   salicylic acid c.
   styptic c.

colloid
   c. acne
   c. bath
   c. bodies
   c. cyst
   c. degeneration
   c. material
   c. milium
   c. pseudomilium

colloidal
   c. iron
   c. oatmeal

colloidalis conglomerata

collum
    c. folliculi pili

coloboma

colonic
    c. adenocarcinoma
    c. carcinoma
    c. polyposis
    c. villous adenoma

colonization
    atypical mycobacterial c.
    Candida parapsilosis c.
    neonatal c.

colonized
    c. skin

colony-forming unit (CFU)

colophony resin

color
    constitutive skin c.
    facultative skin c.
    inducible skin c.
    lesion c.
    pale c.

Colorado
    C. microdissection needle
    C. tick fever
    C. tick fever virus

coloration

colored sweat

colorfast

coloring agent

colorless preparation

ColorZone tape

colostomy

colostrums
    bovine c.

colpotomy

column
    comedoid lamella-like
      parakeratotic c.
    posterior c.

columnar
    c. basal cells
    c. epithelium

coma

combination
    c. skin
    c. therapy

combined
    c. immunodeficiency
    c. immunodeficiency
      disease (CID)
    c. immunodeficiency
      syndrome
    measles, mumps and
      rubella vaccines, c.
    measles and rubella
      vaccines, c.
    rubella and mumps
      vaccines, c.

combining site

combustion
    c./ambustion, first-degree
    c./ambustion, secondary-
      degree
    c./ambustion, third-
      degree
    c. scars

combustionis
    dermatitis c.

comedo *pl.* comedones,
  comedos
    c. acne
    closed c.
    comedones epidermal
      nevus
    c. extraction
    c. extractor
    c. formation
    c. nevus
    open c.
    solar c.

comedocarcinoma

comedogenic

comedones (*plural of* comedo)
   c. extractor
   retroauricular c.

comedonicus
   nevus c.

commercial plastic braces

commissural cheilitis

commissure

committee
   National Vaccine Advisory
    C. (NVAC)

common
   c. acne
   c. baldness
   c. blue nevus
   c. leukocyte antigen
   c. nevus
   c. rice
   c. striped scorpion
   c. striped scorpion sting
   c. variable
    immunodeficiency (CVI)
   c. variable unclassifiable
    immunodeficiency
   c. wart

communicable
   c. disease

compact sclerotic collagen

compactum
   Fonsecaea c.
   Hormodendron c.
   stratum c.

compatibility

compatible

Compeed Skinprotector
  dressing

compensatory
   c. hyperhidrosis
   c. segmental hyperhidrosis

complement
   c. activation

complement (*continued*)
   c. deficiency
   c. fixation (CF)
   c. fixation assay
   c. fixation test
   hemolytic c.
   c. proteins

complementation

complete
   c. excision
   c. nail ablation

complex
   AIDS-related c. (ARC)
   c. cascade
   circulating immune c. (CIC)
   EAHF (eczema, asthma,
    hay fever) c.
   hapten-carrier c.
   membrane attack c. (MAC)
   c. physical therapy
   proteosome c.
   c. reaction
   c. regional pain syndrome
    (CRPS)
   semimembranosus c.
   tertiary c.

Complex 15 Face cream

Complex 15 Hand & Body
  cream

complexion
   T zone c.

complication
   delayed c.
   immunologic c.
   nonimmunologic c.

component
   absent dermal c.
   c. of complement
   matrix c.
   secretory c.
   ultrastructural c.

Compositae

compound

compound (*continued*)
  c. cyst
  c. nevus

compress
  cool c.
  ice c.

compressed air injury

compression
  c. stockings
  c. therapy

compressive
  c. garment
  c. wrap

compromised local integrity

compulsive
  c. neurosis
  c. neurotic habit

computed tomography (CT)

conA
  concanavalin

concave
  c. contour
  c. crust

concavity

concentration
  intradermal test c.
  prick test c.

concentric
  c. area
  c. blanching
  c. lesions
  c. rings
  c. superficial dermal
    infiltrate

concha

concomitant
  c. immunity
  c. topical steroid

concrete seborrhea

condensation

condition
  seborrheic dermatitis-like c.

condyloma *pl.* condylomata
  c. acuminata
  c. acuminatum
  c. acuminatum giganteum
  Buschke-Löwenstein giant
    c.
  flat c.
  giant c.
  c. lata
  c. latum
  c. planus
  pointed c.
  c. subcutaneum

condylomatoid

condylomatosis

condylomatous
  c. lesion

cone
  central c.
  keratosic c.
  c.-shaped epiphysis

conenose, cone-nose
  c. bug
  c. bug bite

conferta
  urticaria c.

confertus

configurate pattern

configuration
  lesion c.

confirmation
  tissue c.

conflagration

confluent
  c. erythema
  c. and reticulate
    papillomatosis

congelation
  c. urticaria

congelationis
    dermatitis c.

congenita
    adermia c.
    aplasia cutis c.
    arthrochalasis multiplex c.
    cutis marmorata
        telangiectasia c.
    dyskeratosis c.
    hyperkeratosis c.
    melanosis diffusa c.
    pachyonychia c.
    type II pachyonychia c.

congenital
    c. absence
    c. adrenal hyperplasia
    c. adrenogenital syndrome
    c. alopecia universalis
    c. 5-alpha-reductase
        deficiency
    c. auricular fistula
    c. AV fistula
    c. baldness
    c. candidiasis
    c. capillary malformation
    c. cataract
    c. circumscribed
        hypomelanosis
    c. constriction
    c. cutaneous candidiasis
    c. deafness
    c. depigmentation
    c. developmental
        abnormality
    c. disorder
    c. dyskeratosis
    c. ectodermal defects
    c. ectodermal dysplasia
    c. elephantiasis
    c. erythrodermic ichthyosis
    c. erythropoietic porphyria
    c. facial melanocytic lesion
    c. fascial dystrophy
    c. fibromatosis
    c. fistula
    c. generalized
        fibromatosis

congenital (*continued*)
    c. generalized
        hypertrichosis
    c. heart defect
    c. hemidysplasia with
        ichthyosiform
        erythroderma and limb
        defects (CHILD)
    c. hemolytic anemia
    c. HIV infection
    c. hypertrichosis lanuginosa
    c. ichthyosiform
    c. ichthyosiform
        erythroderma
    c. ichthyosis
    c. immunodeficiency
    c. infection
    c. isoantibody
    c. lesion
    c. leukemia
    c. leukodermic patches
    c. Lyme disease
    c. lymphedema
    c. malalignment
    c. malformation
    c. melanocytic nevi
    c. melanoma
    c. milk-white skin
    c. mitral stenosis
    c. multiple fibromatosis
    c. myelogenous leukemia
    c. nevocytic nevus
    c. nevus
    c. onychodysplasia
    c. phlebectasia
    c. pigmented nevi
    c. pits
    c. platelet function defect
    c. poikiloderma
    c. predisposition
    c. process
    c. rubella
    c. rubella syndrome
    c. scalp lesion
    c. sebaceous hyperplasia
    c. self-healing
        reticulohistiocytosis
    c. sensory neuropathy

congenital (*continued*)
  c. smooth muscle
    hamartoma
  c. spot
  c. syphilis
  c. telangiectatic erythema
  c. thymic hypoplasia
  c. total lipodystrophy
  c. toxoplasmosis
  c. triangular alopecia
  c. varicella
  c. white leaf-shaped
    macules

congenitale
  erythroderma
    ichthyosiforme c.
  poikiloderma c.

congenitalis
  alopecia c.
  alopecia triangularis c.
  erythroderma
    ichthyosiformis c.

congenitum
  erythroderma
    ichthyosiforme c.

congestivum
  erythema c.

conglobata
  acne c.

conglobate
  c. abscess
  c. acne

conglomerata
  colloidalis c.
  elastosis colloidalis c.

conglomeration

Congo
  C. floor maggot
  A. floor maggot bite
  C.-red positive
  C. red stain

congolensis
  Dermatophilus c.

Congolese

conical
  c. filament
  c. keratinous plus

conidia
  elongated lateral c.

conidiophore

Conidiobolus
  C. coronatus
  C. incongruus

conidium *pl.* conidia

conjunctival
  c. congestion
  c. hemorrhage
  c. neovascularization

conjunctivitis
  acute contagious c.
  acute epidemic c.
  acute follicular c.
  allergic c.
  angular c.
  bacterial c.
  blennorrheal c.
  bulbar c.
  chlamydial c.
  chronic c.
  giant papillary c. (GPC)
  gonococcal c.
  herpes simplex c.
  inclusion c.
  infantile purulent c.
  Lymphogranuloma
    venereum c.
  Moraxella c.
  c. sicca
  tarsal c.
  toxicogenic c.
  vernal c.
  viral c.

connective
  c. tissue capsule
  c. tissue disease (CTD)
  c. tissue panniculitis
  c. tissue septa

connective (*continued*)
    c. tissue sheath
    c. tissue nevus

Conradi
    C's disease
    Conradi-Hünermann
      syndrome
    C.-Hünermann type

consanguineous

consanguinity

consistency
    lesion c.

consolidation
    progressive acinar c.

constant
    c. region

constitutional
    c. hirsutism
    c. illness
    c. reaction
    c. ulcer

constitutive
    c. pigmentation
    c. skin color

consuming ulcer

consumption coagulopathy

Contact
    C. Dermatitis Research
      Group

contact
    allergen c.
    c. allergy
    c. brucellosis
    c. cheilitis
    c. dermatitis
    c. eczema
    c. electrical burn
    c. hypersensitivity
    c. leukoderma
    c. photosensitization
    c. stomatitis
    c.-type dermatitis

contact (*continued*)
    c. urticaria
    c. urticaria syndrome

contactant

contact-type dermatitis

contagion
    immediate c.
    mediate c.

contagiosa
    impetigo c.
    keratosis follicularis c.

contagiosum
    ecthyma c.
    epithelioma c.
    erythema c.
    molluscum c.

contagiosus
    pemphigus c.

contagious
    c. disease
    c. ecthyma
    c. ecthyma (pustular
      dermatitis) virus of sheep
    c. infection
    c. pustular dermatitis
    c. pustular dermatosis
    c. pustular stomatitis virus

contagiousness

contagium

contaminant

contaminate

contamination
    bacterial c.

contiguity

contiguous
    c. inflammatory margin
    c. vesicles

continua
    acrodermatitis c.

continuous-wave mode

contraceptive
c. diaphragm
c. sponge

contraction
wound c.

contracture
Dupuytren c.
flexion c.

contradistinction

contralateral

contrast phlebography

control
mite c.
mold c.
odor c.

controlled
c. anaphylaxis

contusiform
c. nodule

contusiforme
erythema c.

contusion

convalescent
c. carrier
c. serum
c. stage

conversion
peripheral metabolic c.

convertase
C3 proactivator c.

convex
c. border
c. incision
c. nail
c. papules

convoluted
c. foam mattress
c. lobules

convulsion

cookei
Ixodes c.

Cooks syndrome

cool compress

Cooley's anemia

coolie itch

cooling
c. agent
c. blanket
rapid c.

Coombs
C. serum
C. test

Copious sebum

copolymer

copper
c.-binding ion
c. deficiency
c. histidine
c. metabolism
c. sulfate
c. vapor
c. vapor laser

copperhead
c. snake
c. snake bite

Coppertone

copra itch

coproporphyria
hereditary c. (HCP)

coproporphyrin

coproporphyrinogen

COPS
calcinosis cutis, osteoma
cutis, poikiloderma, and
skeletal abnormalities
COPS syndrome

cor pulmonale

coral

coral (*continued*)
    c. bead appearance
    c. cut
    c. dermatitis
    c.-red fluorescence
    c.-reef keratoacanthoma
    c. snake
    c. snake bite

cordlike nodule

Cordran
    C. SP topical
    C. tape
    C. topical

corduroy

Cordylobia anthropophaga

core

corium

corkscrew
    c. hair

corn
    hard c.
    soft c.

cornea
    herpes c.
    ichthyosis c.
    ichthyosis sebacea c.

corneae

corneal
    c. opacification
    c. opacity
    c. scars
    c. ulcer
    c. ulceration

Cornelia de Lange's syndrome

corneocyte
    c. adhesion
    c. desquamation

corneous
    c. plug

corneum

corneum (*continued*)
    Nosema c.
    Stratum c.

corneus
    Aspergillus c.
    c. hypertrophicus
    lichen c. hypertrophicus
    lichen obtusus c.

cornification
    disorder of c. (DOC)
    c. disorder
    normal c.
    type 1-24 c.

cornified
    c. cell envelope
    c. cell layer
    c. keratinocyte
    c. layer

cornoid
    c. lamella

corns

cornstarch

cornu, cornua
    c. cutaneum

cornual

cornuate

corona
    c. phlebectatica
    c. seborrheica
    c. sulcus lymphangitis
    c. veneris

coronae
    zona c.

coronal
    c. sulcus
    c. view

coronary
    c. artery disease (CAD)
    c. occlusion
    c. artery stenosis

Coronavirus

corporis
    pediculosis c.
    Pediculus c.
    pthiriasis c.
    seborrhea c.
    tinea c.
    trichophytosis c.

corps
    c. grains
    c. ronds

corpus
    c. glandulae sudoriferae
    c. unguis

corpuscle
    bridge c.
    molluscum c.

Corque topical

corrosion

corrosive
    c. ulcer

corset

CortaGel

Cortaid
    C. Maximum Strength
    C. with aloe

Cort-Dome

Cortef
    C. Feminine Itch

cortex *pl.* cortices
    deep c.
    c. of hair shaft

Corticaine cream

cortical
    deep c.
    c. trichocytes

corticis (*genitive of* cortex)

corticoid damage

corticosteroid

corticosteroid (*continued*)
    class IV topical c.
    class V topical c.
    c. cream
    c.-induced cataracts
    c. lotion
    c. rosacea
    c. spray
    systemic c.

corticotropin

Cortifair

Cortifoam

Cortin topical

cortisone acetate

Cortisporin
    C. Ophthalmic Ointment
    C. Ophthalmic suspension
    C. Otic
    C. Topical Cream
    C. Topical Ointment

Cortizone-5

Cortizone-10

Cortone
    C. Acetate injection
    C. Acetate oral

Cortril

corymbiform

corymbose
    c. syphilid

corynebacteria

corynebacteriophage
    β c.

Corynebacterium
    C. acnes
    C. diphtheriae
    C. jeikeium
    C. minutissimum

coryneform bacterium

coryza
    allergic c.

Cosmegen

cosmesis

cosmetic
    cheek c.
    c. dermatitis
    eyelash c.
    eyelid c.
    c. intolerance syndrome
    lip c.
    c. treatment
    undercover c.

cosmetica
    acne c.

cosmetician

cosmetologist

cosmetology

Cossus cossus

costal cartilage

Costello syndrome

Cotrim
    C. DS

co-trimoxazole

cotton
    c. dermatitis
    c.-tipped applicator

cottonmouth
    c. moccasin
    c. snake
    c. snake bite

cottonseed

cottonwood
    Arizona/Fremont c.
    c. tree

cotton-wool
    c.-w. patch
    c.-w. spot

Coumadin necrosis

coumarin
    c. necrosis

council
    Medical Research C. (MRC)

counter immunoelectrophoresis
    (CIE)

counteract

counterirritants (*class of drugs*)

counterirritation

coupe
    c. de sabre
    en c. de sabre

coverglass

coverslip

cow dander

cowage

Cowden
    C's disease
    C's syndrome

cow's milk

cowpox
    c. virus

Coxiella
    C. burnetii

Coxsackie
    C. B virus

Coxsackievirus
    c. A10
    c. A16

CPK
    creatinine phosphokinase

CPO
    coproporphyrinogen
        oxidase

crab
    c. grass
    c. hand
    c. louse

crab (*continued*)
  c. yaws

crablike gait

crabs

crack

cracked
  c. heel
  c. lips
  c. skin

crackled
  c. hair
  c. skin

cradle cap

Crandall's syndrome

cranial
  c. arteritis
  c. cleavage planes
  c. fasciitis of childhood
  c. nerve palsy
  c. nerves
  c. osteolysis
  c. penetration
  c. physiognomy

craniocarpotarsal syndrome

craniodiaphysial dysplasia

craniofacial abnormality

craniopharyngioma

craniotubular dysplasia

cranium

craquelé
  eczema c.
  erythema c.
  onychia c.

crateriform
  c. appearance
  c. center
  c. ulcer

craterlike depression

craw-craw (*also* kra-kra)

crazy paving dermatosis

cream
  cleansing c.
  cold c.
  Corticaine c.
  Cortisporin Topical C.
  Elimite C.
  EMLA c.
  Eucerin c.
  facial undercover c.
  Kwell C.
  Lotrimin AF C.
  masoprocol c.
  Maximum Strength
    Desenex Antifungal C.
  Naftin c.
  Neosporin C.
  Pramosone c.
  Psorion C.
  SSD C.
  tretinoin c.
  triamcinolone c. (TAC)
  Zonalon c.

crease
  allergic c.
  earlobe c.
  flexion c.
  genitocrural c.
  palmar c.

creatinine
  c. phosphokinase level

creeping
  c. disease
  c. eruption
  c. myiasis
  c. ulcer
  c. vesiculation

Crème
  Fungoid C.
  Fungoid HC C.
  Gormel C.

creosote dermatitis

creosote bush

crescentic glomerulonephritis

CREST
  calcinosis cutis, Raynaud
    phenomenon, esophageal
    dysfunction/hypermotility,
    sclerodactyly,
    telangiectasia
  CREST syndrome

crest
  c. of matrix of nail

cretinism

cribriform patches

crickled

crinis *pl.* crines

crinium (*genitive plural of*
  crinis)

crinkled flannel moth

crinkly

crisis *pl.* crises
  anaphylactic c.
  anaphylactoid c.

crista
  c. cutis
  c. matrices unguis

Crix belly

Crocq's disease

Crohn's disease

cromolyn sodium

Cronkhite-Canada syndrome

crops
  recurring c.

Cross syndrome

cross
  c. infection
  c. reaction
  c. sensitization

Cross-McKusick-Breen
  syndrome

crotamiton

crotamiton (*continued*)
  c. cream
  c. lotion

crotch itch

Crouzon's disease

Crow-Fukase syndrome

Crowe
  C's sign
  C.-Dickermann syndrome

crown alopecia

crownlike plate

CRPS
  complex regional pain
    syndrome

CRST
  calcification, Raynaud's
    phenomenon,
    scleroderma,
    telangiectasis
  CRST syndrome

crud, the crud

crude
  c. coal tar
  c. petroleum

Cruex topical

crumbling nail plate

crumbly crusting

crural fold

cruris
  tinea c.
  trichophytosis c.

crust
  concave sulfur-yellow c.
  c.-covered
  cup-shaped c.

Crustacea

crustacean

crustaceous

crustaceous (*continued*)
  c. lesion

crusted
  c. erythematous
    papulopustule
  c. lesions
  c. ringworm
  c. scabies
  c. tetter

crux
  cruces pilorum

cryocrystalglobulin
  syndrome

cryofibrinogen

cryofibrinogenemia

cryoglobulin

cryoglobulinemia

cryoprobe

cryoproteinemia

cryosurgery

cryosurgical
  c. procedure
  c. treatment

cryotherapy

cryptococcal
  polysaccharide

cryptococcosis
  cutaneous c.

Cryptococcus
  C. neoformans

cryptorchid

cryptorchidism

Cryptosporidia

cryptotrichotillomania

crystal
  c. rash
  c. violet
  c. violet vaccine

crystallina
  c. deposit
  miliaria c.
  uridrosis c.

crystalloid inclusions

Crysticillin AS injection

CSD
  cat-scratch disease
  CSD skin test

CS/DS
  chondroitin
    sulfate/dermatan sulfate

CSF
  cerebrospinal fluid
  colony-stimulating factor
  CSF nontreponemal titer

CSF-VDRL
  colony-stimulating factor-
    developed by Venereal
    Disease Research
    Laboratory

Csillag's disease

CSS
  Churg-Strauss syndrome

CSSRD
  Cooperative Systematic
    Studies of the Rheumatic
    Disease

CT
  computed tomography
  thin-section CT

CTCL
  cutaneous T-cell lymphoma

CTD
  connective tissue disease

Ctenocephalides
  C. canis
  C. canis bite
  C. felis
  C. felis bite

CTH

CTH (*continued*)
  ceramide trihexoside
CTM
  Chlor-Trimeton
CTS
  carpal tunnel syndrome
Cuban itch
cubitus
  c. valgus
  c. varus
cuboidal
  c. basal cells
  c. epithelial cells
cuirasse
  cancer en c.
  carcinoma en c.
cuirasslike restraint
culdoscope
culdoscopy
Culex
  C. fatigans
  C. mosquito
Culicidae
Culicinae
culicosis bullosa
Culiseta
  C. mosquito
cultivated
  c. barley grass
  c. barley smut
  c. corn grass
  c. corn smut
  c. oat grass
  c. oat smut
  c. rye grass
  c. rye smut
  c. wheat grass
  c. wheat smut
cultural
  c. growth

culture
  fungal c.
  c. medium
cultured epidermal allografts
Cuna moon children
cunicular
cuniculatum
  epithelioma c.
cuniculi
cuniculus
Cunninghamella
Cupid's bow configuration
cuplike depression
"cupping"
cupric
  c. sulfate
cup-shaped crust
curative
curdled
curdling
curettage
curette, curet
curettement
curly hair
currens
  larva c.
current
  fulguration c.
curved linear patterns
curvilinear plane
Curvularia geniculata
Cushing
  C's disease
  C's syndrome
cushingoid

cushingoid (*continued*)
    c. changes
    c. facies

cut
    coral c.

cutanea
    porphyria c. tarda
    sclerosis c.

cutaneous
    c. abscess
    c. absorption
    c. albinism
    c. amyloid
    c. ancylostomiasis
    c. angiitis
    c. anthrax
    c. apoplexy
    c. apudoma
    c. arterioles
    c. basophil hypersensitivity (CBH)
    c. basophil reaction
    c. B-cell lymphoid hyperplasia
    c. B-cell lymphoma
    c. blotching
    c. borreliosis
    c. calcification
    c. candidiasis
    c. candidiasis in Bombay
    c. carcinoma
    c. CD30-positive lymphoproliferative disease
    c. ciliated cyst
    c. coccidioidomycosis
    c. columnar cyst
    c. condition
    c. coxsackievirus infection
    c. Crohn's disease
    c. cylindroma
    c. disease
    c. disorder
    c. dissemination
    c. draining sinus
    c. drug eruption

cutaneous (*continued*)
    c. dyschromia
    c. endometriosis
    c. eruptions of lymphocyte recovery
    c. expressions
    c. findings
    c. focal mucinosis
    c. follicular projections
    c. gangrene
    c. hemangioma
    c. histology
    c. histoplasmosis
    c. Hodgkin's disease
    c. Hodgkin's lymphoma
    c. horn
    c. horn formation
    c. hyperpigmentation
    c. keratocyst
    c. large-vessel vasculitis
    c. larva migrans
    c. laser surgery
    c. lentiginosis
    c. leiomyoma
    c. leishmaniasis
    c. lentiginosis
    c. lesion
    c. lupus
    c. lupus erythematosus
    c. lymphoid hyperplasia
    c. lymphoid infiltrate
    c. lymphoma
    c. malformation
    c. manifestation
    c. marker
    c. mastocytosis
    c. melanoacanthoma
    c. meningocele
    c. meningospinal angiomatosis
    c. metaplastic synovial cyst
    c. morphology
    c. mucinosis
    c. mucinosis of infancy
    c. mucormycosis
    c. myelofibrosis
    c. myxoma
    c. necrotizing vasculitis

cutaneous (*continued*)
- c. neoplasm
- c. nerves
- c. neuroma
- c. nevi
- c. nodule
- c. oncology
- c. ossification
- c. Paget's disease
- c. papilloma
- c. papulation
- c. parameters
- c. plasmacytoma
- c. polyarteritis nodosa
- c. portal
- primary c.
- c. protein
- c. protothecosis
- c. purpura
- c. pustular vasculitis
- c. reaction
- c. Rosai-Dorfman disease
- c. sarcoidosis
- c. sarcoma
- c. schistosomal granuloma
- c. sclerosis
- c. sensitization
- c. sign
- c. sinus histiocytosis
- c. sinus tracts
- c. small-cell lymphoma
- c. small-vessel disease
- c. small-vessel vasculitis
- c. spotty pigmentation
- c. stigmata
- c. strongyloidiasis
- c.-subcutaneous nodule
- c. tag
- c. T-cell lymphoid hyperplasia
- c. T-cell lymphoma (CTCL)
- c. tuberculosis
- c. tumor
- c. ulcer
- c. ulceration
- c. vascular abnormality
- c. vascular anomalies
- c. vasculitis

cutaneous (*continued*)
- c. visceral type
- c. xanthomas

cutaneum
- cornu c.
- sebum c.

cutaneus
- nodulus c.

cutem
- hyperkeratosis follicularis et parafollicularis in c.
- penetrans
- c. penetrans

Cuterebra cuniculi

Cuterebridae

cuticle
- c. of hair
- c. of root sheath
- c. scales

cuticular telangiectases

cuticularization

cutis
- c. anserina
- atrophia maculosa varioliformis c.
- c. elastica
- c. hyperelastica
- c. laxa
- c. laxa acquisita
- c. laxa–like appearance
- c. marmorata
- c. marmorata telangiectasia congenita
- neuroma c.
- osteoma c.
- c. pendula
- c. pensilis
- c. rhomboidalis nuchae
- c. testacea
- c. unctuosa
- c. vera
- c. verticis gyrata
- verrucosa c.

Cutivate
    C. topical

cutting
    c. current
    c. fluid
    c. oils

CVI
    Children's Vaccine Imitative
        common variable
        immunodeficiency

cyanhidrosis

cyanocobalamin
    c. deficiency

cyanosis
    pernio c.

cyanotic

cycle
    hair c.

cyclic
    c. neutropenia
    c. urticaria

cyclical
    c. disease
    c. phase

cyclin-dependent kinase 4

Cyclocort
    C. topical

cycloheximide

cyclomethicone

cyclooxygenase (COX)
    c.-1 (COX-1)
    c.-2 (COX-2)

cyclophosphamide (CTX)
    immunoablative high-dose
        c.
    c. pulse therapy

Cyclops

cyclosporine
    c.-induced nephrotoxicity

cyclosporine (*continued*)
    c. microemulsion
    c. therapy

cylindrical mass

cylindroma

cylindromatous

cyproheptadine
    c. hydrochloride

cyproterone acetate

Cyrano defect

cyst
    adventitious c.
    anogenital epidermal c.
    anogenital pilar c.
    anogenital sebaceous c.
    anogenital vestibular c.
    apocrine retention c.
    atheromatous c.
    Baker c.
    branchial c.
    bronchogenic c.
    colloid c.
    compound c.
    dermoid c.
    desmoid c.
    epidermal c.
    epidermal inclusion c.
    epidermoid c.
    epithelial c.
    false c.
    Favre-Racouchot c.
    follicular infundibular c.
    follicular isthmus c.
    c. formation
    hydatid c.
    implantation c.
    inclusion c.
    keratinizing c.
    keratinous c.
    milia c.
    mucinous c.
    mucous c.
    multilocular thymic c.
        (MTC)

cyst (*continued*)
    myxoid c.
    parasitic c.
    parvilocular c.
    pheomycotic c.
    pilar c.
    piliferous c.
    pilonidal c.
    popliteal c.
    preauricular c.
    proliferating pilar c.
    proliferating trichilemmal c.
    retention c.
    retroauricular c.
    sebaceous c.
    sequestration c.
    subchondral c.
    synovial c.
    thyroglossal c.
    trichilemmal c.
    trichilemmal c.,
      proliferating
    unicameral c.
    unilocular c.
    vestibular c.

cystadenoma
    apocrine c.

Cystamin

cystathionine ß-synthase

cysteine
    c. proteinase
    c. proteinase inhibitor

cystic
    c. acne
    c. basal cell carcinoma
    c. cavities
    c. deformation
    c. dilatation
    c. disease
    c. epithelioma
    c. epithelium
    c. fibrosis (CF)
    c. hidradenoma
    c. hygroma
    c. lymphatic malformation

cystic (*continued*)
    c. sialadenoma
    c. spaces

cystica
    acne c.

cysticerci

cysticercosis cutis

Cysticercus cellulosae

cysticum
    acanthoma adenoides c.
    epithelioma adenoides c.

cystides

cystis

cystitis
    hemorrhagic c.

cystlike protuberance

cystocele

cystoid

cystous

cytochrome
    c. b 558 (gp91-phox)
    c. drug metabolizing system
    c. enzymes
    c. P450 14-*a*-demethylase
    c. P450 system

cytodiagnosis

cytogenic

cytoid body staining

cytokeratin

cytokine
    inhibitory c.
    c. macrophage
    c. production
    regulatory c.

cytologic
    c. appearance
    c. atypia
    c. pleomorphism

cytologically

cytolysin

cytolysis

cytolytic mediators

cytomegalic
c. cells
c. inclusion disease

cytomegalovirus (CMV)
congenital c.
c. disease
c. immune globulin
intravenous, human
c. retinitis

cytopenia

cytophagic
c. histiocyte panniculitis
c. lobular panniculitis

cytoplasm
c. of keratinocytes

cytoplasmic
c. antigen
c. cytochrome oxidase
c. granules
c. inclusion
c. swelling
c. vacuolization

cytosine
c. arabinoside

cytosolic corticoid receptor

cytoskeletal
c. function
c. protein

cytotoxic
c. agent
c. cell
c. defense
c. drug
c. immunologic drug
reaction
c. immunosuppressive
therapy
c. reaction
c. T cells
c. T lymphocyte (CTL)

cytotoxicity
antibody-dependent cell-
mediated c. (ADCC)
lymphocyte-mediated c.
(LMC)

Cytovene

Cytoxan (CTX)
C. injection
C. oral

D
　vitamin D

Dabska's tumor

dacarbazine

Dacron

dacryoadenitis

dacryocystitis

dacryocystorhinostomy

dactinomycin

Dactylaria gallopava

dactyledema

dactylitis
　blistering distal d.
　distal d.
　multidigit d.
　septic d.
　d. strumosa
　syphilitic d.
　d. syphilitica
　d. tuberculosa
　tuberculous d.

dactylolysis spontanea

dactyloscopy

Dalalone
　D. DP
　D. LA

damage
　bacterial-induced vascular
　　d.
　immunologic organ d.
　sun and chemical
　　combination d.

danazol

Danbolt-Closs syndrome

dander

dandruff

Dandy
　D.-Walker syndrome
　D.-Walker deformity

Danielssen
　D. disease

Danielssen
　D.-Boeck disease
　D.-Boeck sarcoidosis

Danlos
　D. disease
　D. syndrome

dapsone (DDS)

Dapsone Pharmacokinetics

dapsone/pyrimethamine

Daraprim

Darier
　D's disease
　D's gene
　morbus D.
　D's sign
　D.-Roussy sarcoid
　D.-White disease

darkened

dark
　d. blue
　d. dot disease
　d. field
　d. red hue
　d. red plaque
　d. skin
　d. staining nodule

darkfield
　d. appearance
　d. condenser
　d. examination
　d. illumination
　d. microscopy
　d. preparation

dartoic
　d. muscle

dartos
    tunica d.

Dasyatidae

date
    d. boil

daunorubicin
    d. hydrochloride

DDEB
    dominant dystrophic
        epidermolysis bullosa

DDS
    dapsone

DDT
    dichlorodiphenyltrichloroet
        hane

de
    d. Quervain disease
    d. Quervain tenosynovitis

dead finger

deaf-mutism

deafness
    keratitis d.
    lentigines,
        electrocardiographic
        defects, ocular
        hypertelorism, pulmonary
        stenosis, abnormalities of
        genitalia, retardation of
        growth, e. (LEOPARD)

deallergize

death-dealing

DEBRA
    Dystrophic Epidermolysis
        Bullosa Research
        Association of America

debridement
    enzymatic d.
    surgical d.

debris
    necrotic d.
    tissue d.

Debrisan
    D. beads
    D. paste

debulking

Decaderm

Decadron
    D. elixir
    D.-LA
    D. Phosphate
    D. with Xylocaine

Decaject
    D.-LA

decalvans
    acne d.
    folliculitis d.
    keratosis follicularis
        spinulosa d.
    porrigo d.

decalvant

decapitation
    d. secretion

Decaspray

decay

deciduous
    d. skin
    d. teeth

deck-chair sign

Declomycin

decompensation

decomposition

decompression sickness

decongestant
    topical d.

decongestive
    d. physiotherapy

decontamination

decreased
    d. fertility, short stature

decubation

decubital
    d. gangrene
    d. ulcer

decubitus
    d. ulcer

DEDLE

distinctive exudative discoid
    and lichenoid dermatitis

deep
    d. bruise
    d. fascia
    d. fungi
    d. granuloma annulare
    d. hemangioma
    d. incisional biopsy
    d. lateral nooks
    d. mycosis
    d. shave excision
    d. vascular plexus
    d. vein thrombosis
    d. venous system
        malformation
    d. venous thrombosis

deep-seated
    d.-s. blister
    d.-s. nodule
    d.-s. paraumbilical
        nodule
    d.-s. pustule
    d.-s. vesicle

deer
    d. fly
    d. fly bite
    d. fly disease
    d. tick

deet
    diethyltoluamide

defatting action

defect
    congenital ectodermal d.
    neuroectodermal d.

defective
    d. bacteriophage
    d. cell-mediated immune
        function
    d. intermediate filament

defects
    congenital hemidysplasia
        with ichthyosiform
        erythroderma and limb d.
        (CHILD)
    host d.

defense mechanism

defensin

defibrination syndrome

deficiency
    immune d.
    immunity d.
    immunological d.
    riboflavin d.
    secretory component d.
    vitamin D d.

deficient
    d. cell-mediated immunity
    d. platelet production

deflorescence

defluvium
    d. capillorum
    d. unguium

defluxio
    d. capillorum
    d. ciliorum

defluxion

deformation
    cystic d.

deformity
    angel wing d.
    arthritis without d.
    boutonnière d.
    clawing d.
    cock-up d.
    opera-glass d.

deformity (*continued*)
    pencil and cup d.
    saddle nose d.
    swan-neck d.

defurfuration

degeneration
    amyloid d.
    ballooning d.
    basophilic d.
    colloid d.
    elastoid d.
    elastotic d.
    epithelial d.
    fatty d.
    granular d.
    hydropic d.
    liquefaction d.
    malignant d.
    mucinous d.
    mucoid d.
    myxomatous d.
    d. of epidermal cells
    reticular d.
    suppurative d.

degenerativa
    melanosis corii d.

degenerative
    d. collagenous plaque
    melanosis corii d.
    d. neurologic syndrome
    d. retinitis

Degos
    D's acanthoma
    D's disease
    malignant papillomatosis of D.
    D's syndrome

degradative
    d. pathway
    d. phase

degranulation

dehematized condition

dehiscence

dehydration

dehydroepiandrosterone

Delaxin

delayed
    d. blanching
    d. complication
    d. cranial suture closure
    d. hypersensitivity (DH)
    d.-hypersensitivity immunologic drug reaction
    d. hypersensitivity reaction
    d. hypersensitivity skin testing
    d. patch test reading
    d. pressure urticaria
    d. reaction
    d. systemic reaction
    d. tanning
    d. telogen release
    d.-type hypersensitivity (DTH)
    d. wound healing

Delcort

deleterious
    d. effects

deletion
    clonal d.

delitescence

Del-Mycin topical

delta-aminolevulinic acid

Delta
    D.-Cortef
    D.-Tritex

Deltasone
    D. Dosepak
    D. Oral

delusion of parasitosis

demarcated
    d. border
    d. cellulitis

demarcated (*continued*)
    d. inflammatory process
    d. reaction

demarcation

Dematiaceae

dematiaceous
    d. fungi
    d. fungus

d'emblée
    d. form
    mycosis fungoides d.
    syphilis d.

demeclocycline hydrochloride

dementia

demethylchlortetracycline

demodectic
    d. acariasis
    d. mange

Demodex
    D. brevis
    D. canis
    D. equi
    D. folliculitis
    D. folliculorum
    D. mites

Demodicidae

demodicidosis

demodicosis

De Morgan's spots

demyelination

demyelinating

dendriform

dendrite

dendritic
    d. cell
    d. corneal ulcer
    d. macrophage
    d. melanocyte
    d. morphology
    d. secretory cell

dendritiform

dendrocyte
    dermal d.

denervation

dengue
    d. facies
    d. fever
    hemorrhagic d.
    d. hemorrhagic fever
    d. virus

Dennie
    D's infraorbital fold
    D's line
    D's sign
    D.-Morgan infraorbital
        fold
    D.-Morgan line
    D.-Morgan sign

Denorex

densa
    lamina d.
    sublamina d.

dense
    d. bands of hyalinized
        collagen
    d. infiltrate
    d. linear cortical
        hyperostosis
    d. neutrophilic infiltrate

dental
    d. amalgam
    d. anomaly
    d. caries
    d. fistula
    d. radiography
    d. silver
    d. sinus

dentigerous cyst

dentigenous cyst

dentition

denudation

denude

denuded
    d. area
    d. surface

deodorant

deoxyribonucleic acid (DNA)
    d. a. synthesis

dependent
    d. areas
    d. edema
    d. rubor

depigmentation
    congenital d.

depigmenting process

depilate

depilation

depilatory
    d. agent
    chemical d.

depMedalone injection

Depoject injection

Depo-Medrol
    D.-M. injection

Depopred injection

deposition
    immunoelectron
      microscopy d.

deposit

depressed
    d. nasal bridge
    d. scars

depression

Dercum's disease

derma

Derma
    D.-Smoothe/FS Oil
    D. Viva lotion

Dermabond

dermabraded

dermabrader
    Iverson d.
    sandpaper d.

dermabrasion

Dermacentor
    D. andersoni
    D. occidentalis
    D. variabilis

Dermacoat

Dermacomb topical

Dermacort

Dermaflex Gel

Dermagraft

dermagraphy

dermahemia

dermal
    d. connective tissue
    d. curette
    d. dendrocyte
    d. duct tumor
    d. duct nevus
    d. eccrine cylindroma
    d. edema
    d. elastorrhexis
    d. fibroblast
    d. fibrosis
    d. granuloma
    d. hypoplasia
    d. infiltrate
    d. inflammation
    d. leishmanoid
    d. lesion
    d. lymphatics
    d. melanin
    d. melanocytic hamartoma
    d. melanocytic lesion
    d. microfibril
    d. microfibril bundle
    d. microvascular unit
    d. mononuclear pustule
    d. mucinosis

dermal (*continued*)
  d. mucin
  d. noncaseating granuloma
  d. nonepidermotropic
    infiltrate
  d. papilla
  d. stroma
  d. sweat duct tumor
  d. system
  d. tuberculosis
  d. tumor
  d. vascular plexus
  d. venular
    hyperpermeability
  d. vessel

Dermal-Rub

dermalaxia

dermametropathism

dermamyiasis
  d. linearis migrans oestrosa

Dermanyssus gallinae

Derma-Pax

Dermarest
  D. Dricort Creme
  D. gel
  D. Plus

Dermasept Antifungal

Dermasil

Derma-Smoothe/FS topical

dermatalgia

dermatan sulfate

dermatic

dermatica
  zona d.

dermatite papulosquameuse
  atrophiante

dermatitic epidermal nevus

dermatitides

dermatitidis

dermatitidis (*continued*)
  Ajellomyces d.
  Blastomyces d.

dermatitis *pl.* dermatitides
  acetone d.
  acneform d.
  actinic d.
  d. actinica
  adhesive d.
  d. aestivalis
  allergic d.
  allergic contact d.
  allergic eczematous
    contact-type d.
  d. ambustionis
  ammonia d.
  ancylostoma d.
  antimicrobial contact d.
  arsenical d.
  arsphenamine d.
  d. artefacta
  ashy d.
  atopic d.
  d. atrophicans
  d. autophytica
  autosensitization d.
  avian mite d.
  axillary d.
  bather's d.
  berlock d.
  berloque d.
  bhiwanol d.
  blastomycetic d.
  d. blastomycotica
  blistering d.
  brown-tail moth d.
  brucella d.
  bubble gum d.
  d. bullosa
  d. bullosa striata pratensis
  d. calorica
  Calycophora d.
  carcinomatous d.
  caterpillar d.
  cement d.
  cercarial d.
  chemical d.

dermatitis (*continued*)
    chigger d.
    chromate d.
    chrome d.
    chromium d.
    chronic acral d.
    chronic actinic d.
    chronic bullous d.
    chronic papular d.
    chronic purpura d.
    circumoral d.
    clothing d.
    cobalt d.
    d. combustionis
    condom d.
    d. congelationis
    contact d.
    contact-type d.
    contagious pustular d.
    d. contusiformis
    copra mite d.
    cosmetic d.
    d. cruris pustulosa et
        atrophicans
    cumulative insult d.
    deodorant d.
    desquamative d.
    dhobie mark d.
    diaper d.
    dried fruit d.
    dust d.
    d. dysmenorrhoeica
    earlobe allergic d.
    eczematous d.
    endogenous d.
    eosinophilic d.
    d. epidemica
    d. erythematosa
    erythematous macular d.
    d. escharotica
    d. estivalis
    ethylenediamine d.
    excoriativa infantum d.
    d. exfoliativa
    d. exfoliativa infantum
    d. exfoliativa epidemica
    d. exfoliativa neonatorum
    exfoliative d.

dermatitis (*continued*)
    exudative discoid and
        lichenoid d.
    eyelid d.
    d. factitia
    factitial d.
    familial rosacea-like d.
    fiberglass d.
    follicular nummular d.
    footwear d.
    formaldehyde resin d.
    d. gangrenosa
    d. gangrenosa infantum
    gas d.
    genital atopic d.
    ginkgo tree d.
    gold d.
    gonococcal d.
    hatband d.
    head d.
    d. hemostatica
    d. herpetiformis (DH)
    d. hiemalis
    hydrocarbon d.
    d. hypostatica
    industrial d.
    d. infectiosa eczematoides
    infectious eczematous d.
    insect d.
    interdigital d.
    interface d.
    io moth d.
    irritant d.
    irritant contact d.
    irritant hand d.
    Jacquet's d.
    Jacquet's erosive diaper d.
    lacquer d.
    Leiner d.
    lichenified d.
    lichenoid d.
    lichenoid contact d.
    livedoid d.
    mango d.
    marine d.
    meadow d.
    meadow grass d.
    d. medicamentosa

dermatitis (*continued*)
    mercury d.
    metal d.
    metal salt d.
    moth d.
    d. multiformis
    mycotic d.
    nail polish d.
    d. nails
    napkin d.
    nasal solar d.
    neck d.
    neomycin d.
    nickel d.
    d. nodosa
    d. nodularis necrotica
    nonspecific d.
    nummular d.
    nummular eczematous d.
    occupational d.
    ocular atopic d.
    onion mite d.
    oozing d.
    d. papillaris capillitii
    papular d.
    papulosquamous d.
    paraphenylenediamine d.
    d. pediculoides ventricosus
    pellagra-associated d.
    pellagroid d.
    Pelodera d.
    perfume d.
    perianal d.
    periocular d.
    perioral d.
    periorbital d.
    periumbilical d.
    petrolatum d.
    photoallergic contact d.
    photocontact d.
    photoingestant d.
    photosensitive nonscarring
     d.
    photosensitivity d.
    phototoxic d.
    phototoxic contact d.
    phytophototoxic d.
    pigmentary atopic d.

dermatitis (*continued*)
    pigmented purpuric
     lichenoid d.
    plant d.
    plantar d.
    platinum d.
    poison ivy d.
    poison oak d.
    poison sumac d.
    d. pratensis striata
    precancerous d.
    prepatellar d.
    primary irritant d.
    primrose d.
    proliferative d.
    protein contact d.
    psoriasiform d.
    d. psoriasiformis nodularis
    purpuric pigmented
     lichenoid d.
    radiation d.
    ragweed d.
    ragweed oil d.
    rat mite d.
    rebound d.
    d. repens
    rhabditic d.
    rhus d.
    roentgen-ray d.
    rosaceaform d.
    rubber d.
    rubber additive d.
    sabra d.
    sandal strap d.
    Schamberg d.
    schistosomal d.
    schistosome d.
    seaweed d.
    seborrheic d.
    d. seborrheica
    shoe d.
    d. simplex
    d. skiagraphica
    solar d.
    d. solaris
    solvent d.
    spongiotic d.
    stasis d.

dermatitis (*continued*)
d. stasis
d. striata pratensis bullosa
subacute d.
subcorneal pustular d.
swimmer's d.
systematized allergic
contact d.
T-cell mediated delayed
type hypersensitivity d.
tear gas d.
tinea d.
toxicodendron d.
traumatic d.
d. traumatica
trefoil d.
d. ulcerosa
uncinarial d.
d. vegetans
d. venenata
d. verrucosa
verrucose d.
verrucous d.
vesicular d.
weeping d.
x-ray d.

dermatitis-arthritis-tenosynovitis
syndrome

dermatoalloplasty

dermatoarthritis
lipid d.
lipoid d.

dermatoautoplasty

Dermatobia
D. cyaniventris
D. hominis

dermatobiasis

dermatoblepharitis

dermatocele

dermatocellulitis

dermatochalasia

dermatochalasis

dermatochalazia

dermatoconiosis

dermatocyst

dermatodynia

dermatodysplasia
d. verruciformis

dermatofibroma
d. lenticulare
d. protuberans

dermatofibrosarcoma
d. protuberans

dermatofibrosis
d. lenticularis disseminata

dermatogenic torticollis

dermatoglyph

dermatoglyphics

dermatograph

dermatographia
black d.
urticarial d.
white d.

dermatographic

dermatographism
black d.
white d.

dermatography

dermatoheliosis

dermatoheteroplasty

dermatohistopathologist

dermatohistopathology

dermatohomoplasty

dermatoid

dermatologic
d. cognoscenti
d. laser
d. pharmaceutics
d. punch
d. therapy

dermatological

Dermatologic Diagnostic
  Algorithm

dermatologist

dermatology
  d. department
  d. research

dermatolysis
  d. palpebrarum

dermatoma

dermatomal
  d. distribution
  d. superficial telangiectasia
  d. trichoepithelioma
  d. zoster

dermatome

dermatomegaly

dermatomic area

dermatomycosis
  blastomycetic d.
  d. furfuracea
  d. microsporina
  d. pedis
  d. trichophytina

dermatomyiasis

dermatomyoma

dermatomyositis (DM)
  childhood d. (CDM)
  juvenile d. (JDM)

dermatoneurosis

dermatonosology

Dermatop

dermatopathia
  d. pigmentosa reticularis

dermatopathic
  d. anemia
  d. lymphadenopathy

dermatopathologist

dermatopathology

dermatopathy

dermatophagia

Dermatophagoides
  D. farinae
  D. microceras
  D. pteronyssinus
  D. scheremetewskyi

dermatophiliasis

dermatophilosis

Dermatophilus congolensis

dermatophone

dermatophylaxis

dermatophyte
  anthropophilic d.
  d. fungal infection
  d. test medium (DTM)

dermatophytic fungi

dermatophytid, dermatophytide
  erysipelas-like d.
  d. monilid
  d. reaction

dermatophytosis *pl.*
  dermatophytoses
  d. complex
  d. furfuracea

dermatoplastic

dermatoplasty
  Thompson d.

dermatopolymyositis

dermatopolyneuritis
  erythredema

dermatorrhagia

dermatorrhea

dermatorrhexis

dermatosclerosis

dermatoscopy

dermatosis *pl.* dermatoses
  acantholytic d.
  acarine d.
  acquired d.
  acute febrile neutrophilic d.
  adult bullous d.
  angioneurotic d.
  ashy d. of Ramirez
  Auspitz d.
  benign papular acantholytic d.
  Bowen's precancerous d.
  d. cenicienta
  childhood bullous d.
  cholinogenic d.
  chronic bullous d. of childhood
  chronic hemosideric d.
  d. cinecienta
  contact d.
  crazy paving d.
  dermolytic bullous d.
  digitate d.
  flaky paint d.
  Gougerot-Blum d.
  hormone-induced d.
  ichthyosiform d.
  IgA d.
  Industrial d.
  inflammatory d.
  intraepidermal neutrophilic IgA d.
  juvenile plantar d.
  lichenoid d.
  lichenoid chronic d.
  linear IgA d. of adulthood
  linear IgA d. of childhood
  linear IgA bullous d.
  meadow grass d.
  d. medicamentosa
  menstrual d.
  neutrophilic d.
  neutrophilic intraepidermal IgA d.
  occupational d.
  palmoplantar d.
  d. palmoplantaris juvenilis
  d. papulosa nigra

dermatosis (*continued*)
  papulosa nigra d.
  persistent acantholytic d.
  pigmented purpuric lichenoid d.
  precancerous d.
  progressive pigmentary d.
  pruritic d.
  purpuric d.
  pustular d.
  radiation d.
  reactive neutrophilic d.
  rhythmical d.
  Schamberg's d.
  Schamberg's progressive pigmented purpuric d.
  seborrheic d.
  stasis d.
  subcorneal pustular d.
  temperature-dependent d.
  transient acantholytic d. (TAD)
  ulcerative d.
  Unna d.
  vulvar d.

dermatosparaxis

dermatotherapy

dermatothlasia

dermatothlasis

dermatotropic
  d. fungi

dermatoxenoplasty

dermatozoiasis

dermatozoon *pl.* dermatozoa

dermatozoonosis

dermatrophia

dermic

Dermicel tape

DermiCort

dermis
  adventitial d.

dermis (*continued*)
    papillary d.
    reticular d.
    superficial d.
    upper d.

dermite

dermitis

dermoepidermal
    d. junction

dermographia

dermographic urticaria

dermographism
    cold-dependent d.
    white d.

dermoid
    d. cyst
    inclusion d.
    sequestration d.

Dermolate

dermolysis

dermolytic
    d. bullous dermatosis
    d. form

dermonecrosis

dermonecrotic

dermoneurosis

dermonosology

dermopathic

dermopathy
    diabetic d.

dermophlebitis

dermoplasty

dermostenosis

dermostosis

dermosynovitis

dermosyphilopathy

dermotoxin

dermotropic

dermotuberculin reaction

dermovascular

Dermoxyl

Dermtex HC with aloe

Derm-Vi Soap

De Sanctis-Cacchione syndrome

desaturation

Descemet's membrane

Desenex

desensitization
    heterologous d.
    homologous d.
    penicillin d.

desensitize

desert
    d. sore

desetope

desferrioxamine

desiccant

desiccate

desiccation
    electric d.
    mucous d.

desiccative

Design
    Clear by D.

desipramine

Desitin topical

desmin filaments

desmoglein
    d.-1
    d.-3

desmoid

desmoid (*continued*)
  d. cyst
  d. tumor

desmolysis

desmon

desmoplasia

desmoplastic
  d. form
  d. malignant melanoma
  d. melanoma
  d. squamous cell
    carcinoma
  d. stromal reaction
  d. trichilemmoma
  d. trichoepithelioma

desmorrhexis

desmosine

desmosomal
  d. glycoprotein
  d. plaque

desmosome
  half d.

desonide

DesOwen
  D. topical

desoximetasone

desquamans
  herpes d.

desquamate

desquamating area

desquamation
  branny d.
  corneocyte d.
  furfuraceous d.
  generalized d.
  lamellar d. of the newborn
  membranous d.
  peribronchial d.
  plantar d.
  siliquose d.

desquamative
  d. dermatitis
  d. gingivitis

desquamativum *pl.*
  desquamativa
  erythema d.
  erythroderma d.

desquamatory

Desquam-X

detergent
  anionic d's
  superfatted synthetic d.
  synthetic d. (syndet)

detergicans
  acne d.

determinant
  antigenic d.

detersive

detoxicate

detoxication

detoxification

detoxified toxin

detoxify

detritus
  tissue d.

developing
  color film d.

developmental delay

Devergie
  D. disease

device
  Flexi-Trak skin anchoring d.
  Handisol phototherapy d.
  SkinTech medical tattooing
    d.

dew itch

dexamethasone (DXM)
  d. acefurate

dexamethasone (*continued*)
 d. acetate
 d. dipropionate
 d. & neomycin sulfate &
  polymyxin B sulfate
 d. sodium phosphate
 d. suppression test
 tobramycin and d.

DEXA scan

Dexasone
 D. LA

Dexchlor

dexchlorpheniramine maleate

Dexone
 D. LA

dexpanthenol

dextranomer
 d. granule

dextrin

dextrocardia

dextrose

Dey-Wash skin wound clean

DFAT
 direct fluorescent antibody
  test

DF-2 septicemia

DFSP
 dermatofibrosarcoma
  protuberans

DH
 delayed hypersensitivity
 dermatitis herpetiformis

DHA
 dihydroxyacetone

DHAP
 dihydroxyacetone
  phosphate

DHEA
 dehydroepiandrosterone

DHEA (*continued*)
   DHEA sulfate

dhobie
 d. itch
 d. mark
 d. mark dermatitis

DHS
 D. Sal shampoo
 D. Tar
 D. zinc

diabetes
 d. insipidus
 d. mellitus

diabetic
 d. blister
 d. bullosis
 d. dermadrome
 d. dermopathy
 d. dermoplasty
 d. foot ulcer
 d. gangrene
 d. hand syndrome
 d. neuropathy
 d. stiff-hand syndrome
 d. ulcer

diabeticorum
 bullosis d.
 eczema d.
 necrobiosis lipoidica d.
 xanthoma d.

diabetid

diabrotic

diacetylmorphine (*heroin*)

Diadema

diadermic

diagnosis
 differential d.
 problem-oriented d.

diagnostic
 d. armamentarium
 d. feature
 d. surgical therapy
 d. test

Dial

dialyzable

Diamanus
    D. montanus

Diamine TD Oral

diaminodiphenylsulfone

diamond
    d.-shaped exfoliation
    d.-shaped patch
    d. skin

diaper
    d. dermatitis
    d. granuloma
    d. rash
    d. rash intertrigo

diaphoresis

diaphoretic

diaphragmatic weakness

diaphyseal proliferation

diapnoic

diascope

diascopic pressure

diascopy

diaspironecrobiosis

diastase
    d. labile
    d. resistant

diathermy

diathesis *pl.* diatheses
    allergic d.
    atopic d.
    hemorrhagic d.

diazepam

diazolidinyl urea

diazoxide

Dibenzyline

dibromodinitrofluorescein
    sodium

dibucaine

DIC
    disseminated intravascular
    coagulation

dicarboxylic acid

dichloroacetic acid

dichlorobenzene
    10-d.

dichlorodifluoromethane and
    trichloromonofluoromethane

dichlorophen

dichromate

Dick
    D. method
    D. reaction
    D. test
    D. test toxin

diclofenac
    d. sodium

dicloxacillin
    d. sodium

dieffenbachia

diethylcarbamazine (DEC)

diethyltoluamide

differential diagnosis

differentiation

Differin gel

diffusa
    leishmaniasis tegumentaria
    d.
    psoriasis d.

diffuse
    d. alimentary tract
    ganglioneuromatosis
    d. angiokeratoma
    d. atrophy

diffuse (*continued*)
    d. cutaneous leishmaniasis
    d. cutaneous mastocytosis
    d. eosinophilic fasciitis
    d. erythema
    d. hyperkeratotic tissue
    d. idiopathic cutaneous
      atrophy
    d. idiopathic skeletal
      hyperostosis (DISH)
    d. infantile fibromatosis
    d. inflammation
    d. lipomatosis
    d. neonatal
      hemangiomatosis
    d. nonepidermolytic
      palmoplantar
      keratoderma
    d. phlegmon
    d. plane xanthoma
    d. progressive systemic
      sclerosis
    d. scleroderma
    d. xanthomatous infiltration

diffusion of the lunula

diffusum
    angiokeratoma corporis d.
    atrophoderma d.
    papilloma d.

diflorasone diacetate

Diflucan
    D. injection
    D. Oral

diflucortolone valerate

digalloyl trioleate

DiGeorge syndrome

digger wasp

digit
    sausage d.
    supernumerary d.

digital
    d. asymmetry

digital (*continued*)
    d. cutaneous perivascular
      nerve
    d. fibrokeratoma
    d. fibromatosis
    d. ischemic ulceration
    d. mucinous cyst
    d. mucinous pseudocyst
    d. mucous cyst
    d. pitted scar
    d. video microscopy
    d. whorl

digitalis
    herpes d.

digitata
    verruca d.

digitate
    d. dermatosis
    d. wart

digoxin

dihydrofolic acid

dihydrotestosterone

dihydroxyacetone

dihydroxyanthranol

diiodohydroxyquin

dikwakwadi

Dilantin
    d. hypersensitivity
      syndrome

dilated
    d. cystic sweat ducts
    d. pore
    d. pore of Winer
    d. ventricle

dilation
    vascular d.

DILE
    drug-induced lupus
      erythematosus

dill

Dilocaine

DILS
   diffuse infiltrative
      lymphocytosis syndrome

diltiazem

diluent

dilute Russell viper venom time

dilution

dimeric

dimethicone cream

Dimetane
   D. Oral

dimethyl
   d. carbamate
   d. glyoxime
   d. phthalate
   d. siloxy
   d. sulfoxide

diminution

dimorphic
   d. fungus

dimorphous leprosy

dimple
   d. sign
   d. wart

dimpling

dinitrochlorobenzene (DNCB)
   d. challenge

dinoflagellate toxin

dioxin

DIP
   distal interphalangeal

dipeptide

Dipetalonema
   D. perstans
   D. streptocerca

diphenhydramine

diphenhydramine (*continued*)
   acetaminophen and d.
   d. hydrochloride
   parenteral d.

Diphenylan Sodium

diphenylhydantoin

diphosphonate

diphtheria
   cutaneous d.
   d. cutis
   d. toxin

diphtheritic
   d. infection
   d. membrane
   d. ulcer

diphtheroid

Diplococcus pneumoniae

diplopia

Diplopoda

Diprolene
   D. AF cream

Diprosone

Diptera

dipterous (fly) larvae

dipyridamole

direct
   d. current
   d. cutaneous
      immunofluorescence
   d. fluorescent antibody test
   d. immunofluorescence
   d. inoculation
   d. lymphography
   d. smear

Dirofilaria immitis

dirofilariasis
   subcutaneous d.

dirty base

Disc
    Clear Away D.

disc-shaped

disciform
    d. keratitis
    d. thickening

disciformis
    granulomatosis d. et
      progressiva

discoid
    chronic d. lupus
      erythematosus
    distinctive exudative d.
    d. LE
    d. lupus
    d. lupus erythematosus
      (DLE)
    d. lupus scars
    d. patch
    d. supernumerary breasts

discoidal eczema

discoidea
    psoriasis d.

discoloration

discolored

discontinuous sterilization

discrete
    d. lesion
    d. nodule
    d. pit
    d. puncta
    d. umbilicated papule

disease
    Addison's d.
    Addison-Gull d.
    Anders' d.
    autodestructive d.
    Bannister's d.
    Barcoo d.
    Bazin's d.
    Beigel's d.
    Besnier-Boeck d.

disease (*continued*)
    Boeck's d.
    Bourneville's d.
    Bowen's d.
    Buerger's d.
    Carrión's d.
    Chlamydia d.
    Christian-Weber d.
    creeping d.
    Darier's d.
    Darier-White d.
    Degos' d.
    Dercum's di.
    Duhring's d.
    Dukes' d.
    early (primary and
      secondary) d.
    erosive d.
    erosive mucous membrane
      d.
    extramammary Paget d.
    Favre-Durand-Nicolas d.
    fifth d.
    Filatov's d.
    Filatov-Dukes d.
    Fordyce's d.
    Fox-Fordyce d.
    Frei's d.
    Gaucher's d.
    Gilbert's d.
    Gilchrist's d.
    grass d.
    Grover's d.
    Habermann's d.
    Hailey-Hailey d.
    hand-foot-and-mouth d.
    Hand-Schüller-Christian d.
    Hansen's d.
    Hartnup d.
    Hebra's d.
    Herlitz' d.
    Hodgkin's d.
    Hutchinson's d.
    immunodeficiency d.
    Johnson-Stevens d.
    Kimura's d.
    knight's d.
    Kyrle's d.

disease (*continued*)
    Landouzy's d.
    Lane's d.
    late (tertiary) d.
    Leiner's d.
    Letterer-Siwe d.
    Lewandowsky-Lutz d.
    Lipschütz's d.
    Lobo's d.
    Lutz-Splendore-Almeida d.
    Lyell's d.
    Madelung's d.
    Majocchi's d.
    Malibu d.
    margarine d.
    Meleda d.
    Milton's d.
    Mitchell's d.
    Mucha's d.
    Mucha-Habermann d.
    mule-spinners' d.
    Nicolas-Favre d.
    Niemann's d.
    Niemann-Pick d.
    oid-oid d.
    Osler's d.
    Osler-Vaquez d.
    ox-warble d.
    Paget's d.
    pink d.
    primary d.
    Pringle's d.
    Quincke's d.
    Raynaud's d.
    Recklinghausen's d.
    Ritter's d.
    Robles' d.
    sandworm d.
    Schamberg's d.
    Schönlein's d.
    secondary d.
    Sjögren's d.
    Sneddon-Wilkinson d.
    Sticker's d.
    Sutton's d.
    Symmers' d.
    tertiary d.
    Underwood's d.

disease (*continued*)
    Unna-Thost d.
    ulcerative d.
    vagabonds' d.
    vagrants' d.
    Weber's d.
    Weber-Christian d.
    Werlhof's d.
    white spot d.
    Winkler's d.
    Witkop's d.
    Witkop-Von Sallmann d.
    Woringer-Kolopp d.
    Zahorsky's d.

disease-modifying
    d.-m. drugs

diseased tissue

disfiguring
    d. scar
    d. ulceration

DISH
    diffuse idiopathic skeletal
      hyperostosis

disinfect

disinfectant
    phenolated d.
    Sactimed-I-Sinald d.

disinfection

disintegrated neutrophil nuclei

disintegrating tissue

disintegration

disk
    hair d.

disodium cromoglycate

disorder
    acquired d.
    acquired cornification d.
    autoimmune d.
    cornification d.
    d. of cornification (DOC)
    Curth-Maklin cornification d.

disorder (*continued*)
    immune complex d.
    immunodeficiency d.
    keratitis-deafness
      cornification d.
    lymphoreticular d.
    National Institute of
      Arthritis, Musculoskeletal
      and Skin D's (NIAMS)
    papulosquamous d.
    severe combined
      immunodeficiency d.
      (SCID)
    unilateral hemidysplasia
      cornification d.

disorientation

dispersion
    amphotericin B colloidal d.
    colloidal d.
    d. effect

disproportionate predilection

disproportionately large-
  appearing head

dissecting
    d. cellulitis
    d. cellulitis of the scalp
    d. perifolliculitis of the scalp

dissection
    blunt d.
    d. cellulites of scalp
    sharp d.

disseminata
    alopecia d.
    dermatofibrosis lenticularis
      d.
    osteitis fibrosa cystica d.
    tuberculosis cutis
      follicularis d.

disseminated
    d. candidiasis
    d. cutaneous gangrene
    d. cutaneous herpes
      simplex
    d. cutaneous leishmaniasis

disseminated (*continued*)
    d. cutaneous types
    d. essential telangiectasia
    d. gonococcal infection
    d. granuloma annulare
    d. herpes simplex
    d. herpes simplex
      infection
    d. intravascular coagulation
      (DIC)
    d. lipogranulomatosis
    d. localized scleroderma
    d. lupus erythematosus
      (DLE)
    d. maculopapular
      exanthema
    d. neurodermatitis
    d. pagetoid reticulosis
    d. porokeratosis
    d. pruriginous
      angiodermatitis
    d. recurrent
      infundibulofolliculitis
    d. rosacea
    d. strongyloidiasis
    d. superficial actinic
      porokeratosis
    d. tuberculosis
    d. vaccinia
    d. vesiculopustular
    d. xanthoma
    d. xanthosiderohistio-
      cytosis

dissemination
    skin d.
    xanthoma d.

disseminatum
    keratoma d.
    xanthoma d.

disseminatus
    lupus miliaris d. faciei

parapsoriasis en plaques
  disseminées

dissociation

dissolution

distal
 d. arthrogryposis
 d. dactylitis
 d. hyperemic bands
 d. ileum
 d. interphalangeal (DIP)
 d. nail matrix
 d. subungual
  onychomycosis
 d. trichorrhexis nodosa

distensae
 striae cutis d.

distension

distichia

distichiasis

distinctive
 d. bleached appearance
 d. exudative discoid
 d. features

distribution
 asymmetric d.
 dermatomal d.
 lesion d.
 linear d.
 pattern of d.
 shawl d.

districhiasis

distrix

disulfide
 d. bond

disulfiram

dithranol

diutinum
 erythema elevatum d.
 scleredema d.

Division (I–IV) lesion

Dizac injection

DLE
 discoid lupus
  erythematosus

DM
 dermatomyositis

D-Med injection

DML Forte cream

DMP
 dimethylphthalate

DMSO
 dimethyl sulfoxide

DNA
 deoxyribonucleic acid
  D. autosensitivity
  D. buoyancy
  D. helicase mutation
  D.-histone
  D. homology
  D. hybridization
   technique
  D. probe test
  D. repair mechanism
  double-stranded D.
  single-stranded D.

DNCB
 dinitrochlorobenzene

DOC
 disorder of cornification

Docramira vinula

dog
 d.-faced boy
 d. flea
 d. flea bite
 d. tapeworm

dolens
 phlegmasia alba dolens

dolichocephalic skull

dolichocephaly

Dolichorespula
 D. sting

dolor

dolorosa
 adiposis d.
 tubercula d.

Domeboro
  Otic D.
  D. packets

dome-shaped
  d.-s. lesion
  d.-s. papule

dominant
  d. disorder
  d. feature

Donohue's syndrome

donor
  d. marrow
  universal d.

donovani
  Leishmania d.

Donovania granulomatis

donovanosis

dopa
  3,4-dihydroxyphenylalanine
  dopa-oxidase
  dopa reaction

dopamine

dopaquinone

Doppler
  D. study
  D. ultrasonography
  D. ultrasound

d'orange
  peau d.

Dormin Oral

Dorothy Reed-Sternberg cell

dorsal
  d. hands
  d. kyphosis
  d. nerve roots
  d. pedis pulse
  d. surface
  d. roots

dorsi
  elastofibroma d.

Doryx Oral

dose
  booster d.
  effective d. (ED)
  infecting d. (ID)
  maintenance d.
  sensitizing d.

Dosepak
  Deltasone D.
  Medrol D.

dose-related effect

dose-response curve

dosing
  once-daily d. (ODD)

dots
  Trantas d.

Douche
  Yeast-Gard Medicated D.

double
  d. athetosis syndrome
  d. groove

double-stranded DNA (dsDNA)

Douglas
  D. fir
  D. fir tree
  D. fir tussock moth

Dove soap

Dovonex

dowager hump

Dowling
  D.-Degos disease
  D.-Meara epidermolysis
    bullosa

down

Down syndrome

Downey cells

downgrading

doxepin (*Sinequan*)
  d. HCl

doxorubicin
    liposomal d.

Doxy Oral

Doxychel
    D. injection
    D. Oral

doxycycline

dracontiasis

dracunculiasis

dracunculosis

Dracunculus medinensis

drainage
    postural d.
    seropurulent d.

Draize Repeat Insult patch test

dressing
    Acticel wound d.
    alginate d.
    Algisorb wound d.
    Band-Aid d.
    Biopatch antimicrobial d.
    Compeed Skinprotector d.
    hydrocolloid d.
    hydrogel d.
    hydrophilic polymer d.
    Kaltostat alginate d.
    LYOfoam d.
    nonocclusive d.
    occlusive d.
    Op-Site semipermeable d.
    plastic adhesive d.
    polymer film d.
    polymer foam d.
    Roly-Derm wound hydrogel
        d.
    semipermeable d.
    Siloskin d.
    Sorbsan alginate d.
    Tegaderm semipermeable d.
    d. therapy
    Vigilon d.
    water-impermeable,
        non–silicone-based
        occlusive d.

dressing (*continued*)
    wet d.

Dricort
    Dermarest D.

Drithocreme

Dritho-Scalp

drop form

dropacism

droplike psoriasis

drop-sized lesions

Dr Scholl's Athlete's Foot

Dr Scholl's Maximum Strength
    Tritin

drug
    d. allergy
    d. anaphylaxis
    d. eruption
    d. hypersensitivity
    d. intolerance
    d. metabolism
    d. rash
    d. reaction

drug-associated erythema
    multiforme

drug-induced
    d.-i. acanthosis nigricans
    d.-i. alopecia
    d.-i. bullous
        photosensitivity
    d.-i. lipofuscinosis
    d.-i. lupus
    d.-i. lupus erythematosus
        (DILE)
    d.-i. melanocyte activation
    d.-i. photosensitivity
    d.-i. pigmentation
    d.-i. progressive symptom
        sclerosis
    d.-i. pruritus
    d.-i. pseudolymphoma
    d.-i. purpura
    d.-i. systemic lupus

DRESS = drug reaction with eosinophilia and systemic symptoms

drug-induced (*continued*)
    d.-i. systemic lupus
      erythematosus
    d.-i. telogen effluvium
    d.-i. thrombocytopenia
    d.-i. ulcer
    d.-i. urticaria

drumstick fingers

drusen of Bruch's membrane

dry
    d. cutaneous leishmaniasis
    D. Eyes solution
    D. Eye Therapy solution
    d. flush
    d. gangrene
    d. ice
    d. leprosy
    d. lips
    d. mouth
    d. skin
    d. tetter

Drysol

DSAP
    disseminated superficial
      actinic porokeratosis

dsDNA
    double-stranded DNA

DTIC-Dome

DTM
    dermatophyte test medium

dual coloration

Dubreuilh
    D's circumscribed
      precancerous melanosis
    circumscribed
      precancerous melanosis
      of D.
    D's elastoma
    D's precancerous
      melanosis

Ducrey
    D. bacillus
    D. test

duct
    sudoriferous d.
    sweat d.

ductal
    d. ectasia
    d. sweat gland carcinoma

ductus
    d. sudoriferus

Duhring
    D's disease
    D's pruritus
    D.-Brocq disease

Dukes disease

Dumdum fever

Duncan
    D's disease
    D's syndrome

DuoDerm
    D. CGF
    D. Extra Thin
    D. Hydroactive

Duofilm solution

Duo-Trach

Duplex
    D. scanning
    D. T

Dupuytren
    D's contracture
    D's disease

dura ganglia

Duralone injection

Duralutin injection

Duranest injection

duration of treatment

Duricef

Durrax

durum
    fibroma d.

durum (*continued*)
    heloma d.
    papilloma d.
    ulcus d.

dwarfism

Dycill

Dyclone

dyclonine
    d. HCl

dye
    azo d.
    d. discoloration
    extravasated d.
    d. sensitivity

Dyna-Hex topical

dynamometer
    Collins d.

Dynapen

dysacousia

dysbetalipoproteinemia
    familial d.
    normocholesterolemic d.

dyschondroplasia

dyschromatosis symmetrica
  hereditaria

dyschromia
    cutaneous d.

dyschromic
    d. lesion
    d. stage

dyschromicum

dysesthesia

dysfibrinogenemia

dysgammaglobulinemia

dysgenesis
    reticular d.

dyshesion

dyshidria

dyshidrosiform
    d. pattern
    d. pemphigoid

dyshidrosis, dyshydrosis,
  dysidrosis *pl.* dyshidroses
    lamellar d.
    d. lamellosa
    d. lamellosa sicca
    sole d.
    trichophytic d.

dyshidrotic
    d. eczema
    d. lesions

dysidria

dysidrosis (*variant of*
  dyshidrosis)

dyskeratinization

dyskeratoma
    acantholytic d.
    focal acantholytic d.
    warty d.

dyskeratosis *pl.* dyskeratoses
    acantholytic d.
    benign d.
    d. congenita
    congenital d.
    focal acantholytic d.
    d. follicularis
    isolated d. follicularis
    malignant d.
    transient acantholytic d.

dyskeratotic
    d. cells
    d. keratinocyte
    d. process

dysmorphic hair

dyspareunia

dysphagia

dyspnea

dyspigmentation

dyspigmentation (*continued*)
  postinflammatory d.

dysplasia
  anhidrotic ectodermal d.
  congenital ectodermal d.
  ectodermal d.
  fibrous d.
  hidrotic ectodermal d.
  hypohidrotic ectodermal d.
  mesodermal d.

dysplastic
  d. clavicle
  d. complex
  d. genetic anomaly
  d. nevus
  d. nevus syndrome
  d. process

dysproteinemia

dysproteinemic purpura

dysregulated homotypic fusion

dyssebacea

dyssebacia

dysseborrheic dermatitis

dystopia canthorum

dystrophia
  d. mediana canaliformis
  d. myotonica
  d. unguis mediana
    canaliformis
  d. unguium

dystrophic
  d. calcinosis
  d. calcinosis cutis
  d. epidermolysis bullosa
  d. form
  d. palmoplantar
    hyperkeratosis
  d. variant

dystrophica
  elastosis d.
  epidermolysis bullosa d.

dystrophy
  median canaliform d. of the
    nail
  twenty-nail d.

E

E
　vitamin E

EAC
　erythema annulare
　　centrifugum

EACD
　extrinsic allergic contact
　　dermatitis

EAHF
　eczema, asthma, hay fever

earlobe
　e. allergic dermatitis
　e. crease
　e. dermatitis

early
　e. catagen follicle
　e. latent syphilis
　e. lesions
　e. reaction
　e. yaws

early-phase response

Easprin

East African form

eastern
　e. coral snake
　e. coral snake bite
　e. tickborne rickettsiosis

easy bruising syndrome

eaten-out ulcer

Eaton agent

EB
　epidermolysis bullosa

EBA
　epidermolysis bullosa
　　acquisita

EBS
　epidermolysis bullosa
　　simplex

EBV
　Epstein-Barr virus
　　EBV genome

eccentric
　e. foci
　e. nucleus

eccentrica
　hyperkeratosis e.
　keratoderma e.

ecchymoma

ecchymosed

ecchymosis *pl.* ecchymoses
　multiple e's
　old e.
　Roederer e.
　scattered e's

ecchymotic
　e. halo
　e. mark
　e. rash

eccrine
　e. acrospiroma
　e. adenocarcinoma
　e. angiomatous hamartoma
　e. bromhidrosis
　e. carcinoma
　e. chromhidrosis
　e. differentiation
　e. ducts
　e. epithelioma
　e. gland
　e. hidradenitis
　e. hidrocystoma
　e. nevus
　e. porocarcinoma
　e. poroma
　e. poromatosis
　e. secretory coils
　e. spiradenoma
　e. sweat ducts
　e. sweat gland
　e. sweat gland adenoma

eccrine (*continued*)
　e. sweat-macerated stratum
　　corneum
　e. syringofibroadenoma

eccrisis

echinococcosis

Echinococcus
　E.

granuloma
　E. granulosus
　E. multilocularis

echinococcus

echinoderm

Echinothrix

echoviral exanthema

echovirus (*serotypes 1–7, 9,
　11–18, 20–27, 29–34*)

ECM
　erythema chronicum
　　migrans

econazole
　e. nitrate

Ecotrin

ECP
　erythropoietic
　　coproporphyria

ecstatic
　e. vascular structures
　e. vessels

ectasia
　papillary e.
　senile e.

ecthyma
　e. contagiosum
　contagious e.
　extragenital gonococcal e.
　e. gangrenosum
　e. infectiosum
　e. simplex
　e. syphiliticum

ecthymatiform

ecthymatous syphilid

ecthymiform

ectoderm

ectodermal
　e. defect
　e. disorder
　e. dysplasia
　e. embryogenesis
　e. structures
　e. tissue

ectodermatosis

ectodermosis
　e. erosiva pluriorificialis

ectopia lentis

ectopic
　e. calcification
　e. cutaneous
　　schistosomiasis
　e. keratinization
　e. mongolian spots
　e. pregnancy
　e. respiratory epithelia
　e. sebaceous gland

ectothrix
　e. infection
　e. spores

ectotoxin

ectozoon *pl.* ectozoa

ectromelia
　e. virus

ectropion

eczema
　adolescent e.
　adult e.
　allergic e.
　e. articulorum
　asteatotic e.
　atopic e.
　baker's e.
　e. barbae

eczema (*continued*)
    breast e.
    e. capitis
    childhood e.
    chronic e.
    contact e.
    e. craquelé
    e. crustosum
    e. diabeticorum
    dyshidrotic e.
    ear e.
    e. epilans
    e. epizootica
    e. erythematosum
    flexural e.
    follicular e
    follicular nummular e.
    hand e.
    e. herpeticatum
    e. herpeticum
    e. hiemalis
    e. hypertrophicum
    idiopathic late-onset e.
    infantile e.
    e. intertrigo
    lichenoid e.
    linear e.
    e. madidans
    e. marginatum
    e. nails
    e. neuriticum
    nipple e.
    nummular e.
    e. nummulare
    nutritional deficiency e.
    orbicular e.
    e. papulosum
    e. parasiticum
    pustular e.
    e. pustulosum
    e. rubrum
    e. scrofuloderma
    seborrheic e.
    e. seborrheicum
    e. siccum
    e. solare
    e. squamosum
    stasis e.

eczema (*continued*)
    tropical e.
    e. tyloticum
    e. vaccinatum
    varicose e.
    e. verrucosum
    e. vesiculosum
    weeping e.
    winter e.
    xerotic e.

eczematide

eczematization

eczematize

eczematodes
    impetigo e.

eczematogenic
    e. allergen
    e. event

eczematogenous
    e. allergen

eczematoid
    e. dermatitis
    e. pruritic plaques
    e. seborrhea

eczematous
    e. clinical appearance
    e. delayed-type
      hypersensitivity reaction
    e. dermatitis
    e. lesion
    e. neurodermatitis
    e. patch
    e. polymorphous light
      eruption (PMLE)
    e. reaction

ED

effective dose

edema
    acute hemorrhagic e.
    angioneurotic e.
    brawny e.
    bullous e.

edema (*continued*)
    circumscribed e.
    cyclic e.
    dependent e.
    epidermal e.
    giant e.
    hemorrhagic e.
    hereditary angioneurotic e.
     (HANE)
    indolent nonpitting e.
    e. indurativum
    inflammatory e.
    intercellular e.
    intracellular e.
    laryngeal e.
    marked solid e.
    Milton e.
    e. neonatorum
    noninflammatory e.
    nonpitting e.
    e. of feet
    e. of hand
    palmar e.
    palpebral e.
    pedal e.
    penile venereal e.
    periodic e.
    periorbital e.
    persistent e.
    pitting e.
    Quincke e.
    Yangtze e.

edematous
    e. epidermal cells
    e. fibroblastic proliferation
    e. plaques

edge
    elevated e.
    ulcer e.

Edge

EDTA
    ethylenediaminete-
     traacetic

Edwardsiella lineata

EEC

EEC (*continued*)
    ectodermal dysplasia,
     ectrodactyly and cleft
     lip/palate
      EEC syndrome

EED
    erythema elevatum
     diutinum
    E.E.S. oral

EFA
    essential fatty acid

effect
    beneficial e.
    Deelman e.
    isomorphic e.
    Köbner (Koebner) e.
    secondary e.
    tattooing e.

effective dose (ED)

effector
    e. cell
    e. lymphocyte
    e. T cell

efferent
    e. limb
    e. phase

efficacious agent

efficacy

efflorescence

effluvium
    anagen e.
    short anagen telogen e.
    telogen e.

Efidac/24
    E. chlorpheniramine

eflornithine
    e. hydrochloride

Efodine

Efudex
    E. cream
    E. topical

EGF
    epidermal growth factor

egg shell nail

EGMEA
    ethylene glycol
        monomethyl ether acetate

egress

Ehlers
    E.-Danlos disease
    E.-Danlos syndrome

Ehrlichia
    E. canis
    E. chaffeensis
    E. sennetsu

ehrlichiosis

EI
    erythema infectiosum

EIA
    enzyme immunoassay

eicosanoid
    e. inhibition

eicosapentaenoic acid

Eikenella
    E. corrodens

EKV
    erythrokeratodermia
        variabilis

elacin

Elajalde syndrome

ELA-MAX cream

elapid

Elapidae

Elase-Chloromycetin topical

Elase topical

elastic
    e. fibers
    e. membrane of Bruch
    e. nodules of anthelix

elastic (*continued*)
    e. skin
    e. tissue
    e. wrap

elasticity

elasticum
    pseudoxanthoma e.

elastin
    e. orientation

elastofibroma dorsi

elastoidosis
    e. cutanea nodularis et
        cystica
    nodular e.
    nodular e. of Favre-
        Racouchot

elastolysis
    generalized e.
    perifollicular e.
    postinflammatory e.

elastolytic giant cell granuloma

elastoma
    juvenile e.
    Miescher e.

elastorrhexis generalisata et
    systemica

elastosis
    actinic e.
    e. colloidalis conglomerata
    cutaneous e.
    e. dystrophica
    linear focal e.
    nodular e. of Favre and
        Racouchot
    e. perforans serpiginosa
    perforating e.
    senile e.
    e. senilis
    solar e.

elastotic
    e. degeneration
    e. stria

elbow
  golfer e.
  Little League e.
  tennis e.

Eldecort

elective culture

electrocauterization

electrocautery

electrocoagulated

electrocoagulation
  pinpoint e.

electrodermal testing

electrodermatome

electrodesiccation

electroencephalographic

electroencephalography

electrofulguration

electrolysis

electrolytic

electrolyzable

electromagnetic
  e. energy
  e. radiation

electromyography (EMG)

electron
  e. beam
  e. beam radiation
  e. beam therapy
  e. microscope (EM)
  e. microscopy
  e. probe microanalysis

electrophoretic
  e. patterns

electrophototherapy

electroplating silver

electrosection

electrostatic

electrosurgery
  bipolar e.

eleidin

Elejalde syndrome

element
  thermostatically controlled
    heating e.

elemental
  e. iron
  e. mercury

elementary
  e. lesion

elephant
  e. leg
  e. man
  e. skin

elephantiac

elephantiasic

elephantiasis
  e. arabum
  e. asturiensis
  congenital e.
  filarial e.
  e. filariensis
  e. graecorum
  e. leishmaniana
  lymphangiectatic d.
  e. neuromatosa
  nevoid e.
  e. nostras
  e. nostra verrucosa
  secondary e.
  e. telangiectodes
  e. tropica

elephantoid
  e. fever

elevated
  e. border
  e. suppressor T cells

elevation

elevation (*continued*)
    blanched cutaneous e.
    rest, ice, compresses, e.
      (RICE)
    tactile e.

elevatum
    erythema e. diutinum

elicitation stage

Elimite
    E. Cream

ELISA
    enzyme-linked
      immunosorbent assay

ellipsoid

ellipsoidal inclusion

elliptic
    e. biopsy
    e. excision

elliptical
    e. biopsy
    e. excision
    e. incision
    e. wound

elm
    e. tree

ELND
    elective lymph node
      dissection

Elocon
    E. topical

elongated
    e. cells
    e. dendritic dermal
      melanocyte
    e. "grain shaped" nucleus
    e. spindle cells

elongation

EM
    electron microscope
    erythema migrans

emaciation

emaculation

embedded

embolia cutis medicamentosa

embolic
    e. gangrene
    e. infarction
    e. phenomenon

embolism

embryogenesis

embryologic
    e. development
    e. malformation

embryonal
    e. cavity
    e. cells
    e. neural crest
    e. periderm
    e. type

embryonic endothelium

emetine

EMG
    electromyography

Emgel topical

EMH
    extramedullary
      hematopoiesis

emigration

EMLA
    E. cream
    E. topical

emollients (*class of drugs*)

emotional
    e. flushing
    e. hyperhidrosis
    e. instability

emphlysis

emphractic

emphraxis

emphysema
    cutaneous e.
    subcutaneous e.

empiric therapy

Empirin

empyema

empyesis

emulsifier

emulsion
    Pusey e.

E-Mycin Oral

EN
    erythema nodosum
        EN septal fibrosis

en
    e. coup de sabre
    e. masse
    parapsoriasis e. plaques
    e. plaques

enamel
    e. hypoplasia
    e. paint spot appearance

enanthem

enanthema

enanthematous

enanthesis

encapsulated
    e. cord
    e. mass
    e. nest
    e. sheet

encased embryo

encephalitis

encephalocele

encephalocraniocutaneous
    lipomatosis

encephalopathy

encephalotrigeminal
    angiomatosis

enchondroma

enchondromatous
    e. change

encircling hair shafts

encode

encompass

encystments

end
    Fab e.
    Fc e.

endangiitis obliterans

endemia

endemic
    febrile disease e.
    e. fungal infection
    e. regions
    e. Reiter's disease
    e. syphilis
    e. typhus

endemica
    urticaria e.

endemicum
    granuloma e.

endemoepidemic

endermic

endermism

End Lice

endocarditis

endocrine
    e. anomaly
    e. dysfunction
    e. neoplasia type I
    e. overactivity
    e. pancreas

endocrinologic

endocrinologic (*continued*)
    e. alopecia
    e. disorder

endocrinologist

endocrinopathy

endoderm

endodermal
    e. elements
    e. origin

Endodermophyton

endoepidermal

endogenous
    e. antigen
    e. circulating vasodilating
      agent
    e. dermatitis
    e. eczema
    e. familial
      hypertriglyceridemia
    e. pathway
    e. porphyrin
    e. triglycerides

endometritis

endomysium

end-organ sensitivity

endoparasitism

endophthalmitis

endophytic proliferation

endoplasmic reticulum

endoscopy

endosome

endothelial
    e. cell
    e. cell culture
    e. cell swelling
    e. dysfunction
    e. proliferation
    e. thrombomodulin
      expression
    e. vascular markers

endothelin

endothelioma
    e. capitis
    e. cutis

endothelium

endothrix
    e. infection
    e. type

endotoxin

endovascular
    e. papillary
      angioendothelioma
    e. surface

ENDRB gene

end-stage
    e.-s. dystrophic calcinosis
    e.-s. lesions
    e.-s. liver disease

Engman
    E. dermatitis
    E. disease

engorged

engraftment

enkephalin

ENL
    erythema nodosum
    leprosum

enoxacin

enoxaparin

ensulizole

Entamoeba histolytica

Enterobacter cloacae

Enterobacteriaceae

enterobiasis

Enterobius
    E. vermicularis

enterochromaffin cells

enterococci
vancomycin-resistant e.
(VRE)

Enterococcus faecalis

enterohepatic circulation

enteropathica
acrodermatitis e.

enteropathy
gluten-sensitive e.

enterotoxin

Enterovirus

enterovirus (EV)
e. infections
e. type 71

enthesitis

enthetic

entirety

Entomophthorales

entomophthoramycosis
basidiobolae

entropion

enucleation

enuresis

envenomation

environment progressive
symptom sclerosis

environmental
e. allergen
e. factors
e. illness
e. mite infestation
e. scabies
e. scleroderma

enzacamene

enzymatic
e. degradation
e. reaction

enzyme
e. catalase
e. deficiency
hepatocellular e.

eosin

eosinophil major basic protein

eosinophilia
recurrent granulomatous
dermatitis e.

eosinophilic
e. abscess
e. adenoma
e. cellulitis
e. coloration
e. cytoplasm
e. dermatitis
e. elastic fiber
e. exudate
e. fasciitis
e. fasciitis syndrome
e. fine fibrillar material
e. folliculitis
e. granuloma
e. granulomatosis
e. inclusion
e. keratin
e. leukocytes
e. lymphofolliculitis
e. myalgia syndrome
e. panniculitis
e. precursor
e. pustular folliculitis
e. sleeve
e. spongiosis
e. ulcer

EpDRF
epithelium-derived
relaxation factor

EPF
eosinophilic pustular
folliculitis

ephelides
nevi, atrial myxoma,
myxoid neurofibromas,
and e. (NAME)

ephelis *pl.* ephelides

ephidrosis
  e. cruenta

epicanthus

Epicauta
  E. fabricii
  E. fabricii sting
  E. vitlata
  E. vitlata sting

Epicel skin graft material

epicutaneous
  e. reaction
  e. (TRUE) test

epicuticle

epidemic
  e. acne
  e. arthritic erythema
  e. dropsy
  e. exanthema
  e. follicular eruption
  e. follicular keratosis
  global e.
  e. keratoconjunctivitis
  e. keratoconjunctivitis virus
  e. myositis
  e. neoplasia
  e. outbreaks
  e. roseola

epidemicity

epidemicum
  erythema arthriticum e.

epidemiography

epidemiologic

epidemiology

epiderm

epidermal
  e. acanthosis
  e. allergen
  e. appendage
  e. atrophy
  e. autograph

epidermal (*continued*)
  e. basal cell fragility
  e. basement membrane
  e. cell
  e. cell kinetics
  e. cyst
  e. desquamation
  e. grafting
  e. horny layer
  e. hyperpigmentation
  e. hyperplasia
  e. inclusion cyst
  e. invagination
  e. keratinosome
  e. Langerhans cell
  e. melanin-bearing
    organelle
  e. melanin unit
  e. melanocytic lesion
  e. multinucleated giant
    cells
  e. necrosis
  e. nuclear staining
  e. nevus
  e. nevus syndrome
  e. nuclear pattern
  e. proliferation
  e. rete ridges
  e. spongiosis
  e. stratification

epidermatitis

epidermatoplasty

epidermic
  e.-dermic nevus

epidermicula

epidermidalization

epidermides (*plural of*
  epidermis)

epidermidis
  Staphylococcus e.

epidermidosis

epidermis *pl.*
  epidermides

epidermides (*continued*)
    hyperkeratotic e.
    hyperplastic e.
    mammalian e.
    viable e.

epidermitis

epidermization

epidermodysplasia
    e. verruciformis
    e. verruciformis of
      Lewandowski-Lutz

epidermoid
    e. cancer
    e. carcinoma
    e. cyst

epidermolysis
    e. bullosa (EB)
    e. bullosa, acquired
    e. bullosa acquisita (EBA)
    e. bullosa acquisita antigen
    e. bullosa atrophicans
    e. bullosa, dermal type
    e. bullosa dystrophica,
      albopapuloid
    e. bullosa dystrophica,
      dominant
    e. bullosa dystrophica,
      dysplastic
    e. bullosa dystrophica,
      hyperplastic
    e. bullosa dystrophica,
      polydysplastic
    e. bullosa dystrophica,
      recessive
    e. bullosa, epidermal type
    e. bullosa hereditaria
    e. bullosa, junctional
    e. bullosa lethalis
    e. bullosa scar
    e. bullosa simplex
    e. bullosa simplex,
      generalized
    e. bullosa simplex,
      herpetiformis
    e. bullosa simplex, localized

    e. simplex
    toxic bullous e.

epidermolytic
    e. acanthoma
    e. exotoxin
    e. hyperkeratosis
    e. keratosis palmaris et
      plantaris
    e. palmoplantar
      keratoderma
    e. type

epidermomycosis

epidermophytid

Epidermophyton
    E. floccosum
    E. inguinale

epidermophytosis
    e. cruris
    e. interdigitale

epidermosis

epidermotropic
    e. cell
    e. lymphocyte
    e. reticulosis

epidermotropism

epididymitis

epidural
    e. lipomatosis

Epifoam

epiglottal lesion

epiglottis

epilans
    eczema e.

epilate

epilating
    e. laser
    e. wax

epilation

epilatory

epilepsanoia

epilepsy

epileptic convulsion

epileptiform seizure

epiloia

epiluminescence microscopy

epinephrine

EpiPen
E. Jr.

epiphora

epiphysitis

episcleritis

episodic
e. angioedema
e. angioedema with
eosinophilia
e. malnutrition

epistasis

epistatic

epistaxis

epithelia (*plural of* epithelium)

epithelial
e. atypia
e. cadherins
e. covering
e. cyst
e. debris
e. degeneration
e. elements
e. hyperplasia
e. keratitis
e. keratopathy
e. lined cavity
e. lining fluid (ELF)
e. migration
e. nests
e. nevus
e. sinus
e. strands
e. tumor

epithelialization

epithelialize

epithelialized

epitheliitis

epitheliogenesis
e. imperfecta

epithelioid
e. blue nevus
e. cell
e. cell nevus
e. cell tubercle
e. hemangioendothelioma
e. melanocyte
e. nevus
e. sarcoma

epithelioma
e. adenoides cysticum
basal cell e. (BCE)
e. basocellulare
benign calcifying e.
Borst-Jadassohn type
intraepidermal e.
calcified e.
calcifying e.
calcifying e. of Malherbe
e. capitis
e. contagiosum
e. cuniculatum
Ferguson-Smith e.
Jadassohn e.
Malherbe calcifying e.
e. of Malherbe
e. mixtum
e. molluscum
multiple benign cystic e.
multiple self-healing
squamous e.
prickle-cell e.
sebaceous e.
self-healing
squamous e.
e. spinocellulare
squamous cell e.
superficial basal cell e.
trichoepithelioma

epitheliomatosis

epitheliomatous

epitheliopathy

epitheliotrophic

epithelium *pl.* epithelia
  lower infundibular e.
  superficial follicular e.
  tegumentary e.

epithelium-derived relaxation factor (EpDRF)

epithelization

epithelize

epitope

epitrichium

epitrochlea

epizootic

eponychia

eponychium

epoxy
  e. resin
  e. resin vapor

EPP
  erythropoietic protoporphyria

EPS
  elastosis perforans serpiginosa

Epsom salts

Epstein-Barr (EB)
  E.-B. exanthema
  E.-B. virus (EBV)

epulis
  e. fissurata

equestrian panniculitis

equi
  Demodex e.

equinia

equinovarus foot deformity

eradicate

eradication

erbium:yttrium-aluminum-garnet laser

ergocalciferol

ergot poisoning

ergotism

erisipela de la costa

eroded
  e. gray center
  e. lesions

erosio interdigitalis blastomycetica

erosion

erosiva
  ectodermosis e. pluriorificialis

erosive
  e. lichen planus
  e. pustular dermatosis of the capillitium
  e. scalp dermatitis

erubescence

erubescent

eruption
  acneform e.
  bullous e.
  bullous pemphigoid-like e.
  butterfly e.
  creeping e.
  cutaneous drug e.
  crustaceous e.
  drug e.
  eczematous polymorphous light e.
  erythematous e.
  erythematous psoriasiform e.
  evanescent e.

eruption (*continued*)
    fixed drug e.
    Kaposi varicelliform e.
    lichenoid e.
    linear e.
    maculopapular e.
    morbilliform e.
    papulosquamous e.
    pemphigus-like e.
    petechial e.
    pityriasis rosea-like e.
    polymorphous light e.
        (PMLE)
    post-traumatic pustular e.
    psoriasiform e.
    purpuric e.
    pustular e.
    scarlatiniform e.
    scleroderma-like e.
    self-limited e.
    serum e.
    skin e.
    squamous e.
    summertime actinic
        lichenoid e.
    tubercular e.
    variola site e.
    vesicopustular e.
    vesicular e.

eruptiva
    telangiectasia macularis e.
        perstans

eruptive
    e. angioma
    e. collagenoma
    e. hidradenoma
    e. histiocytoma
    e. keratoacanthoma
    e. nevus
    e. pseudoangiomatosis
    e. syringoma
    e. vellus hair cyst
    e. xanthoma
    e. xanthomata

Er:YAG laser

Eryc Oral

Erycette topical

EryDerm topical

Erygel topical

Erymax topical

EryPed Oral

erysipelas
    abdominal e.
    ambulant e.
    e. bullosum
    e. carcinomatosum
    chronic recurrent e.
    coast e.
    facial e.
    e. gangrenosum
    gangrenous e.
    e. grave internum
    idiopathic e.
    ignis sacer e.
    e. internum
    e. migrans
    migrant e.
    necrotizing e.
    perineal e.
    e. perstans
    e. perstans faciei
    e. phlegmonosum
    phlegmonous e.
    e. pustulosum
    St. Anthony's fire e.
    surgical e.
    e. verrucosum
    e. vesiculosum
    wandering e.
    zoonotic e.

erysipelas-like
    e.-l. dermatophytid
    e.-l. erythema
    e.-l. skin lesion
    e.-l. reaction

erysipelatous

erysipeloid
    e. of Rosenbach

Erysipelothrix rhusiopathiae

erysipelotoxin

Ery-Tab Oral

erythema
    e. a calore
    e. ab igne
    e. acneforme
    acral e.
    acrodynic e.
    acute infectious e.
    annular e.
    e. annulare
    e. annulare of infancy
    e. annulare centrifugum
        (EAC)
    e. annulare centrifugum
        Darier
    e. annulare rheumaticum
    e. a pudore
    e. arciforme et palpabile
        migrans
    e. arthriticum
    e. arthriticum epidemicum
    bright e.
    e. bullosum
    e. caloricum
    chilblain-like e.
    e. chronicum
    e. chronicum figuratum
        melanodermicum
    e. chronicum migrans
    circinate syphilitic e.
    e. circinatum
    e. circinatum rheumaticum
    cold e.
    congenital telangiectatic e.
    e. congestivum
    e. contagiosum
    e. contusiforme
    e. contusiformis
    e. craquelé
    cyanotic e.
    e. desquamativum
    diaper e.
    diffuse e.
    e. dyschromicum perstans
    e. elevatum diutinum
    e. endemicum

erythema (*continued*)
    exanthematic e.
    e. exfoliativum
    e. exposure
    e. exudativum
    e. exudativum multiforme,
        major form
    e. exudativum multiforme,
        minor form
    facial e.
    figurate e.
    e. figuratum
    e. figuratum perstans
    e. fugax
    gyrate e.
    e. gyratum
    e. gyratum perstans
    e. gyratum repens (EGR)
    hemorrhagic exudative e.
    e. induratum
    e. induratum Bazin
    e. indurativum
    e. infectiosum (EI)
    e. intertrigo
    e. iris
    Jacquet's e.
    e. keratodes
    macular e.
    malar e.
    e. marginatum
    e. marginatum of rheumatic
        fever
    e. marginatum
        rheumaticum
    e. migrans (EM)
    e. migrans linguae
    migratory e.
    Milian's e.
    e. multiforme
    e. multiforme bullosum
    e. multiforme exudativum
    e. multiforme gestationis
    e. multiforme-like eruptions
    e. multiforme major
    e. multiforme minor
    e. multiforme of von Hebra
    e. necrolyticum migrans
    e. multiforme

erythema (*continued*)
- e. multiforme minor
- e. multiforme with mucosal involvement
- necrolytic migratory e.
- e. necrolyticum migrans
- necrolytic migratory e.
- e. necroticans
- e. neonatorum
- e. neonatorum toxicum
- ninth-day e.
- e. nodosum (EN)
- e. nodosum leprosum
- e. nodosum migrans
- e. nodosum syphiliticum
- nonblanching e.
- e. nuchae
- nummular e.
- palmar e.
- e. palmare
- e. palmare hereditarium
- e. papulatum
- papuloerosive e.
- e. papulosum
- e. paratrimma
- pellagroid e.
- periungual e.
- e. pernio
- e. perstans
- e. polymorphe
- e. pudicitiae
- e. pudoris
- punctate e.
- e. punctatum
- recurrent toxin-mediated perianal e.
- rheumatic e.
- e. scarlatiniform
- scarlatiniform e.
- e. scarlatinoides
- e. simplex
- e. solare
- e. subitum
- e. streptogenes
- symptomatic e.
- telangiectatic e.
- e. threshold
- toxic e.

erythema (*continued*)
- e. toxicum
- e. toxicum neonatorum
- e. traumaticum
- e. tuberculatum
- e. typhosum
- e. urticans
- e. venenatum
- violet-blue e.

erythematic

erythematodes
- lupus e.

erythematoedematous

erythematopapular

erythematosa
- acne e.

erythematosum
- eczema e.

erythematosus
- acute cutaneous lupus e. (ACLE)
- acute lupus e.
- chilblain lupus e.
- chronic discoid lupus e.
- cutaneous lupus e.
- discoid lupus e. (DLE)
- disseminated lupus e.
- drug-induced lupus e. (DILE)
- drug-induced systemic lupus e.
- lupus e. (LE)
- neonatal lupus e. (NLE)
- pemphigus e.
- subacute cutaneous lupus e. (SCLE)
- subacute lupus e.
- systemic lupus e. (SLE)
- tumid lupus e.

erythematous
- e. base
- e. follicular papule
- e. halo
- e. hardening

erythematous (*continued*)
  e. macular dermatitis
  e. macule
  e. mark
  e. morbilliform
  e. papular dermatitis
  e. patch
  e. pigmentary disease
  e. plaque
  e. psoriasiform eruption
  e. scaling "discoid" plaque
  e. scaling plaque
  e. skin
  e. subcutaneous nodules
  e. syphilid

erythematovesicular

erythemogenic

erythermalgia

erythralgia

erythrasma
  Baerensprung e.

erythredema

erythredemic polyneuropathy

erythremia

erythrism

erythristic

erythroblastosis
  fetal e.
  e. fetalis

Erythrocin

erythrocyanosis
  e. crurum puellaris
  e. frigida
  e. frigida crurum puellarum
  e. supramalleolaris

erythrocyte
  antibody-coated e.
  e. protoporphyrins
  e. sedimentation rate (ESR)
  e. stroma evoked typical
    lesion

erythroderma
  (*varianterythrodermia*)
  atopic e.
  atypical ichthyosiform e.
  bullous congenital
    ichthyosiform e.
  congenital ichthyosiform e.
  e. desquamation
  e. desquamativum
  exfoliative e.
  e. exfoliativum
  ichthyosiform e.
  e. ichthyosiforme
    congenitale
  e. ichthyosiforme
    congenitum
  lamellar congenital
    ichthyosiform e.
  lymphomatous e.
  e. mastocytosis
  nonbullous congenital
    ichthyosiform e.
  primary e.
  e. psoriaticum
  Sézary e.
  e. squamosum
  e. Wilson-Brocq

erythrodermas

erythrodermatitis

erythrodermia (*variant of*
  erythroderma)
  e. desquamativa in infants
  e. exfoliativa Leiner
  e. ichthyosiformis
    congenitalis
  e. ichthyosiformis
    congenitalis bullosa
    Brocq
  e. ichthyosiformis
    congenitalis nonbullosa

erythrodermic
  e. eruption
  e. neonates
  e. pemphigoid
  e. psoriasis
  e. sarcoidosis

erythrodontia

erythrogenic
e. toxin

erythroid
e. precursor
e. progenitor cells

erythrokeratodermia
e. figurate et variabilis
e. figurate variabilis
Mendes da Costa type e.
e. progressive symmetrica
progressive symmetrical
verrucous e.
e. variabilis

erythrokeratolysis hiemalis

erythroleukoplakia

erythromelalgia
secondary e.

erythromelanin

erythromelanosis follicularis
faciei et colli

erythromelia

erythromycin
e. and benzoyl peroxide
e. and sulfisoxazole
e. estolate
e. ethylsuccinate (EES)
e. propionate lauryl sulfate
e. stearate
e. topical

erythromycin-sulfisoxazole

erythrophagocytosis

erythrophore

erythroplakia

erythroplasia
e. of Queyrat
Zoon e.

erythropoietic
e. porphyria
e. protoporphyria (EPP)

erythropoietin
e. therapy

erythroprosopalgia

érythrose
e. péribuccale pigmentaire
of Brocq
e. pigmentaire péribuccale

erythrosis
e. of Bechterew
e. interfollicularis colli

eschar
black e.
burn e.
necrotizing e.

escharotic

escharotica
rupia e.

Escherichia coli

escutcheon

E-Solve-2 topical

esophageal
e. carcinoma
e. dilation
e. diverticula
e. dysmotility
e. hypomotility
e. manometry
e. stricture
e. varices
e. web

esophagitis dissecans
superficialis

esophagogram

espundia

ESR
erythrocyte sedimentation
rate

ESS
excited skin syndrome

essential

essential (*continued*)
    e. cold urticaria
    e. fatty acid deficiency
    e. mixed cryoglobulinemia
    e. oils
    e. progressive telangiectasia
    e. pruritus
    e. shrinkage of the
      conjunctiva
    e. telangiectasia
    e. thrombocytopenic
      purpura

Estar
    E. Gel

esterification

esthiomene

estival

estivale (*alternative* aestivale)
    hydroa e.

estivalis (*alternative* aestivalis)
    acne e.
    dermatitis e.
    prurigo e.
    pruritus e.

estradiol
    ethinyl e.

estrogen
    e. binding
    e. receptor

ethambutol
    e. hydrochloride

ethanol injection sclerotherapy

Ethilon suture

ethinyl estradiol

ethionamide

ethionine

ethmoid sinuses

ethyl
    e. chloride

ethyl (*continued*)
    e. chloride and
      dichlorotetrafluoroethane
    e. cyanoacrylate adhesive
    e. cyanoacrylate glue
    e. hexanediol

ethylenediamine
    e. dermatitis

ethylenediaminetetraacetate

ethylestrenol

ethylmalonic-adipicaciduria

etidocaine
    e. hydrochloride

etiolation

etiologic

etiology
    unknown e.
    viral e.

etoposide

etretinate

ETS-2% topical

etymologically

etymology

Eubacterium

eucalyptus oil

Eucerin
    E. cream
    E. for face SPF 25
    E. moisturizer
    E. Plus moisturizer

eudiaphoresis

eugenol

eugonic fermenting bacteria

eukaryotic cell

eukeratin

eumelanin

eumycetoma

eunuchoidism

Euproctis
    E. chrysorrhoea
    E. chrysorrhoea sting
    E. flava

Eurax
    E. topical

European
    E. blastomycosis
    E. blister beetle sting

eutrichosis

Eutrombicula alfreddugesi

EV
    enterovirus
    epidermodysplasia
        verruciformis

evaluation
    acute physiology and
        chronic health e.
        (APACHE)

evanescent
    e. eruption
    e. herniation
    e. macule
    e. plaque
    e. vesicle

Evans blue

event
    isolated superficial e.

E-Vista

evolution
    eruption e.
    lesion e.

evulsion

Ewing tumor

exacerbation

Exact skin product

examination

examination (*continued*)
    full-body cutaneous e.
    KOH e.
    Wood light e.

exanthem
    Boston e.
    e. subitum
    vesicular e.
    viral e.

exanthema *pl.* exanthemas,
    exanthemata
    Boston e.
    echoviral e.
    enteroviral e.
    epidemic e.
    Epstein-Barr e.
    keratoid e.
    ordinal designation of the
        exanthemata
    polymorphous e.
    e. subitum
    syphilitic e.
    vesicular e.
    viral e.

exanthemata-like erythema
    infectiosum

exanthematic disease

exanthematicus
    ichthyismus e.

exanthematous
    e. disease
    e. febrile eruption of
        pustules
    e. fever
    e. viral disease

exanthesis
    e. arthrosia

excessive
    e. coloration
    e. dryness
    e. hairiness
    e. perspiration
    e. secretion
    e. sunlight exposure

excessive (*continued*)
    e. sweating
    e. wound edge tension

exchange transfusion

excision
    fusiform e.
    wide e.

excisional
    e. biopsy
    e. removal

excited
    e. skin syndrome (ESS)

exclamation point hairs

excoriate

excoriated

excoriation
    neurotic e.

excrescence
    platelike e.
    wartlike e.

excreta

Exelderm
    E. topical

exercise-induced urticaria

exfoliant

exfoliate

exfoliated
    e. keratin

exfoliatio
    e. areata linguae
    e. manuum areata

exfoliation
    lamellar e. of newborn

exfoliativa
    cheilitis e.
    dermatitis e.
    glossitis areata e.
    keratolysis e.

exfoliative
    e. cheilitis
    e. dermatitis
    e. dermatosis
    e. erythroderma
    e. psoriasis
    e. stage
    e. state
    e. toxin

exfoliativum
    erythema e.
    erythroderma e.

Exidine Scrub

exocrine

exocytosis

exogenous
    e. circulating vasodilating
        agents
    e. ochronosis
    e. pathway
    e. substance
    e. triglycerides

Exophiala
    E. jeanselmei
    E. phaeoannellomyes
    E. spinifera
    E. werneckii

exophthalmos

exophytic
    e. lesion
    e. mass

exoserosis

exoskeleton

exostosis *pl.* exostoses
    subungual e.

exothermal pads

exotic
    e. granuloma
    e. woods

exotoxic

exotoxin
    bacterial e.
    streptococcal pyrogenic e.
        (SPE)

expansion
    clonal e.

exophytic neoplasm

exposure
    allergen e.
    cold e.
    heat e.
    light e.
    occupational e.
    prior drug e.
    repeated e.
    sun e.

Exsel

Exserohilum
    E. genera
    E. rostratum

extensive
    e. skin sloughing
    e. striae

extensor surface

extensum
    hemangioma planum e.

exteriorization

exteriorized tumor

externa
    otitis e.

external
    e. auditory canal (EAC)
    e. auditory canal secretions
    e. auditory meatus
    e. otitis
    e. root sheath

extirpation

extracellular
    e. cholesterosis
    e. collagen domain
    e. granules

extracellular (*continued*)
    e. hyaline deposits
    e. lipid deposit
    e. macromolecules
    e. proteins

extracorporal
    immunoabsorption

extracorporeal
    e. chelation
    e. membrane oxygenation
        (ECMO)
    e. photochemotherapy
    e. photophoresis

extract
    allergenic e.
    allergic e.
    aqueous e.
    venom e.

extraction
    comedo e.

extractor
    Amico e.
    comedo e.
    Schamberg e.
    Schamberg comedo e.
    Unna e.
    Unna comedo e.
    Walton e.

extracutaneous
    e. disease
    e. involvement
    e. juvenile
        xanthogranuloma

extrafacial
    e. disease
    e. swelling

extragenital
    e. chancre
    e. primary lesion

extraglandular
    lymphoproliferative process

extramammary Paget's
    disease

extramedullary
    e. erythropoiesis
    e. hematopoiesis
    e. involvement
    e. plasmacytoma

extranodal
    e. B-cell
    e. involvement
    e. lymphoma

Extra Strength Bayer Enteric 500
  Aspirin

extravasation

extravascular granulomatous
  features

extrinsic
    e. coagulation system
    e. pressure

extruded hair shafts

exuberant cicatrization

exudate
    eosinophilic e.
    neutrophilic e.
    purulent e.

exudation

exudative
    e. chorioretinitis
    e. discoid

exudative (*continued*)
    e. discoid and lichenoid
      dermatitis
    distinctive e. discoid
    e. papulosquamous disease

exudativum
    erythema multiforme e.

exude

exuding pus

exulceratio
    e. simplex

eye
    black e.
    e. makeup
    raccoon e's
    red e.
    e. worm

eyebrow loss

eyelash
    e. cosmetic
    e. loss

eyelid
    e. cosmetic
    e. dermatitis
    e. edema
    e. tumors

eyeline tattoo

eye shadow cosmetics

F

F
    F pilus

Fab
    F. end

Faba
    F. faba
    F. vulgaris

fabism

fabric

Fabry
    F's disease
    F.-like angiokeratomas
    F's syndrome
    F.-Anderson disease

FACE
    Facial Afro-Caribbean
        Childhood Eruption
    FACE syndrome

face
    adenoid f.
    bovine f.
    cleft f.
    cox f.
    dish f.
    dished f.
    frog f.
    Hippocratic f.
    moon f.
    moon-shaped f.
    f. peel

face-lift

faceometer

facial
    f. anomaly
    f. cellulitis
    f. dermatitis
    f. edema and eosinophilia
    f. erythema
    f. foundation
    f. granuloma with
        eosinophilia

facial (*continued*)
    f. herpes simplex
    f. milia
    f. moisturizer
    f. necrobiosis lipoidica
    f. nerve palsy
    f. palsy
    f. paralysis
    f. pore
    f. port-wine stain
    f. powder
    f. undercover cream
    f. vitiligo

faciale
    granuloma f.
    pyoderma f.

facialis
    herpes f.
    pyodermia f.
    zona f.

faciei (*genitive of* facies)
    atrophoderma reticulatum
        symmetricum f.
    chloasma f.
    erysipelas perstans f.
    keratosis pilaris atrophicans
        f.
    lupus miliaris disseminatus f.
    seborrhea f.
    tinea f.

facies
    f. abdominalis
    adenoid f.
    adenoidal f.
    allergic f.
    cushingoid f.
    dengue f.
    f. hepatica
    Hippocratic f.
    f. Hippocratica
    hound-dog f.
    leonine f.
    f. leontina
    moon f.

facies (*continued*)
    myxedematous f.

FACIT
    fibril-associated collagen
        with interrupted triple
        helices

factitia
    dermatitis f.
    urticaria f.

factitial
    f. dermatitis
    f. disease
    f. lymphedema
    f. panniculitis
    f. pseudoainhum
    f. trauma

factitious
    f. dermatitis
    f. purpura
    f. urticaria

factor
    chemotactic f.
    cobra venom f.
    epidermal growth f. (EGF)
    epithelium-derived
        relaxation f. (EpDRF)
    lethal f.

macrophage migration
    inhibitory factor (MIF)
    protective f.
    provocative f.
    sun protection f. (SPF)
    tumor lysis f.
    tumor necrosis f. (TNF)

factor beta
    tumor necrosis f. b.

facultative
    f. bacterium
    f. gram-negative bacillus
    f. myiasis
    f. pathogenicity
    f. pathogens
    f. pigmentation
    f. skin color

fagopyrism

fair skinned

FALDH
    fibroblast and leukocytes
        deficiency in fatty
        aldehyde dehydrogenase

fall
    hair f.

false
    f. knuckle pads

false-negative
    f.-n. patch test
    f.-n. reaction

false-positive
    f.-p. patch test
    f.-p. reaction
    f.-p. syphilis serology
    f.-p. syphilis test

falx cerebri

famciclovir

familial
    f. acanthosis nigricans
    f. alpha-lipoprotein
        deficiency
    f. amyloidotic
        polyneuropathy syndrome
    f. apoprotein CII deficiency
    f. atypical multiple mole
        melanoma syndrome
        (FAMMM)
    f. autosomal dominant
        disorder
    f. benign chronic
        pemphigus
    f. benign pemphigus of
        Hailey-Hailey
    f. combined hyperlipidemia
    f. continuous skin peel
    f. cutaneous collagenoma
    f. dysautonomia
    f. dysbetalipoproteinemia
    f. epidemic aphthosis
    f. histiocytic dermatoarthritis

familial (*continued*)
f. hypercholesterolemia
f. hypermobility syndrome
f. hypertriglyceridemia
f. joint hypermobility
  syndrome
f. keratoderma with
  carcinoma of the
  esophagus
f. Mediterranean fever
f. melanoma
f. multiple lipomatosis
f. myxovascular fibroma
f. nonhemolytic jaundice
f. pancytopenia
f. panmyelophthisis
f. paroxysmal
  polyserositis
f. polymorphous light
  eruption
f. presenile sebaceous
  hyperplasia
f. progressive
  hyperpigmentation
f. reticuloendotheliosis
f. rosacea-like dermatitis
f. urticaria pigmentosa
f. white folded mucosal
  dysplasia
f. woolly hair

FAMMM
familial atypical multiple
  mole melanoma
  syndrome

famotidine

Famvir

Fanconi
F. syndrome
F. type

Fansidar-R

Farber's disease

farcy
bovine f.
f. buds

farinae
  Dermatophagoides f.

farmer's skin

farmyard pox

fascia
f. lata
palmar f.
plantar f.
Scarpa's f.
superficial f.
f. superficialis

fascial hernia

fascicles of spindle cells

fasciitis
eosinophilic f.
exudative f.
necrotizing f.
nodular f.
f. nodularis
  pseudosarcomatosa
proliferative f.
pseudosarcomatous f.

fascioliasis

fastidious

fat
atrophy of f.
f. cell
f.-laden histiocytes
f. malabsorption
f. necrosis
f.-replacement atrophy
subcutaneous f.

fatty
f. acrochordon
f. degeneration
f. material
f. substance

fauces

faucial pillar

faun tail nevus

favid

favism

favosa
porrigo f.
tinea f.

Favre
F. disease
F.-Durand-Nicolas disease
F.-Racouchot cyst
F.-Racouchot disease
F.-Racouchot nodular
elastosis syndrome
F.-Racouchot skin
F.-Racouchot syndrome

favus
f. circinatus
f. herpeticus
f. herpetiformis
mouse f.
f. murium
f. pilaris

FB
foreign body

Fc
Fc end
Fc epsilon RI
Fc receptor

FCP
florid cutaneous
papillomatosis

feather
f. pillow dermatitis
f. sensitivity

feature
extravascular
granulomatous f's
histologic f's
immunologic f.
immunopathologic f's
pathologic f.

febricitans
pes f.

febricula

febrifuge

febrile
f. disease
f. urticaria

febrilis
herpes f.
urticaria f.

fecal
f. protoporphyrin

Feer's disease

feet
cold f.
burning f.
edema of f.
reddening of soles of f.

Fegeler syndrome

feigned eruption

felis

fell

fellatio

felodipine

felon
bone f.
deep f.
f. mactans
subcutaneous f.
subcuticular f.
subperiosteal f.
thecal f.

felting

Felty's syndrome

female pattern alopecia

female pseudo-Turner
syndrome

feminization

fenfluramine hydrochloride

fennel
dog f.

fenticlor

Ferguson Smith
    F. S's epithelioma
    F. S's keratoacanthoma
    F. S. type epithelioma
    F. S. type of multiple self-
        healing keratoacanthomas
    F. S. type of self-healing
        squamous epithelioma

fermentation products

Fernandez reaction

ferox
    prurigo f.

ferret
    f. epithelium

ferrochelatase

fester

festering

festoon

festooned appearance

festooning

fetal
    f. alcohol syndrome
    f. damage
    f. hydantoin syndrome

fetalis
    erythroblastosis f.
    ichthyosis f.
    keratosis diffusa f.

fetid
    f. exudate
    f. odor
    f. sweat

Feuerstein
    F.-Mims syndrome
    F.-Mims-Schimmelpenning
        syndrome

fever
    Aden f.
    f. blister
    boutonneuse f.

fever (*continued*)
    deer fly f.
    epidemic hemorrhagic f.
    eruptive f.
    exanthematous f.
    Fort Bragg f.
    Haverhill f.
    hemorrhagic f.
    herpetic f.
    Mediterranean f.
    pappataci f.
    Phlebotomus f.
    pretibial f.
    relapsing f.
    sandfly f.
    San Joaquin f.
    f. sores
    trench f.
    typhoid f.
    valley f.

fexofenadine

FGF
    fibroblast growth factor

FGFR
    fibroblast growth factor
        receptor

fiber
    A alpha nerve f.
    hair f.
    Herxheimer f's

fiberglass
    f. dermatitis

fibril
    anchoring f.
    collagen f.

fibrillar
    f. appearance
    f. collagen
    f. matrix
    f. protein keratin

fibrillarin

fibrillation

fibrillin

fibrin
    f. degradation product
    f. deposition
    f. dust
    f. plug
    f. thrombi

fibrinogenopenia

fibrinoid
    f. change
    f. necrosis

fibrinolysin and
    deoxyribonuclease

fibrinolysis syndrome

fibrinolytic
    f. activity
    f. anomaly
    f. purpura

fibrinopurulent exudate

fibroblast
    f. fissure
    f.-like cell
    f. proliferation

fibroblastic
    f. infiltration
    f. proliferation
    f. tissue

fibrocystic
    f. breast disease
    f. dysmucopolysaccharidosis

fibrodysplasia

fibroelastic

fibroelastolytic
    f. papulosis

fibroepithelial
    f. neoplasm
    f. polyp

fibroepithelioma
    f. basal cell carcinoma
    f. of Pinkus

fibroepithelioma (*continued*)
    premalignant f.
    f. tumor

fibrofolliculoma

fibrogenesis imperfecta ossium

fibrokeratoma
    acquired acral f.
    acquired digit f.
    digital f.

fibrolipoma

fibrolipomatous

fibroma
    aponeurotic f.
    f. areolare
    cutaneous f.
    f. cutis
    f. durum
    infantile digital f.
    irritation f.
    f. linguae
    f. lipomatodes
    f. molle
    f. molle gravidarum
    f. molluscum
    f. mucinosum
    f. myxomatodes
    f. of the mucosa
    f. pendulans
    f. pendulum
    perifollicular f.
    peripheral ossifying f.
    periungual f.
    senile f.
    f. simplex
    soft f.
    telangiectatic f.
    f. xanthoma

fibromatogenic

fibromatoid

fibromatosis
    f. colli
    gingival f.

fibromatous

fibromectomy

fibromyxoma

fibronectin

fibroplasia
  papular f.

fibrosa
  osteitis f.

fibrosarcoma
  f.-like tissue

fibrosing alopecia

fibrosis
  cystic f. (CF)
  lamellar perifollicular f.
  nodular subepidermal f.
  obliterative granulomatous
    f.
  f. of the septa
  subepidermal nodular f.

fibrosum
  molluscum f.

fibrosus
  nevus f.

fibrotic tract

fibrous
  f. chordee
  f. collagen
  f. connective tissue
  f. dysplasia
  f. hamartoma of infancy
  f. histiocytoma
  f. papule
  f. papule fibroxanthoma
  f. stroma
  f. subcutaneous nodules
  f. synovium (FS)
  f. thickening
  f. tissue
  f. tissue abnormality
  f. trabeculae
  f. tract
  f. tumors
  f. xanthoma

fibroxanthoma
  atypical f.

fiddle-back
  f.-b. spider
  f.-b. spider bite

fiddler neck

field fire epithelioma

Fiessinger
  F.-Leroy syndrome
  F.-Leroy-Reiter syndrome
  F.-Rendu syndrome

fifth
  f. decade of life
  f. disease
  f. phakomatosis

fig
  f. wart

figurata
  keratosis rubra f.

figurate

figuratum
  erythema f.

figuratus

figure
  flame f.
  mitotic f.

filamentary keratitis

Filaria
  F. bancrofti
  F. loa

filaria *pl.* filariae

filarial
  f. elephantiasis
  f. nematode
  f. orchitis
  f. parasites

filariasis
  Bancroftian f.
  Loiasis f.
  Malayan f.

Filatov
    F's disease
    F's spot
    F.-Dukes disease

filiform
    f. adnatum
    f. horny spine
    f. hyperkeratosis
    f. lesion
    f. tumor
    f. warts

filiformis
    verruca f.

filles
    acné excoriée des jeunes f.

filter
    Wood's f.

filtered flashlamp pulsed light
    source

finasteride

fine
    f. epilating needle
    f. hairs
    f. needle aspiration (FNA)
    f. papules

finely
    f. granular
    f. stippled basophilic
        material

Finevin

finger
    blubber f.
    bolster f.
    clubbed f.
    dead f.
    Hippocratic f.
    f.-pebbling
    sausage f.
    seal f.
    snapping f.
    spade f.
    speck f.
    trigger f.

finger (*continued*)
    tulip f.
    waxy f.
    f. webs
    whale f.
    white f.

finger-in-glove appearance

fingernail
    half-and-half f.
    f. ridging pattern

fingerprint
    f. folds
    Galton system of
        classification of f.

Finkelstein's disease

Finn chamber

fire
    f. ant
    f. ant anaphylaxis
    f. ant sting
    f. coral
    f. coral sting
    St. Anthony's f.

firm
    f. lesion
    f. plaque

first
    f. degree burn
    f. degree frostbite
    f. disease

Fischer unit

fish
    f. skin
    f.-mouth wound
    f. odor syndrome
    f. tank granuloma

fishy condition

fissurata
    epulis f.

fissuratum
    acanthoma f.

fissuratum (*continued*)
    granuloma f.

fissure
    interpalpebral f.
    f.-prone

fissured tongue

fissuring plaque

fistula *pl.* fistulae, fistulas
    anal f.
    f. in ano
    aural f.
    f. auris congenitalis
    dental f.
    f. of the ear
    pilonidal f.
    rectal f.
    urethral f.
    vesical f.

fistulous tracts

fixed
    f. cutaneous
        sporotrichosis
    f. drug eruption
    f. drug photoeruption
    f. drug reaction
    f. tissue
    f.-tissue technique

FLA-ABS
    florescent lepromin
        antibody-absorbed

flaccid
    f. bullae
    f. pustules
    f. quadriplegia

flag sign

flagella (*plural of* flagellum)

flagellate erythematous
    urticarial wheals

Flagyl

flaking

flaky paint dermatosis

flame
    f. figure
    f. nevus

flammeus
    nevus f.

flannel moth

flare
    wheal and f.

flash
    f. burn

flashlamp
    f.-pumped pulsed dye laser
    f. pulsed dye laser (FPDL)

flask-shaped

flat
    f. condyloma
    f. papular syphilid
    f.-topped
    f. wart

flattened keratinocytes

flatworm

flavedo

Flaviviridae

flea
    f. bites
    cat f.
    chigger f.
    dog f.
    sand f.
    f. venom

fleck

Flegel's disease

flesh
    f.-colored
    goose f.
    proud f.

flesh-colored

fleshy mass

flexible plastic tube

flexion contracture

Flexi-Trak skin anchoring device

flexor
   f. aspects
   f. wrists

flexural
   f. area
   f. aspect
   f. eczema
   f. lichenification
   f. psoriasis

floccosum
   Epidermophyton f.

flood fever

florid
   f. cutaneous papillomatosis
      (FCP)
   f. oral papillomatosis
   f. skin lesions

Florida
   F. holly
   F. jellyfish-induced eruption

Florinef acetate

Florone
   F. E Topical
   F. Topical

fluconazole

fluctuant

fluctuation

5-flucytosine

fludarabine phosphate

fludrocortisone acetate

fluid
   ascitic f.
   edema f.
   epithelial lining f. (ELF)
   free f.

fluid-filled
   f.-f. cysts
   f.-f. sacs

flumen
   f. pilorum

fluocinolone
   f. acetonide

fluocinonide
   f. cream
   f. gel
   f. ointment

Fluonex topical

Fluonid topical

fluoresce

fluorescein-labeled antiantibody

fluorescence
   beaded f.
   f. microscope
   f. quenching

fluorescent
   f. antibody
   f. antibody technique
   f. tagged antibody

fluoridated
   f. dentifrice

fluorides

Fluori-Methane topical spray

fluorinated
   f. corticosteroids
   f. topical steroids
   f. topical steroid cream

fluorine

fluorochrome

fluorometric procedure

Fluoroplex
   F. cream
   F. solution
   F. topical

fluoroquinolone

fluorouracil
   5-f. (5-FU)
   5-f. cream

fluoxetine
  f. HCl
  f. hydrochloride

flurandrenolide

Fluro-Ethyl
  F. aerosol

Flurosyn topical

flush
  f. area
  dry f.
  histamine f.
  wet f.

flushing
  emotional f.
  facial f.
  food-associated f.
  menopausal f.
  neural-mediated f.
  paroxysmal f.
  f. reaction
  thermal f.

flutamide

fluticasone
  f. propionate

fluting

flutter
  f. device
  f. valve purpura

fluvoxamine

flux
  f. allergen
  soldering f.

fly
  f. bite
  f. blister

FMD
  foot-and-mouth disease
  FMD virus

FNA
  fine needle
    aspiration

foam cell
  f. c. of Virchow

foamy
  f. agent
  f. cytoplasm
  f. histiocytes
  f. virus

focal
  f. acantholytic dyskeratoma
  f. acantholytic dyskeratosis
  f. acral hyperkeratosis
  f. dermal hypoplasia
  f. epithelial hyperplasia
  f. extravascular plasma cell
  f. infection
  f. inflammation
  f. lytic bone lesions
  f. mucinosis-type lesion
  f. mucosal hypertrophy
  f. parakeratosis
  f. poliosis
  f. reaction
  f. scale crust
  f. spongiosis with
    exocytosis of
    polymorphonuclear
    leukocytes

focus *pl.* foci
  granulomatous foci
  persistent inflammatory foci

fodrin

fogo
  f. selvagem

folate

fold
  crural f.
  Dennie infraorbital f.
  Dennie-Morgan infraorbital
    f.
  interdigital f.
  lateral nail f.
  Morgan f.
  nail f.
  nasolabial f. (NLF)

fold (*continued*)
   villous f.

Folex PFS

foliaceous
   f. pemphigus

foliaceus
   pemphigus f.

folic acid
   f. a. antagonist
   f. a. deficiency

follicle
   black-dot f.
   hair f.
   hypertrophic lymphoid f.
   patulous f.
   pilosebaceous f.
   sebaceous f.
   tertiary f.

follicular
   f. abscess
   f. accentuation
   f. adenocarcinoma
   f. atrophoderma
   f. center cell
   f. degeneration syndrome
   f. dendritic cells
   f. eczema
   f. epithelium
   f. fusion
   f. germinative cells
   f. hyperkeratosis
   f. ichthyosis
   f. impetigo
   f. infundibulum
   f. infundibular cyst
   f. isthmus cyst
   f. keratosis
   f. level
   f. lichen planus
   f. localization
   f. lymphoblastoma
   f. lymphoma
   f. mange
   f. markings
   f. melanin unit

follicular (*continued*)
   f. mucinosis
   f. mucinosis of infancy
   f. mycosis fungoides
   f. nummular dermatitis
   f. nummular eczema
   f. occlusion triad
   f. openings
   f. orifice
   f. ostia
   f. papule
   f. papulopustules
   f. pattern
   f. plug
   f. plugging
   f. poroma
   f. psoriasis
   f. pustule
   f. pyoderma
   f. rupture
   f. scaling
   f. scar
   f. seborrheide
   f. structure
   f. syphilid
   f. vesicopustules
   f. vulvitis
   f. walls

follicularis
   alopecia f.
   ichthyosis f.
   isolated dyskeratosis f.
   keratosis f.
   lichen planus f.

folliculitis
   f. abscedens et
      suffodiens
   agminate f.
   f. barbae
   Bockhart's f.
   Candida f.
   f. cheloidalis
   f. cruris atrophicans
   f. decalvans
   f. decalvans capillitii
   f. decalvans cryptococcia

folliculitis (*continued*)
  f. decalvans et lichen
    spinulosus
  eosinophilic pustular f.
  f. et perifolliculitis
    abscedens et suffodiens
  f. gonorrhoeica
  gram-negative f.
  hot tub f.
  industrial f.
  keloidal f.
  f. keloidalis
  f. nares perforans
  f. narium perforans
  oil f.
  perforating f.
  Pityrosporum f.
  Pseudomonas aeruginosa
    f.
  pustular f.
  pyogenic f.
  staphylococcal f.
  ulerythema reticulata
  f. ulerythematosa reticulata
  f. varioliformis

folliculocentric
  f. abscess

folliculorum
  Acarus f.
  Demodex f.
  pityriasis f.

folliculosebaceous cystic
  hamartoma

folliculotropism

folliculus
  f. pili

fomes

fomite
  f. contact

Fong's syndrome

Fonsecaea
  F. compactum
  F. pedrosoi

fontanelle
  bulging f.

food
  f. allergen
  f. allergy

foot
  athlete's f.
  Dr Scholl's Athlete's F.
  fungous f.
  Hong Kong f.
  immersion f.
  immersion f., tropical
  Madura f.
  moccasin f.
  mossy f.
  neuropathic f.
  perforating ulcer of f.
  f. ringworm
  ringworm of f.
  sea boot f.
  shelter f.
  tennis shoe f.
  f. tetter
  trench f.
  f. yaws

foot-and-mouth
  f.-and-m. disease (FMD)
  f.-and-m. disease virus
  f.-and-m. disease virus
    vaccine

force
  Van der Waals f.

forceps
  epilating f.

Forschheimer's spots

Fordyce
  angiokeratoma of F.
  F's condition
  F's disease
  F's granule
  F's spots

forefoot

foreign body (FB)

foreign-body
    f.-b. giant cell
    f.-b. granuloma
    f.-b. implantation
    f.-b. reaction

forelock
    white f.
    white frontal f.

forest
    f. epiphyte
    f. yaws

form
    yeast f.

formaldehyde
    ethylene urea melamine f.
    free f.
    melamine f.
    f. resin
    f. textile resin allergy
    urea f.

formalin

formation
    anterior synechia f.
    central scar f.
    immune granuloma f.
    keloid f.
    posterior synechia f.
    scar f.
    web f.

forme
    f. fruste
    f. tardive

formication

formula
    Berkow f.

forniceal conjunctiva

fornix *pl.* fornices
    interior f.

Fortaz

foscarnet
    f. sodium

Foscavir
    F. injection

fossa *pl.* fossae
    antecubital f.
    popliteal f.

Fostex

Fototar

foundation
    anhydrous facial f.
    facial f.
    oil-based facial f.
    water-based facial f.
    water-free facial f.

fountain-spray splatters

Fournier
    F's disease
    F's gangrene
    F's syndrome

fourth disease

foveation

foveolar

foveolate

Fowler's solution

fowlpox
    f. virus

Fox
    F. disease
    F. impetigo
    F.-Fordyce disease

foxglove
    purple f.

FPH
    familial progressive
      hyperpigmentation

fracture
    frequent f.

fractured hair

fragilitas
    f. crinium
    f. unguium

fragility

fragment
Fab f.
protein f.

fragmented nuclei

fragmentation

fragrance

frambesia

frambesiform
f. syphilid

frambesiformis
sycosis f.

frambesioma

framboesioides
mycosis f.

Franceschetti
F's syndrome
F.-Jadassohn syndrome
F.-Klein syndrome

Francisella tularensis

freckle
f. of Hutchinson
melanotic f. of
Hutchinson

freckling
axillary f.

Fredrickson's type II disease

free
f. distal border
f. edge
f. fluid
f. sebaceous glands

Free & Clear shampoo

Freeman-Sheldon syndrome

freeze-thaw cycles

freezing
surface f.

Freezone solution

Frei
F. antigen
F. bubo

frenum

frenzied itching

Freon

frequent infections

fresh
f. crop of pustules

freshwater swimmer's itch

Freund's incomplete adjuvant

Frey
F's hair
F's syndrome

friable

friction
f. blisters
f. bulla

frictional area

Frigiderm

fringe tonsure

frizzy

Fröhlich's syndrome

frond
villous f.

frontal
f. bossing
f. hairline
f. recession
f. scalp margin

frontalis
acne f.
alopecia liminaris f.
f. muscle

frontoparietal baldness

frost
f. itch
urea f.

frostbite
  deep f.
  first degree f.
  superficial f.

frothy leukorrhea

frozen
  f. joints
  f. section

Frullania nisquallensis

FS
  fibrous synovium
  FS Shampoo topical

FTA-ABS
  fluorescent treponemal
    antibody absorption
  FTA-ABS test

5-FU
  5-fluorouracil

fuchsin
  basic f.

fucosidosis

fugax
  erythema f.

fugitive
  f. swelling
  f. wart

fungous infection

fulguration

full
  f.-body cutaneous
    examination
  f.-coverage facial powder
  f. dermal thickness
  f.-thickness burn
  f.-thickness graft

fulminans
  acne f.
  purpura f.

fulminant
  f. illness

fulminant (*continued*)
  f. infection
  f. meningococcemia

fulminating
  f. course
  f. smallpox

Fulvicin
  F. P/G
  F.-U/F

fulvum
  Microsporum f.

fumaric acid

fumigation

function
  primary f.

functional protein

funduscopic examination

fungal
  f. culture
  f. disease
  f. elements
  f. folliculitis
  f. hyphae
  f. id reaction
  f. infection
  f. mycelium
  f. scraping
  f. tests

fungate

fungating
  f. sore
  f. tumor

fungemia

fungi (*plural of* fungus)

Fungi Imperfecti

fungicidal

fungicide

fungiform
  f. papillae

fungistasis

fungistat

fungistatic

fungitoxic

Fungizone
F. intravenous

Fungoid
F. creme
F. HC creme
F. tincture
F. topical solution

fungoid

fungoides
granuloma f.
microabscess of mycosis f.
mycosis f.

fungosity

fungous
f. colonies
f. foot
f. infection

fungus *pl.* fungi
f. ball
beefsteak f.
bracket f.
cutaneous f.
dematiaceous fungi
dematiaceous f.
mosaic f.
nonpathogenic f.
Phoma f.
umbilical f.

funnel-shaped

FUO
fever of unknown origin

Furacin topical

furfur
Malassezia f.
Microsporum f.

furfuracea
alopecia f.
impetigo f.
seborrhea f.

furfuraceous
f. impetigo

furfurans
porrigo f.

furniture beetle

furocoumarin
f.-containing plants

furosemide

furrow
digital f.
skin f.
transverse f.

furrowed
f. depression
f. tongue

furrowing

furuncle
nasal f.

furuncular
f. disease
f. myiasis

furunculoid
f. eruption

furunculosis
chronic f.
hospital f.
f. orientalis

furunculous

furunculus *pl.* furunculi
f. vulgaris

Fusarium
F. oxysporum
F. solani

fusca
lamina f.

fuscoceruleus
  nevus f.
  nevus f. acromiodeltoideus
  nevus f.
    ophthalmomaxillaris

fusi

fusiform
  f. bacillus
  f. cell
  f. ellipse
  f. excision

fusion toxin

fusobacterum

fusospirillary gangrenous
  stomatitis

fusospirochetal
  f. disease
  f. organism
  f. stomatitis

fusus *pl.* fusi
  cortical f.
  fracture f.

Futcher's lines

G

gabapentin

Gaboon ulcer

gadfly

galactidrosis

galactophlysis

galactorrhea

galactosamine-
6-sulfatase

galactosialidosis

gallamine

gallery

gallinae
    Dermanyssus g.

galling

gallium scan

galvanic
    g. current
    g. epilator

Gamasidae

gamasoidosis

Gamastan

Gambian
    G. form
    G. trypanosomiasis

Gamimune N

gamma
    g. globulin
    g. globulin infusion
    g. globulin protein
    g. interferon
    interferon g.
    g. rays

Gammagard S/D

Gammar

gammopathy

ganciclovir

ganglion *pl.* ganglia
    g. cells
    synovial g.

ganglionectomy
    sympathetic g.

ganglioneuroblastoma

gangliosidosis

gangosa

gangrene
    cold g.
    cutaneous g.
    decubital g.
    diabetic g.
    disseminated cutaneous g.
    dry g.
    Fournier's g.
    gas g.
    gaseous g.
    hospital g.
    hot g.
    Meleney's g.
    Meleney's synergistic g.
    moist g.
    nosocomial g.
    postoperative progressive
      bacterial synergetic g.
    pressure g.
    progressive bacterial
      synergistic g.
    progressive synergistic g.
    progressive synergistic
      bacterial g.
    symmetrical g.
    Raynaud g.
    vascular g.
    wet g.
    white g.

gangrenescens
    granuloma g.

gangrenosa
    phagedena g.

gangrenosa (*continued*)
  pyodermia g.
  vaccinia g.
  varicella g.

gangrenosum
  bullous hemorrhagic
    pyoderma g.
  ecthyma g.
  hemorrhagic pyoderma g.
  pyoderma g.

gangrenosus
  pemphigus g.

gangrenous
  g. balanitis
  g. lesions
  g. stomatitis
  g. vaccinia

Garamycin
  G. injection
  G. Ophthalmic
  G. topical

Gardner
  G's syndrome
  G.-Diamond purpura
  G.-Diamond syndrome

gargoylelike features

gargoylism

garment nevus

gas
  g. bubbles
  g. plant

Gasterophilus
  G. intestinalis
  G. nasalis

gastric
  g. achlorhydria
  g. antral vascular ectasia
  g. intrinsic factor
  g. ulcer

gastroenteropathy

gastrointestinal

gastrointestinal (*continued*)
  g. bleeding
  g. disorder
  g. distress
  g. edema
  g. hemangioma
  g. malignancy
  g. tract
  g. venous malformation

gastroscopy

Gaucher
  G's cells
  G's disease

gaussian
  g. curve
  g. distribution

gauze
  nonstick g.

G-CSF
  granulocyte colony-
    stimulating factor

Geheimratswinkeln

gel
  adapalene g.
  Benzac AC g.
  Cann-Ease moisturizing
    nasal g.
  Dermaflex g.
  Differin g.
  g. diffusion
  g. diffusion precipitin test
  Estar g.
  HP Acthar g.
  Keralyt g.
  PreSun lotion and g.
  Vergogel g.

gelatin
  g. waving solutions
  zinc g.

gelatinous capsule

Gelfoam

gelsolin

gemfibrozil

Genahist oral

Genaspor

gene
g. expression

genera

general
g. paresis
g. urticaria

generalis
acne g.

generalisata
alopecia g.

generalisatus
herpes g.
herpes zoster g.

generalized
g. acquired hypertrichosis
g. allergic eczematous
  contact dermatitis
g. anaphylaxis
g. anhidrosis
g. atrophic benign
  epidermolysis bullosa
g. congenital hypertrichosis
g. dermal melanocytosis
g. dermatitis of infants
g. dermatophytosis
g. desquamation
g. discoid lupus
  erythematosus
g. elastolysis
g. epidermolytic
  hyperkeratosis
g. eruption, adult type
g. eruption, childhood type
g. eruptive histiocytoma
g. erythema
g. essential telangiectasia
g. exfoliative erythroderma
g. exfoliative process
g. follicular hamartomas
g. gastrointestinal polyposis

generalized (*continued*)
g. granuloma annulare
g. hair follicle hamartoma
  syndrome
g. hyperhidrosis
g. hyperreflexia
g. ichthyosis
g. lentiginosis
g. maculopapular rash
g. melanosis
g. morphea
g. morphea variant
g. myxedema
g. osteoporosis
g. pustular psoriasis
g. pustular psoriasis of von
  Zumbusch
g. Shwartzman
  phenomenon
g. telangiectasia
g. trichoepithelioma
g. vaccinia
g. vitiligo
g. weakness
g. xanthelasma

gene
g. coding
g. directing synthesis
g. smooth and hedgehog
g. regulating synthesis
V g.

genesis

genetic
g. analysis
g. basis
g. determinant
g. disorder
g. immunodeficiency
  syndrome
g. linkage
g. predisposition
g. recombination
g. studies

geniculate
g. ganglion

genital
- g. anomaly
- g. aphthous ulcer
- g. atopic dermatitis
- g. dermatitis
- g. dysplasia
- g. erosive lichen planus
- g. hair
- g. herpes
- g. herpes simplex infection
- g. herpes simplex virus
- g. hidradenitis suppurativa
- g. hypoplasia
- g. infections
- g. lentigines
- g. lentigo
- g. lichen sclerosus
- g. lichen simplex chronicus
- g. neurodermatitis
- g. papulosquamous lesion
- g. pruritus
- g. psoriasis
- g. Reiter syndrome
- g. squamous cell carcinoma
- g. tumor
- g. ulceration
- g. wart

genitalis
- herpes g.

genitocrural
- g. area
- g. fold

genitourinary lesion

genodermatology

genodermatosis

genome

genotype

Gensan

Gensoul's disease

gentamicin
- prednisolone and g.
- g. sulfate

gentian
- g. violet

genu valgum

geographic
- g. pattern
- g. stippling of nail
- g. tongue

geographica
- lingua g.
- psoriasis g.

geographical distribution

geometric
- g. fissures

geotrichosis

Geotrichum candidum

geraniol

gerbil

Gerhardt
- G. disease
- G. phenomenon
- G. reaction
- G. test for acetoacetic acid

germ
- g. cell
- hair g.
- primary epithelial g.

German
- G. measles
- G. measles virus

germicidal

germicide

germinal centers

germinative
- g. cell

germinativum
- stratum g.

germline
- g. mutation

geroderma

gerodermia

geromarasmus

geromorphism
   cutaneous g.

gestationis
   herpes g.
   hydroa g.
   impetigo g.
   prurigo g.

GF
   granuloma faciale
   growth factor

GFR

glomerular filtration rate

Ghon complex

ghoul hand

GI
   gastrointestinal
   GI carcinoma

Gianotti
   G.-Crosti disease
   G.-Crosti syndrome

giant
   g. cell
   g. cell arteritis
   g. cell epulis
   g. cell granuloma
   g. cell myositis
   g. cell tumor
   g. comedo
   g. condyloma
   g. condyloma acuminatum
   g. condyloma of Buschke
      and Loewenstein
   g. congenital nevus
   g. desert centipede
   g. desert centipede bite
   g. eccrine acrospiroma
   g. epulis
   g. granuloma
   g. hairy nevus

giant (*continued*)
   g. hive
   g. intracytoplasmic
      inclusion body
   g. lichenification
   g. melanocytic nevus
   g. melanosome
   g. multinucleated epithelial
      cell
   g. pigmented nevus
   g. solitary keratoacanthoma
   g. solitary
      trichoepitheliomas
   g. urticaria

giantism

gibbus

gift spot

gigantism

Gila monster
   G. m. bite

Gilbert
   G's disease
   G's pityriasis

Gilchrist
   G's disease
   G's sycosis

Gillette Blue Blade

gingiva

gingival
   g. disease
   g. disorder
   g. fibromatosis
   g. hyperplasia
   g. infiltration
   g. lymphoma
   g. platinum line
   g. sulcus

gingivitis
   acute necrotizing ulcerative
      g.
   desquamative g.
   g. plasmacellularis

gingivitis (*continued*)
    ulcerative g.

gingivolabial sulcus

gingivostomatitis
    acute herpetic g.
    herpetic g.

ginkgo biloba

girth

glabella

glabellar
    g. area
    g. region

glabra
    verruca g.

glabrata
    Candida g.
    Torulopsis g.

glabrate

glabrosa
    tinea g.

glabrous
    g. external genitalia
    g. nails
    g. skin

gladiatorum
    herpes g.

glairy

gland
    apocrine g.
    apocrine sweat g.
    ceruminous g.
    coil g.
    cutaneous g.
    eccrine g.
    eccrine sweat g.
    ectopic sebaceous g.
    holocrine g.
    hyperplasia of sebaceous g.
    large sweat g.
    Moll g.
    oil g.

gland (*continued*)
    sebaceous g.
    sudoriferous g.
    sudoriparous g.
    sweat g.
    Zeis g.

glanderous

glanders

glandula
    g. cutis
    g. sebacea
    g. sudorifera

glandular
    g. adnexal carcinoma
    g. elements
    g. fever
    g. hairs
    g. swelling

glandularis
    cheilitis g.

glans
    g. penis

glass
    Wood's g.

glassy cytoplasm

glaucoma

glazed surface

glenoid labrum

Gliadin

glial
    g. giant cells
    g. tissue

glibenclamide

glioblastoma

gliomatous proliferation

glistening
    g. streaks
    g. surface

global

global (*continued*)
    g. epidemic
    g. rating of pain

globi

globular tumor

globulin
    g. level
    sex-hormone–binding g.
    vaccinia immune g.
    varicella-zoster immune g.
    zoster immune g.

glomangioma

glomangiomatosis

glomangiosarcoma

glomera (*plural of* glomus)

glomeruli

glomeruloid hemangioma

glomerulonephritis
    acute g.

glomerulus
    renal g.

glomus *pl.* glomera
    g. body
    g. cell
    cutaneous g.
    digital g.
    neuromyoarterial g.
    solitary g.
    g. tumor

Glossina
    G. bite
    G. morsitans

glossitis *pl.* glossitides
    g. areata exfoliativa
    atrophic g.
    benign migratory g.
    Candida g.
    g. dissecans
    Hunter's g.
    g. mediana rhombica
    median rhomboid g.
    g. migrans
    migratory g.
    Moeller's g.
    g. Moeller-Hunter
    g. of pellagra
    g. parasitica
    parenchymatous g.
    g. rhombica mediana
    rhomboid g.
    g. rhomboidea
      mediana

glossodynia
    Candida g.

glossopharyngitis

glossopyrosis

glossy
    g. skin
    g. tongue

gloves
    cotton g.
    plastic g.
    rubber g.

gloves and socks syndrome

glowing red lips

glucagon

glucagonoma syndrome

glucocerebroside

glucocorticoid (GC)

glucosamine

gluelike discharge

Gluta

glutamic acid

glutaraldehyde
    topical g.

glutathione
    g. deficiency

gluteal
    g. folds
    g. crease

gluten
    g.-free diet
    g.-sensitive enteropathy

glyburide

glyceride

glycerin

glyceryl

glycine

glycogen
    g.-rich cells
    g.-rich clear cells
    g. particles
    g. storage disease

glycolic acid
    g. a. lotion
    g. a. peel

glycolipid lipidosis

glycoprotein
    g. P component
    g. complex

glycopyrrolate

glycosaminoglycan (GAG)
    g. chain

glycosphingolipid metabolism

glycosphingolipidosis

glycosuria

G-myticin topical

gnat bite

Gnathostoma
    G. dolorosi
    G. spinigerum

gnathostomiasis
    human g.

gnawed-out

gnawing ulcer

goat moth

goatpox

goatpox (*continued*)
    g. virus

Goeckerman
    G. method
    G. therapy
    G. treatment

gold
    g. chloride
    g. salts
    Selsun G.
    Selsun G. for Women
    g. sodium thiomalate
    g. therapy

golf tee hair

golfer
    g. elbow
    g. skin

Golgi
    G. apparatus
    G. zone

Goltz
    G. syndrome
    G.-Gorlin syndrome

Gomori's stains

gonadal dysgenesis

gonadotropin

gonitis
    fungous g.

gonococcal
    acute g. infection of lower
      genitourinary tract
    g. arthritis
    g. conjunctivitis
    g. infection of lower
      genitourinary tract
    g. septicemia
    g. stomatitis

gonococcemia

gonococci

gonorrhea
    acute g.

gonorrhea (*continued*)
    chronic g.

gonorrheal arthritis

gonorrhoica
    macula g.

Good's syndrome

goose
    g. bump
    g. bump appearance
    g. flesh
    g. foot
    g. skin

gooseflesh (*variant of* goose flesh)

Gopalan's syndrome

Gordofilm Liquid

Gorham's disease

Gorlin
    G's disease
    G's sign
    G's syndrome
    G.-Goltz syndrome

Gormel Creme

Gottron
    G's papules
    G's sign
    G's syndrome

Gougerot
    pigmented purpuric
        lichenoid dermatitis of G.
    G. triad
    G.-Blum disease
    G.-Blum dermatosis
    G.-Blum syndrome
    papillomatosis of G.-
        Carteaud
    G.-Carteaud syndrome
    G.-Sjögren disease

goundou

gout
    chronic tophaceous g.

gout (*continued*)
    intercritical g.
    g. nodule
    g. pearls
    tophaceous g.

gouttes
    parapsoriasis en g.

gouty
    g. arthritis
    g. panniculitis
    g. tophus

Gower
    G's panatrophy
    panatrophy of G.

graded
    g. compression stockings
    g. elastic bandages

Gradle scissors

graft
    advancement g.
    Allo-Derm universal dermal
        tissue g.
    flap g.
    full-thickness g.
    partial-thickness g.
    g. versus host (GVH)
    g.-versus-host disease
    g.-versus-host reaction
        (GVHR)
    white g.
    xenogeneic g.

grafting
    hair g.
    skin g.

Graham Little
    G. L. syndrome
    G. L.–Piccardi-Lasseur
        syndrome

Graham Patch

grain
    g. itch

grainlike conglomerations

graininess

gramicidin
- g. & neomycin sulfate & polymyxin B sulfate

gram-negative
- g.-n. bacillus (GNB)
- g.-n. bacteria
- g.-n. bacteremia
- g.-n. folliculitis
- g.-n. infection of the foot
- g.-n. organism
- g.-n. pleomorphic bacterium
- g.-n. toe web infection

gram-positive
- g.-p. bacillus
- g.-p. bacteria
- g.-p. bacteremia
- g.-p. cocci
- g.-p. group A beta-hemolytic streptococci
- g.-p. organism

Gram stain

granule
- Birbeck g.
- Fordyce's g.
- keratohyalin g.
- lamellar g.
- Langerhans' g.
- membrane-coating g.
- trichohyalin g.
- vermiform g.

granular
- g. cell
- g. cell layer
- g. cell myoblastoma
- g. cell tumor
- g. cytoplasm
- g. degeneration
- g. deposit
- g. deposition
- g. horny material
- g. layer
- g. papulation
- g. pyogenicum

granular (*continued*)
- g. vaginitis
- g. zone

granulate

granulation
- red g.
- g. tissue

granule
- azurophil g.
- Birbeck g.
- bismuth g.
- Bollinger g's
- dextranomer g.
- Fordyce g.
- keratohyaline g.
- lamellar g.
- Langerhans cell g.
- membrane-coating g.
- Much g.
- Snaplets-FR G.
- sulfur g.
- rod-shaped cytoplasmic g.

Granulex

granulocyte
- g. colony-stimulating factor (G-CSF)
- g.-macrophage colony stimulating factor
- g.-rich infiltration

granulocytic sarcoma

granuloma
- actinic g.
- g. annulare
- g. annulare-like eruption
- beryllium g.
- bilharzial g.
- *Candida* g.
- candidal g.
- g. candidomycetica
- caseating g.
- coccidioidal g.
- coli g.
- dermal tuberculoid g.

granuloma (*continued*)
- diaper g.
- elastolytic giant cell g.
- g. endemicum
- eosinophilic g.
- g. eosinophilicum faciei
- g. faciale
- fish tank g.
- g. fissuratum
- foreign-body g.
- g. fungoides
- g. gangraenescens
- g. gravidarum
- giant cell g.
- g. gluteale infantum
- g. gravidarum
- Hodgkin g.
- infectious g.
- g. inguinale
- g. inguinale tropicum
- lethal midline g.
- lipoid g.
- lipophagic g.
- lycopodium g.
- Majocchi's g.
- g. malignum
- metastatic g.
- midline lethal g.
- Miescher's g.
- monilial g.
- g. multiforme
- necrotizing g.
- noncaseating g.
- noncaseating epithelioid cell g.
- oily g.
- palisading g.
- paracoccidioidal g.
- parasitic g.
- peripheral giant cell g.
- pseudopyogenic g.
- g. pudendi
- pyogenic g.
- g. pyogenicum
- reticulohistiocytic g.
- sarcoidlike g.
- g. sarcomatodes
- schistosome g.

granuloma (*continued*)
- sea urchin g.
- silica g.
- swimming pool g.
- g. telangiectaticum
- trichophytic g.
- g. trichophyticum
- tuberculoid g.
- g. venereum
- zirconium g.

granulomatosa
- cheilitis g.
- Miescher cheilitis g.

granulomatosis
- allergic g.
- Churg-Strauss g.
- g. disciformis chronica et progressiva
- g. disciformis et progressiva
- g. disciformis progressiva et chronica
- eosinophilic g.
- lethal midline g.
- limited Wegener's g.
- lipid g.
- lymphomatoid g.
- midline g.
- Miescher-Leder g.
- g. rhinitis
- Wegener's g.

granulomatous
- g. bacterial infection
- g. cheilitis
- g. colitis
- g. cutaneous T-cell lymphoma
- g. dermal infiltrate
- g. disease
- g. eruption
- g. foci
- g. inflammation
- g. inflammatory reaction
- g. lobular panniculitis
- g. nodules
- g. papular facial disease
- g. perioral dermatitis

granulomatous (*continued*)
    g. pyoderma
    g. reaction
    g. rosacea
    g. secondary syphilis
    g. slack skin
    g. uveitis
    g. vasculitis

granulosis
    g. rubra nasi

granulosity

granulosum
    stratum g.

grapelike clusters

grasper
    nonsuction g.

grave types

Graves' disease

gravidarum
    chloasma g.
    fibroma molle g.
    melasma g.
    striae g.

gravis
    icterus g.

gravitational
    g. ulcer

gray
    g. hair
    g. patch tinea capitis
    g. scales

greasy
    g. scales

Grecian Formula

green
    g. hair
    g. lynx spider
    g. nail syndrome

Greenhow's disease

Greither

Greither (*continued*)
    G. syndrome

Grenz
    G. rays
    G. zone

Grevillea
    G. banksii
    G. robusta
    G. "Robyn Gordon"

Gridley methenamine silver stain

Griesinger's disease

Griffith's sign

Grifulvin V

Grisactin
    G. Ultra

Griscelli
    G. syndrome
    G. and Chediak-Higashi syndrome

griseofulvin
    ultramicronized g.

Gris-PEG

grocer
    g's eczema
    g's itch

Grönblad-Strandberg syndrome

groove
    double g.
    nail g.

grooving

gross
    g. hypertrophy
    g. lesion
    g. "thorniness"

ground
    g. itch
    g. substance

ground-glass

ground-glass (*continued*)
  g.-g. appearance
  g.-g. cytoplasm
  g.-g. opacification
  g.-g. pattern

grounding electrode

group
  g. A beta hemolytic
    streptococcus
  g. B streptococcus (GBS)
  Contact Dermatitis
    Research G.
  g. D streptococcus
  International Contact
    Dermatitis Research G.
    (ICDRG)
  North American Contact
    Dermatitis G. (NACDG)
  g. 5 topical steroid

grouped
  g. blisters
  g. erosions

Grover's disease

growth
  g. dysregulation
  g. phase
  g. retardation

gryphosis

gryposis
  g. unguium

GSE
  gluten-sensitive enteropathy

Guillain-Barré syndrome

guinea
  g. corn yaws
  g. worm infection

gum
  g. arabic
  g. benjamin
  g. benzoin
  g. camphor
  karaya g.

gum (*continued*)
  g. rash
  sterculia g.
  g. tragacanth
  vegetable g.

gumma
  g. of tertiary syphilis

gummatous
  g. lesions
  g. osteoarthritis
  g. syphilid
  g. syphilis
  g. ulcer

gummosa
  scrofuloderma g.

gummy

Günther
  G's disease
  G's syndrome
  G's variety

gustatory
  g. hyperhidrosis
  g. rhinitis
  g. sweating

guttata
  morphea g.
  parapsoriasis g.
  psoriasis g.

guttate
  g. erythematous macules
  g. hypomelanosis
  g. lesion
  g. macules
  g. parapsoriasis
  g. psoriasis
  g. psoriasis-like
  g. varieties

guttering
  limbal g.

GV
  gentian violet

GVH

GVH (*continued*)
    graft versus host
    GVH disease

GVHR
    graft versus host reaction

G-well
    G. lotion
    G. shampoo

gynandroblastoma

gynecomastia

Gynecort

Gyne-Lotrimin

gypseum
    Microsporum g.

gypsy
    g. moth
    g. moth larva
    g. moth larva sting

gyrata
    cutis verticis g.
    psoriasis g.

gyrate
    g. border
    g. erythema
    g. figure
    g. pattern
    g. serpiginous erythema

gyratum
    erythema g.

gyrose

H

H zone

H1 blocker

H2 blocker

haarscheibe tumor

HAART
    highly active antiretroviral
        therapy

Haber's syndrome

Habermann's disease

habitual
    h. actinic exposure
    h. licking

habitus
    marfanoid h.

HAE
    hereditary angioneurotic
        edema

HAEM
    herpes simplex-associated
        erythema multiforme

Haemophilus
    H. ducreyi
    H. influenzae
    H. influenzae cellulitis
    H. suis

Haemopis sanguisuga

Hailey-Hailey disease

hair
    h. apparatus
    axillary h.
    bamboo h.
    bayonet h.
    beaded h.
    bubble h.
    h. bulb
    burrowing h.
    h. cast
    club h.
    h. collar sign

hair (*continued*)
    h. color
    corkscrew h.
    cortex of h.
    cuticle of h.
    h. cycle
    h. density
    h. disk
    h. dye
    exclamation point h.
    excessive facial h.
    excessive h. loss
    h. fall
    falling h.
    h. follicle
    h. follicle dystrophy
    h. follicle epithelium
    h. follicle mite
    h. follicle mite scabies
    h. follicle nevus
    h. follicle sheath
    h. follicle tumor
    Frey h.
    genital h.
    h. germ
    h. grafting
    hypopigmented h.
    ingrowing h.
    ingrown h.
    kinky h.
    knotted h.
    lanugo h.
    h. loss
    h. lotions
    h. melanin
    moniliform h.
    h.-nest sinus
    nettling h.
    h. patterning
    pubic h.
    resting h.
    ringed h.
    Schridde cancer h.
    h. shaft
    h. snakes
    softening hair

hair (*continued*)
    h. spray
    stellate h.
    h. straightening
    straightening h.
    h. structure defect
    terminal h.
    thinning h.
    h. tonics
    h. transplant
    h. transplantation
    tuft of h.
    twisted h.
    vellus h.
    woolly h.

HAIR-AN syndrome

hairiness
    excessive h.

hairless streaks

hairlessness

hairlike structure

hairline

hairy
    h. cell leukemia
    h. fleas
    h. hamartoma
    h. lesions
    h. leukoplakia, oral
    h. mole
    h. nevus
    h. tongue

halcinonide

Haldrone

Halecium

half-and-half
    h.-and-h. fingernail
    h.-and-h. nail

half-moon
    red h.-m.

Halfprin 81

halide

Hallermann
    H.-Streiff syndrome
    H.-Streiff-Francois
      syndrome

Hallopeau
    acrodermatitis continua of
      H.
    H's acrodermatitis
    H's disease
    H. type
    H.-Siemens epidermolysis
      bullosa
    H.-Siemens syndrome

hallucination

hallux
    h. valgus
    h. varus

halo
    h. melanoma
    h. nevus
    h. phenomenon
    purpuric h.
    red h.
    violaceous h.

halobetasol propionate

halodermia

Halog
    H. topical
    H.-E topical

halogen
    h. acne

halogenoderma

haloperidol
    h. decanoate
    h. LA
    h. lactate

haloprogin

Halotex
    H. topical

Ham's test

Hamamelis

hamamelis

hamartoma *pl.* hamartomata
    Becker hairy h.
    hairy h.
    sclerosing epithelial h.

hamartomatous
    h. hyperplasia
    h. intestinal polyps
    h. polyp
    h. proliferations

Hamilton
    H. bandage
    H. pseudophlegmon
    H. test

hammer toe, hammertoe

Hand
    H.-Schüller-Christian
      disease
    H.-Schüller-Christian
      syndrome

hand
    crab h.
    h. eczema, allergic
    edema of h.
    ghoul h.
    Marinesco succulent h.
    mechanic h.
    pulling boat h.
    trench h.

hand-and-foot syndrome

hand-foot-and-mouth
    h.-f.-and-m. disease
    h.-f.-and-m. disease virus
    h.-f.-and-m. exanthem

handwashing
    meticulous h.

HANE
    hereditary angioneurotic
      edema

HANES
    National Health and Nutrition
      Examination Survey

hang nail, hangnail

hanging
    h. pendulum
    h. skin

Hanot
    H. disease
    H. syndrome

Hansen
    H's bacillus
    H's disease

hapalonychia

haplotype

Happle syndrome

hapten
    h.-carrier complex

Harada
    H. disease
    H. syndrome

harara

hard
    h. chancre
    h. corn
    h. keratin
    h. lesion
    h. papilloma
    h. sore
    h. tick
    h. ulcer

hardened skin

hardening
    h. of skin

harderoporphyria

harlequin
    h. fetus
    h. ichthyosis

harsh skin

Harter's syndrome

Hartnup
    H's disease

Hartnup (*continued*)
H's syndrome

harvest
h. itch
h. mite
h. mite bite

harvester ant

Hashimoto
H's disease
H's thyroiditis
H.-Pritzker disease

Hassall
H's bodies
H's corpuscles

hatband dermatitis

Haverhill fever

Hawaiian
H. scorpion
H. sunfish

Hay-Wells syndrome

hazel
witch h.

HBO
hyperbaric oxygen

HCP
hereditary coproporphyria

HCV
hepatitis C virus

HDL
high-density lipoprotein

head
h. lice
h. louse
white h.

Head and Shoulders shampoo

healed ulcer

healing
fish-mouth h.
wound h.
h. wound

health
National Institute of H.
(NIH)

health maintenance
organization (HMO)

heaped-up scaling

heart
h. defect
h. failure
h. muscle disease

heat
h. desensitization
h. exposure
prickly h.
h. rash
h. urticaria

heavy
h. chain disease
h. chain proteins
h. freckling
h. metal poisoning
h. scaling

Heberden
H's arthritis
H's node

Hebra
H's disease
H's ointment
H's pityriasis
H's prurigo

Heck
H's disease
H's syndrome

heel
basketball h.
black h.
cracked h.

Heelbo decubitus protector

Heerfordt
H's disease
H's syndrome

helical

helicis
  chondrodermatitis
    nodularis chronica h.

Helicobacter
  H. cinaedi
  H. pylori

heliotherapy

heliotrope
  h. eyelids
  h. rash

helix
  triple h.

helminth

helminthiasis
  h. elastica

helminthic
  h. parasitic disease
  h. infestation

Helminthosporium
  H. spiciferum

Heloderma
  H. horridum
  H. suspectum
  H. suspectum bite

heloma
  h. durum
  h. molle

helosis

helotomy

helper
  antigen-specific h.
  antigen-nonspecific h.
  h. cell
  h. T cell
  h. T cell–dominant
    lymphocytic infiltrate

hemagglutination
  assay

hemangiectasia
  hypertrophicans

hemangiectatic hypertrophy

hemangioendothelioma
  malignant h.
  spindle cell h.

hemangioma *pl.* hemangiomata
  h. birthmark
  capillary h.
  cavernous h.
  h. congenitale
  deep h.
  h. hypertrophicum cutis
  involuting flat h.
  mixed h.
  h. planum
  h. planum extensum
  h. racemosum
  sclerosing h.
  senile h.
  h. simplex
  spider h.
  strawberry h.
  superficial h.
  synovial h.
  h.-thrombocytopenia
    syndrome
  verrucous h.

hemangiomatosis

hemangiopericytoma

hemarthrosis

hematemesis

hemathidrosis

hematidrosis

hematin

hematocrit

hematogenous
  h. allergic contact
    dermatitis
  h. allergic contact eczema
  h. dissemination of
    tuberculosis
  h. metastasis
  h. spread

hematogenously

hematohidrosis

hematologic
    h. abnormalities
    h. malignancy

hematoma
    subungual h.

hematophagous arthropods

hematopoietic
    h. disease
    h. stem cell transplantation
    h. system
    h. ulcer

hematoporphyrin

hematoxylin
    h. and eosin (H&E)
    h. eosin stain

heme

Hemenocampa pseudotsugata

Hemerocampa

hemianopia

hemiatrophy
    facial h.
    progressive lingual h.

hemiatrophy
    progressive facial h.

hemicanities

hemidesmosomal protein

hemidesmosome
    rudimentary h.

hemidiaphoresis

hemidrosis

hemifacial
    h. plaque

hemihidrosis

hemihyperhidrosis

hemihypertrophy

hemiparesis

hemiplegia

Hemiptera

hemispherical pitted papules

hemivertebra

hemizygous

hemochromatosis

hemoconcentration

hemodialysis (HD)

hemodiapedesis

hemodynamics

hemoglobin

hemolysis

hemolytic
    h. anemia of newborn
    h. assay
    h. complement
    h. disease
    h. *Staphylococcus albus*
    h. sickle cell disease
    h. uremic syndrome (HUS)

hemophagocytic syndrome

hemophilia
    acquired h.

hemophilus

hemoprotein

hemorrhage
    petechial h.
    punctate h.
    splinter h.

hemorrhagic
    h. bulla
    h. diathesis
    h. edema
    h. exudative erythema
    h. fever
    h. gangrene
    h. gingivitis

hemorrhagic (*continued*)
  h. lesion
  h. macular stain
  h. puncta
  h. pyoderma gangrenosum
  h. rash
  h. signs
  h. smallpox
  h. telangiectasia

hemorrhagica
  purpura h.
  scarlatina h.
  urticaria h.
  variola h.

hemorrhagicus
  lichen h.

hemorrhoid
  third-degree h's

hemosiderin
  h. deposition
  h. hyperpigmentation

hemosiderosis

hemostasis

hemostatics (*class of drugs*)

Henderson-Paterson bodies

Hendersonula
  H. toruloidea

Henoch
  H. disease
  H. purpura
  H. -Schönlein purpura
    (HSP)
  H.-Schönlein purpura
    vasculitis
  H.-Schönlein syndrome
    (HSS)
  H.-Schönlein vasculitis

HEP
  hepatoerythrocytic
    porphyria

heparin
  h. cofactor II

heparin (*continued*)
  h. necrosis
  h. sulfate

heparitin sulfate

hepatic
  h. abscess
  h. disease
  h. dysfunction
  h. hemangiomatosis
  h. porphyria
  h. tubercle
  h. tumor
  h. tyrosine
    aminotransferase
  h. vein thrombosis

hepatitic

hepatitis
  h. B (HB)
  h. B vaccine
  h. B virus
  h. C (HC)
  h. C–associated unilateral
    nevoid telangiectasia
  h. C virus (HCV)
  h. contagiosa canis
    granulomatous h.
  h. serology (B and C)

hepatobiliary
  h. disease
  h. origin

hepatocellular
  h. carcinoma

Hepatocystis

hepatoerythropoietic porphyria

hepatolenticular degeneration

hepatoma

hepatomegaly

hepatorenal
  h. failure

hepatosplenomegaly

hepatotoxic

hepatotoxic (*continued*)
  h. drugs
  h. reaction

hepatotoxicity

hepatotoxin

herald
  h. patch
  h. plaque

herbicides

hereditable phenomenon

hereditaria
  alopecia h.

hereditarium
  erythema palmare h.

hereditary
  h. acrolabial telangiectasia
  h. angioedema (HAE)
  h. angioneurotic edema
    (HANE)
  h. benign telangiectasia
  h. bullous disease
  h. coproporphyria (HCP)
  h. disease
  h. factor
  h. gene mutation
  h. hemorrhagic
    telangiectasia
  h. hemorrhagic
    telangiectasis
  h. hyperglobulinemia
  h. lymphedema
  h. metabolic disease
  h. multiple
    trichoepithelioma
  h. osteo-onychodysplasia
  h. palmoplantar
    keratoderma
  h. polymorphous light
    eruption
  h. process
  h. progressive mucinous
    histiocytosis
  h. sclerosing poikiloderma
  h. sensory neuropathy

hereditary (*continued*)
  h. spherocytosis
  h. syndromes
  h. systemic angiomatosis
  h. thymic dysplasia
  h. vibratory angioedema
  h. woolly hair

heredopathia atactica
  polyneuritiformis

heritable
  h. connective tissue disease
  h. disorder

Herlitz
  H. disease
  H. epidermolysis bullosa
  H. junctional epidermolysis
    bullosa
  H. syndrome

Hermansky-Pudlak syndrome

hernia
  diaphragmatic h.
  h. inguinalis

herniated
  h. nodules
  h. presacral fat pad

herpangina

herpes
  h. auricularis
  h. blattae
  h. catarrhalis
  h. circinatus bullosus
  congenital h. simplex
  h. digitalis
  h. facialis
  h. farinosus
  h. febrilis
  h. generalisatus
  genital h.
  h. genitalis
  h. gestationis
  h. gladiatorum
  h. iris
  h. labialis
  h. menstrualis

herpes (*continued*)
   h. mentalis
   nasal h.
   h. odeus
   h. phlyctaenodes
   h. praepuffalis
   h. progenitalis
   h. recurrens
   h. simplex
   h. simplex conjunctivitis
   h. simplex DNA
   h. simplex genitalis
   h. simplex infection
   h. simplex labialis
   h. simplex oralis
   h. simplex recurrens
   h. simplex virus (HSV)
   h. simplex virus type I
   h. simplex virus type II
   h. tonsurans
   h. tonsurans maculosus
   h. vegetans
   h. virus cytopathic effects
   h. virus infection
   wrestler h.
   h. zoster (HZ)
   h. zoster generalisatus
   h. zoster infection
   h. zoster ophthalmicus
   h. zoster oticus
   h. zoster varicellosus
   h. zoster virus

herpesvirus
   h. DNA polymerase
   herpes whitlow h.

Herpesvirus simiae

herpetic
   h. gingivostomatitis
   h. infection
   h. intranuclear inclusions
   h. keratitis
   h. keratoconjunctivitis
   h. paronychia
   h. pharyngitis
   h. ulcer
   h. vulvovaginitis

herpetic (*continued*)
   h. whitlow
   zoster sine h.

herpeticum
   eczema h.

herpetiform
   h. aphtha
   h. pemphigus

herpetiforme
   hydroa h.

herpetiformis
   dermatitis h. (DH)
   epidermolysis bullosa
     simplex h.
   impetigo h.
   morphea h.

herpetoid

Herplex Ophthalmic

herringbone
   h. nail
   h. pattern

Hertoghe's sign

Herxheimer
   H. fibers
   H. reaction
   H. spirals

HES
   hydroxyethyl starch
   hypereosinophilic
     syndrome

heterochromia iridis

heterodermic

heterogeneity

heterograft

heterokeratoplasty

heterologous
   h. graft

heterophil, heterophile
   h. antibody

heterophil (*continued*)
  h. antigen

heteroplastic
  h. graft

heterospecific
  h. graft

heterotrichosis
  h. superciliorum

heterozygote

heterozygous
  h. deficiency

hexachlorobenzene

hexachlorophene

Hexadrol
  Decadron and H.
  H. phosphate

hexamethyl violet

Hexapoda

hexavalent
  h. chromates
  h. chrome compounds

hexylresorcinol

Hgb
  oxy Hgb
  reduced Hgb

HG
  herpes gestationis
  HG factor

HGPRT
  hypoxanthine guanine
    phosphoribosyltransferase
  HGPRT deficiency

HHT
  hereditary hemorrhagic
    telangiectasia

HHV
  human herpesvirus
  HHV-8 genome
  HHV-8 infection

5-HIAA

hibernoma

Hibiclens topical

Hibistat topical

Hi-Cor
  H.-1.0
  H.-2.5

hickey

hidden nail skin

hidebound
  h. disease

hidradenitis
  h. axillaris
  h. axillaris of Verneuil
  eccrine h.
  neutrophilic h.
  neutrophilic eccrine h.
  h. suppurativa
  suppurative h.

hidradenocarcinoma
  clear cell h.

hidradenoma
  clear cell h.
  cystic h.
  eruptive h.
  h. eruptivum
  nodular h.
  papillary h.
  h. papilliferum
  poroid h.
  solid h.
  solid-cystic h.

hidroa
  h. vacciniforme

hidroacanthoma
  h. simplex

hidroadenoma
  h. papilliferum

hidrocystoma
  apocrine h.
  eccrine h.

hidromeiosis

hidropoiesis

hidropoietic

hidrorrhea

hidrosadenitis

hidroschesis

hidrosis

hidrotic
    h. ectodermal dysplasia

hiemalis
    acrodermatitis h.
    dermatitis h.
    erythrokeratolysis h.
    prurigo h.
    pruritus h.

high
    h.-arched palate
    h. palate

Higoumenaki's sign

hilar
    h. adenopathy
    h. cell tumor
    h. lymphadenopathy

hindfoot
    h. splint

hippocratic
    h. face
    h. facies
    h. finger
    h. nail

hippocratica
    facies H.

hirci (*plural of* hircus)

hircismus

hircus *pl.* hirci

Hirschsprung's disease

hirsute

hirsuties

hirsutism
    Apert h.
    constitutional h.
    idiopathic h.

hirudin

Hirudinaria

Hirudinea

hirudiniasis

hirudinization

hirudinize

Hirudo
    H. aegyptiaca
    H. japonica
    H. javanica
    H. medicinalis
    H. quinquestriata
    H. sangulsorba
    H. troctina

Hismanal

histamine
    h. metabolites
    methylhistamine

histiocyte
    bacilli-laden h.
    lipid-laden h.

histiocytic
    h. cytophagic panniculitis
    h. giant cells
    h. medullary reticulosis
    h. phase

histiocytoma
    benign fibrous h.
    h. cutis
    fibrous h.
    generalized eruptive h.
    lipoid h.
    malignant fibrous h.

histiocytosis
    juvenile xanthogranuloma
     h.

histiocytosis (*continued*)
    Langerhans cell h.
    nodular non-X h.
    non-X h.
    h. X

histochemical

histocompatibility
    h. antigen
    h. complex
    h. molecules

histoid leprosy

histogenesis

histologic
    h. change
    h. evaluation
    h. hallmark
    h. lepromatous process
    h. lesion
    h. pattern
    h. staining

histological

histology

histolytica

histomorphologic

histone
    h. determinant

histone-DNA antibody

histopathology

Histoplasma
    H. capsulatum
    H. duboisii

histoplasmin

histoplasmosis
    primary pulmonary h.

history
    relevant sting h.

HIV
    human immunodeficiency
      virus

hive, hives
    giant h.

HLA
    human leukocyte antigen
    human lymphocyte antigen
        HLA-129
        HLA-A
        HLA-A11
        HLA allele
        HLA-B
        HLA-B8
        HLA-B13
        HLA-B17
        HLA-B27 genetic
          marker
        HLA-C
        HLA class I
        HLA class I associated
          disease
        HLA complex
        HLA Cw6
        HLA-DP
        HLA-DQ
        HLA-DR
        HLA-DR3
        HLA-DR3 gene
        HLA-DR4
        HLA-DRB and -DRQ
          DNA typing
        HLA-DRw4
        HLA-DRw52
        HLA-E
        HLA-F
        HLA-G
        HLA intercellular
          interaction
        HLA typing

HM-175

HMB-45

HMO
    health maintenance
      organization

hMSH2 mismatch repair gene

hobnail tongue

Hodgkin
  H's disease
  H's granuloma

Hofmann violet

Hollister
  H. medial adhesive
    bandage
  H.-Stier Laboratory

hollows

Holmes-Adie syndrome

holocarboxylase synthetase

holocrine
  h. gland

home cleaning product

homeostatic
  h. mechanism

hominis
  Actinomyces h.
  Sarcoptes h.

homme
  h. orange
  h. rouge

homocysteine

homocystinuria

homogeneous
  h. cytoplasm
  h. eosinophilic dermal
    ground substance
  h. eosinophilic material
  h. material
  h. staining pattern
  h. tissue

homogentisic acid

homolateral
  h. leptomeningeal
    angiomatosis

homologous
  h. graft

homology

homonymous
  h. hemianopsia

homoplastic graft

homosalate

homosexual

homozygous
  h. defect
  h. keratin 14
  h. protein C

honeybee

honey-colored crust

honeycomb
  h. appearance
  h. atrophy
  h. lung
  h. ringworm
  h. structure
  h. tetter

honeycomblike structure

Hong Kong
  H. K. foot
  H. K. toe

HOOD
  hereditary osteo-
    onychodysplasia

hoof-and-mouth disease

hookworm
  h. disease

Hopf
  acrokeratosis verruciformis
    of H.

hordeolum

Horder spot

horizontal
  h. fibrosis
  h. growth phase
  h. sectioning

Hormodendron

Hormodendrum

hormonal
   h. changes
   h. factor
   h. manipulation

hormonally-induced acne

horn
   cicatricial h.
   cutaneous h.
   h. cyst
   nail h.
   h. pseudocyst
   sebaceous h.
   h. substance
   warty h.

hornet
   h. sting
   white-faced h.
   yellow h.

hornification

horny
   h. cell layer
   h. center
   h. crusting
   h. follicular lesion
   h. follicular papule
   h. formation
   h. layer
   h. material
   h. plug
   h. projection
   h. spicules
   h. tissue

horripilation

horse-collar appearance

horsefly, horse fly
   h. bite

horsepox
   h. virus

horseradish peroxidase

horseshoe arrangement

Horton
   H's disease

Horton (*continued*)
   H's syndrome

hospital
   h. gangrene

hospital-acquired infectious
   disease

host
   graft versus h. (GVH)
   h. immunity
   h. immunosuppression
   h. specificity

hot
   h. comb alopecia
   h. gangrene

hotfoot

house
   h. dust mite
   h. dust mite antigen
   h. spider

housefly

Howel-Evans' syndrome

HP
   hydroxylysylpyridinole

HP Acthar Gel

HPA
   hypothalamic-pituitary-
      adrenal
         HPA axis

HPV
   human papillomavirus
   human parvovirus
      HPV aerosol
         contamination
      HPV acanthoma
      HPV capsid antigen
      HPV-induced genital
         dysplasia
      HPV-induced
         squamous cell
         carcinoma

HSP
   Henoch-Schönlein purpura

HSP (*continued*)
  hereditary sclerosing
    poikiloderma
HSS
  Henoch-Schönlein
    syndrome
HSV
  herpes simplex virus
    HSV DNA
HTLV-1
  human T-lymphotrophic
    virus type I
HTLV-2
  human T-lymphotrophic
    virus type II
HTLV-III
  human T-cell
    lymphotrophic virus type
    III (*human
    immunodeficiency virus*)
human
  h. adjuvant disease
  h. botfly
  chickenpox immune
    globulin (h.)
  h. dermatosparaxis—EDS
    type VIIC
  h. flea
  h. hair mimics pili
    annulati
  h. heat shock protein
  h. helicase gene
  h. herpes virus 6 (HH6,
    HBLV)
  h. herpesvirus 1–8 (HHV)
  h. infestation
  measles immune globulin
    (h.)
  h. measles immune serum
  h. monkeypox
  h. papilloma virus 16 (HPV-
    16)
  h. parvovirus B19
  h. trypanosomiasis
  h. werewolf

humect
humectant
humectate
humectation
humid
  h. tetter
humidity
humoral
  h. (B cell) reaction
  h. immune response
  h. immunity
  h. immunodeficiency
hump
  buffalo h.
  dowager h.
Hunan hand
hunchbacked
Hünermann
  H. disease
Hunt
  H. syndrome
Hunter
  H's glossitis
  H's syndrome
hunterian
  h. chancre
hunting wasp
Huriez syndrome
Hurler
  H's disease
  H's syndrome
Hutchinson
  H's disease
  H's freckle
  freckle of H.
  H's lentigo
  melanotic freckle of H.
  H's sign
  H's summer prurigo

Hutchinson (*continued*)
  H's syndrome
  H's teeth
  H's triad
  H.-Gilford progeria
  H.-Gilford syndrome

Huxley layer

hyalin
  h. deposits
  h. substance

hyaline
  h. degeneration
  h. papillary bodies
  h. papillary projections

hyalinization

hyalinized
  h. collagen
  h. stroma

hyalinosis
  h. cutis et mucosae

hyalohyphomycosis

hyaluronic acid

hyaluronidase

hybrid cells

Hycort

hydantoin

hydatid
  h. disease
  h. rash

Hyde's disease

Hydeltrasol injection

Hydeltra-TBA injection

hydradenitis

hydradenoma

hydralazine

Hydramyn syrup

hydrate

hydration
  adequate h.
  vigorous h.

Hydrea

hydroa
  h. aestivale
  h. estivale
  h. febrile
  h. gestationis
  h. gravidarum
  h. herpetiforme
  h. puerorum
  h. vacciniforme
  h. vesiculosum

hydrocarbon

hydrocele

hydrocephalus

hydrochlorothiazide (HCTZ)

hydrocolloid
  h. dressing
  h. occlusion

Hydrocort

hydrocortisone
  h. butyrate
  bacitracin, neomycin,
    polymyxin B, and h.
  chloramphenicol,
    polymyxin B, and h.
  colistin, neomycin, and h.
  h. hemisuccinate
  lidocaine and h.
  neomycin, polymyxin B,
    and h.
  polymyxin B and h.
  h. valerate

Hydrocortone
  H. acetate
  H. phosphate

hydrocystoma

hydrogel dressing

hydrogen peroxide mouthwash

hydroid
  marine h.

hydrolase

hydrolytic enzyme

hydrolyze

hydrolyzing

hydrophilic
  h. cream
  h. occlusive dressing
  h. ointment
  h. polymer dressing

hydropic
  h. degeneration
  h. epithelioid cells

hydrops
  fetal h.
  h. fetalis

hydroquinone

HydroSKIN

Hydro-Tex

hydroxocobalamin

hydroxyzine
  h. HCl
  h. pamoate

hydroxychloroquine (HCQ)
  h. sulfate
  h. therapy

5-hydroxyindoleacetic acid
  (5-HIAA)

hydroxylysine
  h. pathway

hydroxylysyl

hydroxyprogesterone caproate

hydroxyquinoline

5-hydroxytryptamine (5-HT)

hydroxyurea

hydroxyvitamin D

hydroxyzine
  h. HCl
  h. hydrochloride

Hy-Gestrone injection

hygienically deprived

hygroma
  h. colli
  cystic h.
  h. cysticum cutis et
    subcutis
  h. cysticum

hygroscopicity

Hylesia

Hylutin injection

Hymenoptera
  H. sting
  H. venom
  H. venom anaphylaxis

Hy-Pam

hyperacanthosis

hyperaminoaciduria

hyperandrogenism

hyperbaric
  h. oxygen (HBO)
  h. oxygen therapy

hyperbilirubinemia

hypercalcemia

hypercarotenemia

hypercatabolism

hypercholesteremic
  xanthoma

hyperchromatic
  h. nucleus

hyperchromatism

hyperchylomicronemia

hyperchylomicronemic
  syndrome (*types I & V*)

hypercoagulable state

hyperemia
   bulbar conjunctival h.

hyperemic

hyperemization

hyperendemic area

hypereosinophilia

hypereosinophilic
   h. dermatitis
   h. syndrome

hyperesthesia

hyperextensibility

hyperextensible joint

hypergammaglobulinemia of
   Waldenström

hypergammaglobulinemic
   purpura

hyperglucagonemia

hypergranulosis

hyperhidrosis
   axillary h.
   emotional h.
   generalized h.
   gustatory h.
   h. lateralis
   h. oleosa
   palmar h.
   palmoplantar h.
   primary h.
   unilateral h.
   h. unilateralis
   volar h.

hyperhidrotic

hyperhydration

hyperidrosis

hyperimmunoglobulinemia
   h. D syndrome
   h. E syndrome

hyperinfection

hyperinsulinemia

hyperirritability

hyperirritable skin

hyperkeratinization

hyperkeratomycosis

hyperkeratosis *pl.*
   hyperkeratoses
   h. condition
   h. congenita
   h. congenitalis palmaris et
     plantaris
   h. eccentrica
   epidermolytic h.
   h. excentrica
   h. figurate centrifuga
     atrophica
   focal acral h.
   follicular h.
   h. follicularis et
     parafollicularis
   h. follicularis et
     parafollicularis in cutem
     penetrans
   h. follicularis in cutem
     penetrans
   h. follicularis vegetans
   generalized epidermolytic
     h.
   h. hemorrhagica
   h. lenticularis perstans
   h. linguae
   h. of palms and soles
   palmoplantar h.
   h. penetrans
   h. process
   progressive dystrophic h.
   h. punctata of the palmar
     creases
   subungual h.
   h. subungualis
   h. universalis congenita

hyperkeratotic

hyperkeratotic (*continued*)
    h. dermatitis of the palms
       and fingers
    h. epidermis
    h. fissured hand and foot
       eczema
    h. form
    h. linear lesion
    h. melanoma
    h. palmoplantar eczema
    h. plaque
    h. scabies
    h. surface

hyperlinear palm

hyperlipemic xanthoma

hyperlipidemia

hyperlipoproteinemia
    multiple-type h.

hyperliposis

hypermelanosis
    linear and whorled nevoid
       h.
    nevoid h.

hypermelanotic

hypermetabolic state

hypernephroma

hyperonychia

hyperorthokeratosis

hyperostosis
    diffuse idiopathic skeletal h.
       (DISH)

hyperparathyroidism

hyperperistalsis

hyperphosphatemia

hyperpigmentation
    central h.
    h. of familial periorbital
       melanosis

hyperpigmented

hyperpigmented (*continued*)
    h. borders
    cutaneous h.
    h. fundus
    h. macules
    postinflammatory h.
    h. scar

hyperplasia
    angiolymphoid h. with
       eosinophilic
    basal cell h.
    congenital sebaceous h.
    congenital sebaceous gland
       h.
    cutaneous lymphoid h.
    epidermal h.
    fibrous h.
    focal epithelial h.
    intravascular papillary
       endothelial h.
    pilosebaceous gland h.
    pseudoepitheliomatous h.
    sebaceous h.
    h. of sebaceous gland
    senile sebaceous h.
    synovial h.
    verrucous h.

hyperplastic
    h. epidermis
    h. foveae
    h. mesodermal stroma
    h. sebaceous glands
    h. synovium (HS)

hyperprebetalipoproteinemia

hyperprolactinemia

hyperpyrexia

hyperreactivity

hyperresponsive

hyperresponsiveness

hypersecretion
    mucus h.

hypersensitiveness

hypersensitivity
  atopic h.
  contact h.
  cutaneous basophil h.
    (CBH)
  drug h.
  food h.
  immediate h.
  h. reaction
  h. skin testing
  h. syndrome
  h. vasculitis

hypersensitization

hypersplenism

hypersteatosis

hyperstretchability

hypersusceptibility

hypertelorism

hypertension

hyperthermia

hyperthermic
  h. circuit
  h. episodes

hyperthyroidism

hypertonic

hypertrichiasis

hypertrichophrydia

hypertrichosis
  h. lanuginosa acquisita
  h. lanuginosa
  nevoid h.
  h. partialis
  h. universalis

hypertrichotic condition

hypertriglyceridemia
  progressive h.

hypertrophic
  h. cardiomyopathy
  h. collagenous tissue

hypertrophic (*continued*)
  h. gums
  h. lichen planus
  h. lupus erythematosus
  h. lymphoid follicle
  h. nails
  h. osteoarthropathy
  h. rosacea
  h. peripheral neuropathy
  h. pigmented actinic
    keratosis
  h. scar
  h. scarring
  h. smooth muscle layer

hypertrophica
  acne h.

hypertrophicum
  eczema h.

hypertrophicus
  corneus h.
  lichen corneus h.
  lichen planus h.
  lupus erythematosus h.

hypertrophy
  gigantic h.

hyperuricemia

hypervascularity

hypervitaminosis
  h. A
  h. C
  h. D
  h. E

hypesthesia

hypesthetic

hypha *pl.* hyphae
  intrafollicular h.
  intrapilary h.

hyphal form

hyphidrosis

hypoalbuminemia

hypocatalasia

hypocellularity

hypochondriacal

hypochondriasis
    h. normocytic anemia

hypochromic anemia

hypochromotrichia

hypocoagulable state

hypocomplementemia

hypocomplementemic
    h. urticarial vasculitis
    h. vasculitis urticarial
        syndrome

hypocorticism

hypoderm

Hypoderma lineatum

hypodermatic

hypodermatitis
    sclerodermiformis

hypodermatomy

hypodermic
    h. needle

hypodermis

hypodermolithiasis

hypodermosis

hypodontia

hypofibrinogenemia

hypogammaglobinemia

hypogammaglobulinemia

hypogeusia

hypoglycemia

hypoglycemic agent

hypogonadism

hypogonadotropic

hypohidrosis

hypohidrotic
    h. ectodermal dysplasia

hypoidrosis

hypomelanism

hypomelanosis
    congenital circumscribed h.
    guttate h.
    hereditary h.
    idiopathic guttate h.
    h. of Ito

hypomelanotic macules

hyponychial

hyponychium

hyponychon

hypoparathyroidism

hypophysial cachexia

hypopigmentation
    postinflammatory h.

hypopigmented
    h. form
    h. hair
    h. lesions
    h. macular eruption
    h. macule
    h. sarcoidosis
    h. scar

hypopigmenter

hypoplasia
    cartilage-hair h.
    h. cutis congenita
    dermal h.
    focal dermal h.
    h. of hemidesmosomes

hypoplastic
    h. limbs
    h. lymphatics
    h. maxilla

hypoproteinemia

hypopyon
    h. iritis

hyporeactive

hyposensitivity

hyposensitization
    oral h.

hyposmia

hypospadias

hypostaticum
    ulcus h.

hypostome

hypotension

hypotensive agent

hypothalamic-pituitary-adrenal
    system

hypothenar eminence

hypothermia

hypothermic

hypothesis

hypothyroidism

hypotonia

hypotrichiasis

hypotrichosis
    h. congenita hereditaria of
        Marie Unna

hypovitaminosis
    h. A
    h. B

hypoxanthine-guanine
    h.-g.
        phosphoribosyltransferase
        (HGPRT)
    h.-g.
        phosphoribosyltransferase
        deficiency

hypoxemia

hypoxia

hypoxic vasoconstriction

Hyprogest injection

Hysone topical

hysterical
    h. edema
    h. reaction

hystrix
    ichthyismus h.
    ichthyosis h.

Hytone

Hyzine-50

HZ
    herpes zoster

I

I
    I pilus

iatrogenic
    i. calcinosis
    i. Cushing syndrome

IBIDS
    ichthyosis plus BIDS
        IBIDS syndrome

IC
    intercellular antibody

ICAM
    intercellular adhesion
        module

ICAM-1
    intercellular adhesion
        molecule-1

ICDRG
    International Contact
        Dermatitis Research
        Group

ice
    i. compress
    i. cube test positive
    dry i.

ice-pick type scar

ichthyismus
    i. exanthematicus
    i. hystrix

ichthyoid

ichthyosiform
    i. change
    i. dermatitis
    i. dermatosis
    i. erythroderma
    i. lesion
    i. sarcoidosis
    i. syndrome

ichthyosis
    acquired i.

ichthyosis (*continued*)
    autosomal dominant
        lamellar i.
    autosomal recessive i.
    i. bullosa of Siemens
    i. congenita
    congenital i.
    congenital erythrodermic i.
    i. congenital neonatorum
    i. cornea
    i. fetalis
    follicular i.
    i. follicularis
    harlequin i.
    i. hystrix
    i. intrauterina
    lamellar i.
    i. lethalis
    linear i.
    i. linearis circumflexa
    i. linguae
    nacreous i.
    nonbullous congenital
        erythrodermic i.
    i. palmaris
    i. palmaris et plantaris
    i. plantaris
    i. plus BIDS (IBIDS)
    recessive X-linked i.
    i. sauroderma
    i. scutulata
    i. sebacea
    i. sebacea cornea
    senile i.
    i. serpentina
    i. simplex
    i. spinosa
    i. syndrome
    i. uteri
    i. vulgaris
    X-linked i.

ichthyotic
    i. appearance
    i. disorders

icosahedral

icteric

icterohaemorrhagiae
  Leptospira i.

icteroid

icterus
  i. melas

id *(secondary skin eruption)*
  id reaction

ID
  infectious disease

I&D
  incision and drainage

idiopathic
  i. atrophoderma
  i. atrophoderma of Pasini
    and Pierini
  i. B-cell lymphoid
    hyperplasia
  i. calcinosis
  i. calcinosis cutis
  i. clubbing
  i. cold urticaria
  i. cutaneous small-vessel
    vasculitis
  i. eczematous disease
  i. form
  i. guttate hypomelanosis
  i. hirsutism
  i. hypereosinophilic
    syndrome (IHES)
  i. hypertrophic osteoarthritis
  i. late-onset eczema
  i. lichen planus
  i. livedo reticularis
  i. nodular vasculitis
  i. plantar hidradenitis
  i. roseola
  i. scrotal calcinosis
  i. shedding
  i. swelling
  i. thrombocytopenic
    purpura (ITP)
  i. urticaria
  i. uveitis

idiopathica
  livedo reticularis i.

idiosyncrasy

idiosyncratic
  i. drug reaction
  i. sensitivity

idiotype
  i. network

IDL
  intermediate-density
    lipoprotein

idoxuridine

idrosis

IDSA
  Infectious Disease Society
    of America

iduronate-2-sulfatase

iduronic acid

IF
  immunofluorescence
    direct IF
    indirect IF

IFAP
  ichthyosis follicularis,
    alopecia, and
    photophobia syndrome

IgA
  immunoglobulin A
    IgA antibody
    IgA antikeratinocyte
      cell
    IgA autoantibody
    IgA deficiency
    IgA deposits
    IgA dermatosis
    IgA immune complex
    IgA multiple myeloma
    IgA nephropathy
    IgA paraproteinemia
    IgA pemphigus
    serum IgA

IgE
    immunoglobulin E
        IgE antibody
        IgE-mediated
            hypersensitivity
        IgE radioallergosorbent
            test
        IgE receptor
        total serum IgE
IgG
    immunoglobulin G
        IgG anti-basement-
            zone antibody
        IgG antibody
        IgG anti-type-II-
            collagen antibody
        IgG autoantibody
        Candida albicans IgG
        IgG complex
        IgG lambda type
        IgG mediated humoral
        IgG myeloma protein
        IgG paraprotein
        IgG RF
        IgG subclass
            determination
        IgG subclass level
        IgG titer
IgM
    immunoglobulin M
        IgM gammopathy
        IgM isotope
        IgM kappa
        IgM mediated humoral
igne
    erythema ab i.
ignea
    zona i.
ignis
    sacer i.
IH
    impetigo herpetiformis
IL
    interleukin

IL-1-15
    interleukin-1-15
ileal disease
ileitis
    terminal i.
ileocolitis
ill-defined
illinition
illness
    environmental i.
    roseola-like i.
iloprost
Ilosone Oral
ILVEN
    inflamed linear verrucous
        epidermal nevus
imbedded
    i. ovipositor
    i. stinger
imbricata
    tinea i.
imbricated
I-Methasone
imidazole
    i. antifungal agent
    i. carboxamide
imipramine
imiquimod cream
immature
    i. granulocyte
    i. metabolic pathway
    i. myeloid cell
    i. pluripotential cell
immaturity
immediate
    i. allergy
    i. contagion
    i. hypersensitivity

immediate (*continued*)
  i. hypersensitivity reaction
  i. reaction
  i. skin reactivity
  i. tanning
  i.-type hypersensitivity
  i. urticarial wheal

immersion
  excessive water i.
  i. foot syndrome
  i. oil
  oil i.

immitis
  Coccidioides i.

immobilization

immobilize

immune
  i. complex
  i. complex deposition
  i. complex disease
  i. complex mediated
  i. complex reaction
  i. complex vasculitis
  i. dysregulation
  i. globulin, intramuscular
  i. globulin, intravenous
  i. granuloma formation
  i. modulators
  i. recognition
  i. response
  i. status
  i. system

immunifacient

immunity
  cell-mediated i. (CMI)

immunization
  passive i.

immunize

immunoblast

immunoblastic
  i. lymphoma

immunoblot

immunoblot (*continued*)
  i. technique

immunoblotting
  i. technique

immunochemical
  i. stain
  i. staining

immunocompetent
  i. cells
  i. host

immunocomplex

immunocompromised
  i. host
  i. patient

immunodeficiency
  i. disease
  i. with hypoparathyroidism

immunodeficient
  i. host

immunodermatology

immunodestruction

immunodiffusion (ID)
  single radial i. (SRID)
  i. test

immunoelectromicroscopy

immunoelectron
  microscope

immunofluorescence
  Izumi direct i.
  i. test

immunofluorescent
  i. mapping

immunogen

immunogenetics
  i. analysis
  i. study

immunogenic
  i. peptides

immunogenicity

immunoglobulin (Ig)
   i. fragment
   i. gene
   measles i.
   i. molecule
   i. production
   varicella-zoster i. (VZIG)

immunohistochemical
   i. analysis
   i. studies

immunohistochemistry

immunoincompetent
   i. host

immunologic
   i. complication
   i. contact urticaria
   i. defense
   i. developments
   i. disorder
   i. drug reaction
   i. feature
   i. high dose tolerance
   i. inflammatory disease
   i. mechanism
   i. response
   i. tolerance
   i. transformations
   i. urticaria

immunological
   i. competence
   i. deficiency

immunologically mediated

immunology

immunomodulator

immunopathogenesis

immunopathologic

immunopathology

immunoperoxidase
   i. stain test
   i. staining
   i. technique

immunophenotype

immunophenotypic
   i. markers
   i. profile
   i. property

immunophenotyping

immunoprecipitation

immunoreactant

immunoreactive

immunoregulation

immunosuppression

immunosuppressive
   i. agent
   i. drug
   i. epidermal cytokines
   i. medication
   i. state
   i. therapy

immunosurveillance

immunotherapy

immunotoxin

impaction

impaired barrier

impairment
   functional i.
   photosensitivity, ichthyosis,
     brittle hair, intellectual i.
   restrictive functional i.

Imperfecti
   Fungi I.

impermeable

impetigines (*plural of* impetigo)

impetiginization

impetiginize

impetiginous
   i. cheilitis
   i. syphilid

impetigo *pl.* impetigines
    Bockhart's i.
    i. bullosa
    bullous i.
    i. circinata
    i. contagiosa
    i. contagiosa bullosa
    i. contagiosa, small-vesicle
    i. contagiosa staphylogenes
    i. contagiosa streptogenes
    i. eczematodes
    follicular i.
    Fox i.
    i. furfuracea
    furfuraceous i.
    i. gestationis
    i. herpetiformis
    i. herpetiformis Hebra-Kaposi
    i. neonatorum
    nonbullous i.
    i. of Bockhart
    i. simplex
    i. staphylococcal i.
    i. staphylogenes
    streptococcal i.
    i. syphilitica
    i. variolosa
    i. vulgaris

implant
    bovine collagen dermal i.
    collagen i.

implantation cyst

importance
    allergic i.

Imuran

in
    i. noma ulcer
    i. situ hybridization
    i. situ squamous cell
      carcinoma
    i. toto

inactivate

inactivated
    i. serum

inactivation

inactivator
    anaphylatoxin i.

inanimate agents

incarnati
    pili i.

incarnatus
    unguis i.

incipient

incision
    elliptical i.

incisional biopsy

incisor

inclusion
    i. body
    i. body disease
    i. cyst
    i. dermoid cyst

incognito
    scabies i.
    tinea i.

incomplete
    i. neurofibromatosis

incontinence
    melanin i.
    melanin pigment i.
    i. of pigment

incontinentia
    i. pigmenti
    i. pigmenti achromians

incrustation

incubation
    i. period

incubative stage

incubatory carrier

Inderal

indeterminate
    i. cell histiocytosis

indeterminate (*continued*)
    i. disease
    i. leprosy

index *pl.* indices, indexes
    i. cases
    endemic i.
    phagocytic i.
    volume thickness i. (VTI)

India
    I. ink
    I. ink stain
    I.-rubber skin

indican

indicanidrosis

indices (*plural of* index)

indifference to pain

indigenous

indigo

indinavir
    i. sulfate

indirect
    i. assays
    i. fluorescent antibody test
    i. fluorescent test
    i. hemagglutination test
    i. hyperbilirubinemia
    i. immunofluorescence
    i. lymphography

indolent
    i. disorder
    i. lesion
    i. nonpitting edema
    i. papule
    i. ulcer

indomethacin

inducible skin color

induction period

indurata
    acne i.
    tuberculosis cutis i.

indurated
    i. area
    i. border
    i. cellulites
    i. lymphangitis
    i. papule
    i. plaque
    i. wart
    i. welt

induration
    brawny i.
    i. of skin
    phlebitic i.

induratio plastica penis

indurativa
    tuberculosis cutis i.

induratum
    erythema i.

industrial hyperpigmentation

inelastic

inertial
    i. suction sampler

infancy
    acropustulosis of i.
    capillary hemangioma of i.

infantile
    i. acropustulosis
    i. acute hemorrhagic
      edema of the skin
    i. atopic dermatitis
    i. digital fibroma
    i. digital fibromatosis
    i. digital myofibroblastoma
    i. disease
    i. eczema
    i. fibromatosis
    i. hemangioma
    i. seborrheic dermatitis
    i. macrostomia
    i. mucocutaneous
      leishmaniasis
    i. myofibromatosis
    i. neuroblastoma

infantile (*continued*)
    i. purulent conjunctivitis
    i. tumor
    i. zoster

infantilis
    prurigo i.
    roseola i.

infantilism

infant's sera

infantum
    acrodermatitis papulosa i.
    dermatitis exfoliativa i.
    dermatitis gangrenosa i.
    granuloma gluteale i.
    lichen i.
    roseola i.

infarctive
    i. lesion

infect

infected
    i. aneurysm
    i. vascular gangrene

infecting
    i. dose (ID)
    i. micro-organism

infection
    atypical mycobacterial i.
    bacterial i.
    Candida i.
    candidal i.
    chlamydial i.
    cryptogenic i.
    dermatophyte fungal i.
    fungal i.
    fungous i.
    herpes simplex i.
    herpes zoster i.
    herpetic i.
    mixed nail i.
    mycobacterial i.
    necrotizing i.
    nondermatophyte fungal i.
    opportunistic i.

infection (*continued*)
    opportunistic systemic
      fungal i.
    primary herpes simplex i.
    pyodermatous i.
    pyogenic i.
    recurrent i.
    scalp i.
    subcutaneous fungal i.
    subcutaneous necrotizing i.
    superficial i.
    sycosiform fungous i.
    systemic fungal i.
    vaccinia i.
    varicella-zoster i.
    vesicular viral i.
    yeast i.
    zoonotic i.

infectiosity

infectiosum
    ecthyma i.
    erythema i. (EI)

infectious
    i. eczematoid dermatitis
    i. enteritis
    i. erythema
    i. granuloma
    i. labial dermatitis
    i. mononucleosis
    i. neutrophilic hidradenitis
    i. wart

Infectious Disease Society of
  America (IDSA)

infectiousness

infective

infectivity

infertility

infest

infestation
    environmental mite i.
    louse i.
    mite i.

infiltrate
bandlike i.
granulomatous dermal i.
inflammatory i.
lymphocytic i.
lymphoid i.
patchy i.

infiltrated
i. patch
i. plaque

infiltration
adipose i.
cellular i.
inflammatory i.
lymphocytic i. of skin

infiltrative basal cell carcinoma

inflame

inflamed
i. linear verrucous
epidermal nevus (ILVEN)
i. scalp
i. ulcer

inflammation
acute i. (AI)
allergic i.
chronic i. (CI)
diffuse i.
focal i.
immune i.
interstitial i.
mucosal i.
perifollicular i.
i. reaction

inflammatory
i. acneiform pustule
i. acquired oral
hyperpigmentation
i. areolae
i. bowel disease (IBD)
i. bowel syndrome (IBS)
i. carcinoma
i. cell
i. conditions
i. dermatosis

inflammatory (*continued*)
i. dermatosis of pregnancy
i. disease
i. edema
i. eicosanoid generation
i. encystment
i. factor of anaphylaxis
(IF-A)
i. infiltrate
i. linear verrucous
epidermal nevus
i. lymphedema
i. mediator
i. melanoma
i. panniculitis
i. plaque
i. proximal myopathy
i. response
i. rosacea
i. tinea capitis
i. ulcer

infolded

inframammary
i. fold
i. region

infriction

infundibular
i. cystic structure
i. formation
i. level

infundibulofolliculitis
disseminated recurrent i.
recurrent i.

infundibulum

ingrowing
i. hair
i. nail

ingrown
i. hair
i. nail

inguinal
i. adenitis

inguinale

inguinale (*continued*)
    Epidermophyton i.
    granuloma i.
    lymphogranuloma i.

inguinalis
    tinea i.

inhalant

inherited
    i. epidermolysis bullosa
    i. pattern lentiginosis
    i. platelet function defect

initial
    i. clinical lesion
    i. episode
    i. exposure
    i. lesion

injectable

injection
    i. site reaction

injury
    thermal i.

innate immunity

inner
    i. canthus
    i. root sheath

innervation

innocuous
    i. stimuli

inoculability

inoculable

inoculate

inoculating

inoculation
    i. cutaneous
      tuberculosis

inoculum

inorganic
    i. arsenic
    i. arsenic poisoning

inscrutable

insect
    i. bite
    i. bite reaction
    biting i.
    i. sting
    i. sting kit
    i. vector
    i. virus

Insecta

insecticide

insensible perspiration

insensitive sweat

insidious
    i. lesion
    i. onset

in situ hybridization technique

inspissated
    i. material
    i. sebum
    i. serum

insula

insulin
    i. resistance
    i. skin test
    i./steroid lipodystrophy

insulinopenic form

insusceptibility

integrin
    i. expression
    i. molecules

integument
    common i.

integumentary
    i. system

integumentum
    i. commune

interaction

intercellular

intercellular (*continued*)
    i. attachment (ICAM-1)
    i. bridge
    i. cement
    i. contacts
    i. edema
    i. epidermal edema
    i. fluid
    i. IgG
    i. serum
    i. viruses

interconnecting sinuses

intercrural
    i. fold

interdental
    i. papilla

interdigital
    i. maceration

interdigitalis
    erosio i. blastomycetica

interdigitating
    i. follicular cells
    i. reticular cells

interdigit

interface
    i. dermatitis
    dermoepidermal i.

interferon (IFN)
    i. alfa (IFN-*a*)
    i. alfa-2a
    i. alfa-2b
    i. alfa polychemotherapy
    i.-beta (IFN-ß)
    gamma i.
    i. gamma (IFN-γ)

interfibrillary
    i. matrix

intergluteal
    i. area
    i. cleft

interleukin (IL) (*specific interleukins are designated by an Arabic numeral, as interleukin-1, interleukin-2, IL-1, IL-2*)

intermediate
    i. carcinoma
    i. filaments
    i. leprosy

intermetacarpal

intermingled
    i. petechiae
    i. scarring

intermittent
    i. hydrarthrosis

intermixed

internal
    i. hair apparatus
    i. malignancy

International
    I. Contact Dermatitis
       Research Group (ICDRG)

internum
    erysipelas i.

interpalpebral fissure

interpapillary ridges

interphalangeal
    i. articulation
    distal i. (DIP)
    i. joint
    proximal i. (PIP)

interplant

interplanting

interpretation
    patch test i.

intersectio

interspace

interspecific graft

interstitial
    i. calcinosis
    i. hemorrhage

interstitial (*continued*)
  i. keratitis
  i. mucin
  i. pattern

intertrigines (*plural of* intertrigo)

intertriginous
  i. area
  i. psoriasis
  i. region
  i. spaces
  i. weeping eruption

intertrigo *pl.* intertrigines
  Candida i.
  diaper rash i.
  eczema i.
  erythema i.
  i. labialis
  i. saccharomycetica
  i. with ulceration

intertwined

interwoven

intestinal
  i. amebiasis
  i. parasite
  i. polyposis
  i. virus

intimitis
  proliferative i.

intolerance
  drug i.

intoxication
  anaphylactic i.
  bromide i.
  metal i.

intra-abdominal

intra-articular (IA)
  i.-a. hemorrhage

intracellular
  i. antigens
  i. diplococci
  i. edema
  i. hyaline globules

intracerebral
  i. calcification

intracranial
  i. arteriovenous aneurysm
  i. communication
  i. hemorrhage
  i. mass
  i. meningioma

intractable
  i. pyoderma

intracutaneous
  i. deposition
  i. nevus
  i. reaction

intracytoplasmic
  i. eosinophilic granules

intradermal
  i. anesthetic
  i. eccrine ducts
  i. melanocyte
  i. nevus
  i. reaction
  i. skin test
  i. skin testing
  i. test
  i. test concentration
  i. wheal

intraepidermal
  i. abscess
  i. acanthoma
  i. basal cell carcinoma
  i. basal cell epithelioma of
    Borst-Jadassohn
  i. bulla
  i. carcinoma
  i. epithelioma
  i. epithelioma of
    Judassohn
  i. form
  i. inflammatory cell
  i. keratin-filled space
  i. lacunae
  i. microabscess
  i. microabscess of psoriasis
  i. nest

intraepidermal (*continued*)
 i. neutrophilic IgA
    dermatosis
 i. nevus
 i. pustules
 i. spongiform pustules
 i. squamous cell carcinoma
 i. vesicle formation
 i. vesicles
 i. vesiculation

intraepithelial
 i. growth
 i. spongiform pustule
 i. vesicle

intrafollicular
 i. abscess
 i. androstenedione
 i. hyphae
 i. mucin deposition

intrahepatic
 i. bile ductular atresia
 i. cholestasis of pregnancy

intralesional
 i. corticosteroid injection
 i. cytotoxic agents
 i. emetine hydrochloride
 i. infection
 i. injection
 i. sodium stibogluconate
    antimony
 i. steroid
 i. therapy
 i. tumor necrosis
 i. vinblastine

Intralipid

intraluminal
 i. deposit
 i. papillary endothelial
    proliferation

intramuscular
 i. hemorrhage
 i. injection
 i. iron dextran complex
 i. tobramycin

intranasal
 i. foreign body
 i. pyogenic infection

intranuclear
 i. inclusions
 i. viral particles

intraoperative
 i. bleeding
 i. hemostasis
 i. lymphatic mapping

intraoral
 i. candidiasis
 i. squamous cell carcinoma

intraosseous
 i. disease
 i. epidermoid cyst

intrathoracic
 i. lesion

intratumoral
 i. chemotherapy with
    fluorouracil/epinephrine
 i. hemorrhage
 intrauterine ichthyosis i.

intraurethral
 i. condylomata

intrauterine
 i. anemia
 i. herpes simplex
 i. infection
 i. viral infection

intravascular
 i. fibrinolytic activity
 i. large B-cell lymphoma
 i. lymphoma
 i. papillary endothelial
    hyperplasia
 i. papillary proliferation
 i. thrombosis
 i. thrombotic disorder

intravenous
 i. anti-D
 i. contrast material
 i. drug abuse

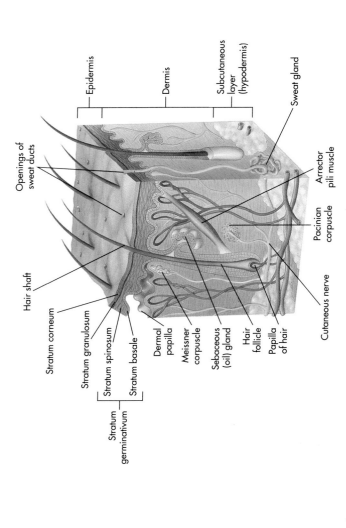

Microscopic diagram of the skin. The epidermis, shown in longitudinal section, is raised at one corner to reveal the ridges in the dermis. (From Thibodeau GA, Patton KT: Anatomy & Physiology, ed 4. St. Louis, 1999, Mosby.)

Epidermis

Dermis

Subcutaneous layer (hypodermis)

Sweat gland

Openings of sweat ducts

Arrector pili muscle

Pacinian corpuscle

Cutaneous nerve

Hair shaft

Stratum corneum

Stratum granulosum

Stratum spinosum

Stratum basale

Stratum germinativum

Dermal papilla

Meissner corpuscle

Sebaceous (oil) gland

Hair follicle

Papilla of hair

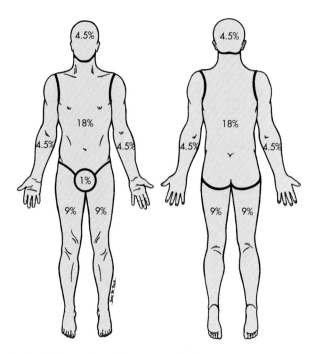

"Rule of nines." "Rule of nines" is one method to estimate amount of skin surface burned in an adult. (From Thibodeau GA, Patton KT: Anatomy & Physiology, ed 4. St. Louis, 1999, Mosby.)

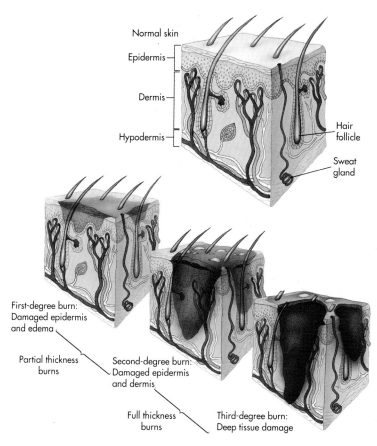

Normal skin

Epidermis

Dermis

Hypodermis

Hair follicle

Sweat gland

First-degree burn:
Damaged epidermis
and edema

Partial thickness
burns

Second-degree burn:
Damaged epidermis
and dermis

Full thickness
burns

Third-degree burn:
Deep tissue damage

Classification of burns. (From Thibodeau GA, Patton KT: Anatomy & Physiology, ed 4. St. Louis, 1999, Mosby.)

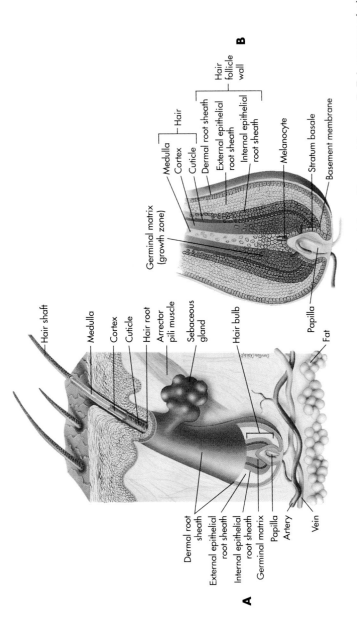

Hair follicle. **A,** Relationship of a hair follicle and related structures to the epidermal and dermal layers of the skin. **B,** Enlargement of a hair follicle wall and hair bulb. (From Thibodeau GA, Patton KT: Anatomy & Physiology, ed 4. St. Louis, 1999, Mosby.)

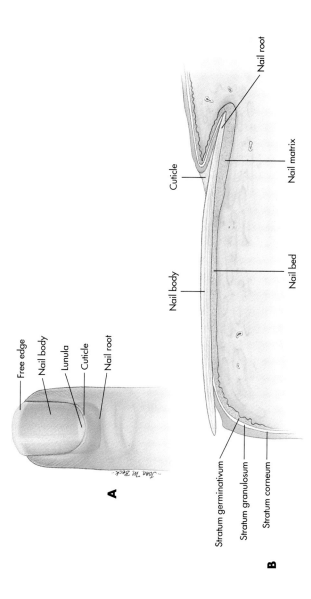

Structure of nails. **A,** Fingernail viewed from above. **B,** Sagittal section of fingernail and associated structures. (From Thibodeau GA, Patton KT: Anatomy & Physiology, ed 4. St. Louis, 1999, Mosby.)

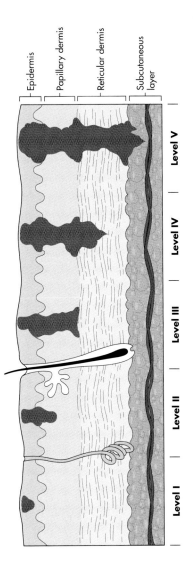

Staging of melanoma by depth of invasion (Clark levels). A progressively worse prognosis is associated with increasing invasion of the dermis and subcutaneous layers of the skin. (From Chabner DE: The language of medicine, ed 6. Philadelphia, 2001, WB Saunders.)

Epidermis

Papillary dermis

Reticular dermis

Subcutaneous layer

Level I   Level II   Level III   Level IV   Level V

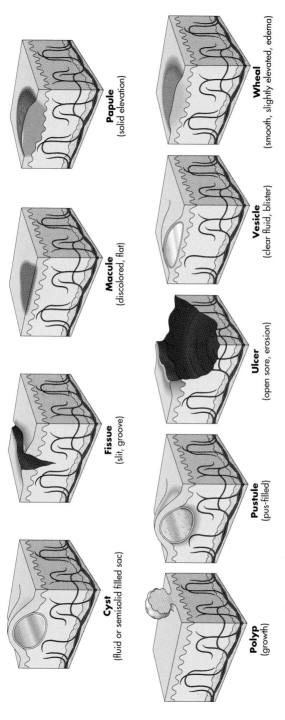

Cutaneous lesions. (From Chabner DE: The language of medicine, ed 6. Philadelphia, 2001, WB Saunders.)

Papule
(solid elevation)

Macule
(discolored, flat)

Fissue
(slit, groove)

Cyst
(fluid or semisolid filled sac)

Wheal
(smooth, slightly elevated, edema)

Vesicle
(clear fluid, blister)

Ulcer
(open sore, erosion)

Pustule
(pus-filled)

Polyp
(growth)

intravenous (*continued*)
    i. gamma globulin
    i. infusion
    i. lipid therapy

Intravenous
    Fungizone I.

intrinsic
    i. coagulation system
    i. factor
    i. melanin-like pigmentation

intromission

Intron A

intubation

intussusception

inunct

inunction

inundation fever

invaccination

invaginata
    trichorrhexis i.

invaginate

invagination

invasion
    bacterial i.

invasive
    i. aspergillosis
    i. candidiasis
    i. squamous cell carcinoma

inversa
    acne i.

inverse
    i. anaphylaxis
    i. distribution
    i. psoriasis

inverted follicular keratosis

inveterata
    i. patch
    psoriasis i.

involucrum

involute

involuting flat hemangioma

involution

involvement
    skin i.

ioderma

Iodex Regular

iodica
    purpura i.

iodide
    i. acne

iodine

iodochlorhydroxyquin

iododerma

iodoform
    i. gauze

iodoquinol
    i. and hydrocortisone

ion
    i. exchange resin

ionization

ionizing
    i. electromagnetic energy
    i. radiation
    i. radiation therapy

ionotherapy

iontophoresis medium

IPD
    immediate pigment
      darkening

ipsilateral
    i. focal paralysis
    i. limb hypoplasia
    i. lipodermoids
    i. poliosis
    i. port-wine stain
    i. vitiligo

irides

iridocyclitis
    acute diffuse i.

iris
    erythema i.
    herpes i.
    i. lesion
    lichen i.
    i. pearls

iritis
    chronic granulomatous i.

iron
    i. chelation
    i. deficiency
    i. deposition

irradiate

irradiation
    therapeutic i.
    i. therapy

irregular
    i. acanthosis
    i. border
    i. menses
    i. undulation

irritability

irritable

irritant
    i. contact dermatitis
    i. contact urticaria
    i. hand dermatitis
    mild i.
    i. patch-test reaction
    i. patch-test response
    primary i.

irritate

irritation
    i. fibroma

irritative

ischemia

ischemic

ischemic (*continued*)
    i. necrosis
    i. pallor
    i. ulcer

ischidrosis

island disease

isoamyl methoxycinnamate

Isocaine HCl injection

isoconazole

isodesmosine

Isodine

isoenzyme
    i. electrophoresis

isoeugenol

isogeneic
    i. graft

isograft

isohemagglutinin antibodies

isohemagglutination

isolated
    i. collagenoma
    i. dyskeratosis follicularis
    i. elastomas
    i. IgA deficiency
    i. limb perfusion
    i. primary IgM deficiency

isologous
    i. graft

Isometrus maculatus

isomorphic
    i. effect
    i. phenomenon
    i. response

isoniazid

isoplastic
    i. graft

isopropyl alcohol

isosporiasis

isotope
    radioactive i.

isotopic lymphoscintigraphy

isotransplantation

isotretinoin
    i. therapy

isotype

isradipine

isthmus

itch
    Absorbine Jock I.
    azo i.
    bakers' i.
    barbers' i.
    barn i.
    bath i.
    Boeck i.
    clamdigger's i.
    coolie i.
    copra i.
    Cortef Feminine I.
    Cuban i.
    dew i.
    dhobie i.
    dhobie mark i.
    frost i.
    grain i.
    grocers' i.
    ground i.
    jock i.
    jock strap i.
    kabure i.
    lumberman's i.
    mad i.
    Malabar i.
    i. mite
    Moeller i.
    Norway i.
    poultryman's i.
    prairie i.
    rice i.
    Saint Ignatius i.
    seven-year i.

itch (*continued*)
    straw i.
    summer i.
    swamp i.
    swimmers' i.
    i. threshold
    toe i.
    warehouseman's i.
    washerwoman's i.
    water i.
    winter i.

itching
    i. purpura

itchy
    i. red bump disease

Ito
    hypomelanosis of I.
    nevus of I.
    I's nevus

itraconazole

ivermectin

IVGG
    intravenous gamma
        globulin

IVIG
    intravenous immune serum
        globulin

ivy
    poison i.

Ixodes
    I. cookie
    I. dammini
    I. pacificus
    I. persulcatus
    I. ricinus
    I. scapularis
    I. spinipalpis

ixodiasis

ixodic

ixodid
    i. ticks

Ixodidae

J

jacket
  yellow i.

Jackson-Sertoli syndrome

Jacob
  J. ulcer

Jacquet
  J's dermatitis
  J's erythema

Jadassohn
  anetoderma of J.
  J. anetoderma
  J. disease
  J. epithelioma
  J. nevus
  nevus sebaceus of J.
  J. sebaceous nevus
  J. test
  J.-Lewandowski law
  J.-Lewandowski syndrome
  J.-Pellizzari anetoderma
  J.-Tièche nevus

Jadelot
  J. furrows
  J. lines

Janeway
  J's lesion
  J's spots

Japanese
  J. lacquer tree
  J. river fever

Jarisch-Herxheimer reaction

jaundice

jaw cyst

JCML
  juvenile chronic
    myelogenous leukemia

JDMS
  juvenile dermatomyositis

JDMS/PM

JDMS/PM (*continued*)
  juvenile
    dermato/polymyositis

Jeanselme nodule

jeanselmei
  Exophiala *j.*

JEB
  junctional epidermolysis
    bullosa

jejunal
  j. mucosa

jejunoileal
  j. bypass

jelly
  mineral j.
  petroleum j.
  Vaseline petroleum j.

jellyfish
  j. dermatitis
  thimble j.

Jenamicin injection

Jessner
  lymphocytic infiltrate of J.
  J's lymphocytic infiltration
  J's solution
  J.-Kanof disease

jigger

Job's syndrome

jock
  j. itch
  j. strap itch

Johnson's Ultra Sensitive Baby
  Shampoo

Johnson-Stevens disease

joint
  Charcot j.
  Clutton's j.
  syphilitic j.

jojoba
  j. oil

Jones-Mote reaction

Jonston
  J. alopecia
  J. area

JRA
  juvenile rheumatoid
    arthritis
  JRA rash

juccuya

junction
  dermoepidermal j.
  gap j.
  mucocutaneous j.
  j. nevus

junctional
  j. epidermolysis bullosa
    (JEB)
  j. epidermolysis bullosa
    with pyloric atresia
  j. nevus
  j. proliferation

jungle
  j. rot

Juniperus

juvenile
  j. aponeurotic fibroma
  j. cataracts
  j. chronic myelogenous
    leukemia

juvenile (*continued*)
  j. dermatomyositis (JDMS)
  j. dermato/polymyositis
    (JDMS/PM)
  j. elastoma
  j. gout
  j. hyalin fibromatosis
  j. lentigo melanoma
  j. melanoma
  j. Niemann-Pick disease
  j. palmo-plantar
    fibromatosis
  j. papillomatosis
  j. pityriasis rubra pilaris
  j. plantar dermatosis
  j. posterior subcapsular
    lenticular opacity
  j. rheumatoid arthritis
    (JRA)
  j. spring eruption
  j. xanthogranuloma
  j. xanthogranuloma
    histiocytosis

juveniles
  verrucae planae j.

juvenilis
  verruca plana j.

juxta-articular
  j. node
  j. nodule

juxtacrine

JXG
  juvenile xanthogranuloma

K

kabure
    k. itch

Kaffir pox

kala azar

Kalcinate

Kalischer
    K. disease

kallak

Kaltostat alginate dressing

kanamycin
    k. sulfate

Kandahar sore

kangaroo tick

Kanzaki's disease

Kapetanakis type

Kaposi
    K's disease
    K's hemorrhagic sarcoma
    K's sarcoma (KS)
    K's varicelliform eruption
    K's xeroderma

kappa light chain

karaya

karyolysis

karyolytic

karyorrhexis

Kasabach-Merritt
    K.-M. syndrome
    K.-M. phenomenon

Katayama fever

Kathon CG

Kawasaki
    K's disease (KD)
    K's syndrome

Kayser-Fleischer ring

ked
    k. itch
    sheep k.

kedani fever

Keflex

Kefzol

Keller ultraviolet test

Kelly's medium

keloid
    acne k.
    Addison k.
    k. formation

keloidal
    k. basal cell carcinoma
    k. blastomycosis
    k. folliculitis
    k. papule
    k. plaque
    k. scarring
    k. type scar

keloidalis
    acne k.
    folliculitis k.

keloidosis

Kenacort
    K. syrup
    K. tablet

Kenalog
    K. injection
    K. in Orabase
    K.-10
    K.-40

Kenonel

Kentucky coffee tree

Keralyt Gel

keratiasis

keratic

keratin
    alpha k.
    k. complex
    k. cyst
    k. damp
    k. fibrils
    k. filaments
    k. gene mutations
    hard k.
    nail k.
    k. plug
    k. polypeptides
    soft k.
    k. sulfate

keratinase

keratinization
    central k.
    ectopic k.
    faulty k.
    premature k.

keratinize

keratinized
    k. epidermal cells
    k. lining
    k. mucosa
    k. squamous epithelium

keratinocyte
    activated k.
    basal k.
    dyskeratotic k.
    epidermal k.
    k. hyperproliferation
    k. necrosis
    necrotic k.

keratinocytic adhesion

keratinosome

keratinous
    k. cyst
    k. debris
    k. mass
    k. material
    k. sheet
    k. sleeve

keratitis
    amebic k.
    epithelial k.
    filamentary k.
    herpetic k.
    interstitial k.
    nonsyphilitic interstitial k.
    k. rubra figurata

keratitis-ichthyosis-deafness
  (KID)

keratoacanthoma
    k. centrifugum
    k. centrifugum marginatum
    k. dyskeratoticum et
      segregans
    eruptive k.
    giant k.
    multiple k.
    solitary k.
    subungual k.

keratoatrophoderma

keratoconjunctivitis
    epidemic k.
    herpetic k.
    k. sicca
    vernal k.
    virus k.

keratoconus

keratoderma
    k. blennorrhagica
    k. blennorrhagicum
    k. climacteria
    k. climactericum
    k. disseminatum palmare et
      plantare
    k. eccentrica
    k. eccentricum
    epidermolytic palmoplantar
      k.
    glucan-induced k.
    lymphedematous k.
    mutilating k.
    k. palmare et plantare
    palmoplantar k. (PPK)

keratoderma (*continued*)
  palmoplantar k., diffuse
  plantar k.
  k. plantare sulcatum
  k. punctata
  punctate k.
  punctate porokeratotic k.
  k. punctatum
  senile k.
  k. symmetrica
  symmetric k.
  Unna-Thost k.
  Vorner variant of Unna-
    Thost k.

keratodermatitis

keratodermia

keratodermic sandal

keratodes
  erythema k.

keratoelastoidosis
  k. marginalis
  k. verrucosa

keratogenesis

keratogenetic

keratogenous
  k. zone

keratohyalin

keratohyaline
  k. granules

keratoid
  k. exanthema

keratolysis
  k. exfoliativa
  k. exfoliativa areata
    manuum
  k. neonatorum
  pitted k.
  k. plantare sulcatum

keratolytics (*class of drugs*)

keratoma
  k. diffusum

keratoma (*continued*)
  k. disseminatum
  k. hereditaria mutilans
  k. hereditarium mutilans
  k. hereditarium dissipatum
    palmare et plantare
  k. malignum
  k. malignum congenitale
  k. palmare et plantare
  k. plantare sulcatum
  k. senile
  senile k.

keratomalacia

keratomata

keratomycosis
  k. linguae
  k. nigricans

keratonosis

keratopachyderma

keratoplastic

keratosa
  acne k.

keratose

keratosis *pl.* keratoses
  k. actinica
  actinic k.
  arsenic k.
  arsenical k.
  aural k.
  k. blennorrhagica
  k. climactericum
  k. diffusa fetalis
  follicular k.
  k. follicularis
  k. follicularis contagiosa
  k. follicularis spinulosa
    decalvans
  gonorrheal k.
  inverted follicular k.
  k. labialis
  lichenoid k.
  k. lichenoides chronica
  lichen planus–like k.

keratosis (*continued*)
  nevoid k.
  nevus follicularis k.
  k. nigricans
  k. obliterans
  oral k.
  k. palmaris et plantaris
  k. palmaris et plantaris of
    the Meleda type
  k. palmaris et plantaris of
    Unna-Thost
  k. palmoplantaris
  k. palmoplantaris
    disseminata
  k. palmoplantaris punctata
  k. pilaris
  k. pilaris atrophicans
  k. pilaris atrophicans faciei
  k. pilaris follicularis
    spinulosa decalvans
  k. pilaris rubra
  k. pilaris rubra atrophicans
    faciei
  k. pilaris rubra congenita
  k. punctata
  k. punctata of the creases
  k. punctata of the palmar
    creases
  k. punctata palmaris et
    plantaris
  roentgen k.
  k. rubra figurata
  seborrheic k.
  k. seborrheica
  senile k.
  k. senilis
  solar k.
  k. solaris
  k. spinulosa
  stucco k.
  k. suprafollicularis
  tar k.
  k. universalis congenita
  k. vegetans
keratotic
  k. angioma
  k. deposits

keratotic (*continued*)
  k. material
  k. papule
  k. pits of the palmar
    creases
  k. plug
  k. scabies
  k. wall

Keri moisturizer

kerion
  k. celsi
  Celsus k.
  tinea k.

kerionic

kernicterus

keroid

kerotherapy

ketoacidosis

ketoconazole

ketotifen

Ketron-Goodman disease

Kettle's syndrome

Key-Pred
  K.-P. injection
  K.-P.-SP injection

KFSD
  keratosis follicularis
    spinulosa decalvans

KHE
  kaposiform
    hemangioendothelioma

KID
  keratitis-ichthyosis-deafness
  KID syndrome

kidney transplantation

Kienböck-Adamson points

killer
  k. cell (K cell)

killer (*continued*)
  natural k. (NK)

Kimura's disease

kinetoplast

kinin peptide

kininase II

kinky
  k. hair
  k. hair disease
  k. hair syndrome

kissing
  k. bug
  k. lesion

Kitamura's reticulate
  acropigmentation

Klauder
  K. syndrome

Klebsiella
  K. pneumoniae

Klein-Waardenburg syndrome

Kligman
  K's combination
  K's formula

Klinefelter's syndrome

Klippel
  K.-Feil syndrome
  K.-Trenaunay syndrome
  K.-Trenaunay-Weber
    syndrome

Knapp
  K's streaks
  K's striae

knife
  chalazion k.

knob
  surfers' k.

knobby skin

knock knee

knot
  surfers' k.

knotted hair

knuckle pad
  false k. p.

Köbberling
  K.-Duncan disease
  K.-Dunnigan syndrome

Köbner (Koebner)
  K. disease
  K. effect
  K. epidermolysis bullosa
  K. phenomenon
  K. reaction

Koch
  K's bacillus
  K's postulate

Koebner (*see* Köbner)

Kocnen's tumor

Kogoj
  K's pustule
  spongiform pustule of K.

KOH
  potassium chloride
    KOH examination
    KOH preparation
    KOH stain

Kohlmeier-Degos syndrome

Kohn pore

koilocytosis

koilonychia

Kondoleon operation

Koplik's spots

Korean yellow moth
  dermatitis

kra-kra (*variant of* craw-craw)

kraurosis
  k. penis
  k. vulvae

Krazy Glue

krusei

krusei (*continued*)
    Candida k.

KS
    Kaposi sarcoma

KTP
    potassium titanyl phosphate
        crystal

Kupffer's cells

kuru

Kurunegala ulcer

Kveim
    K. antigen
    K. reaction
    K. test

Kveim (*continued*)
    K.-Siltzbach antigen
    K.-Siltzbach test

kwashiorkor
    marasmic k.
    k. red children

Kwell
    K. Cream
    K. Lotion
    K. Shampoo

kynurenine
    k.-niacin pathway

kyphoscoliosis

Kyrle's disease

L

LA
    long acting
    lupus anticoagulant

"la bonita" type

Laband syndrome

labia
    l. majora
    l. minora

labial
    l. commissure
    l. fistula
    l. fusion
    l. herpes simplex virus
    l. melanotic macule
    l. stenosis

labialis
    herpes l.
    keratosis l.
    myxadenitis l.

labioalveolar
    l. surface

labium

laboratory
    Medical Research Council
        L's (MRCL)
    l. parameters
    Venereal Disease Research
        L. (VDRL)
    l. vortex vibration

lacerate

lacerated

laceration

Lac-Hydrin
    L.-H. Five

lacrimal
    l. glands
    l. puncta

lacrimation

lacrimator

lactic
    l. acid
    l. acidosis
    l. acid with ammonium
        hydroxide
    l. dehydrogenase

LactiCare
    L.-HC

lactose

lacuna

lacunae
    osteocyte l.

lacunula *pl.* lacunulae

lacunule

LAD
    leukocyte adhesion
        deficiency

lady slipper

Lafora
    L's disease
    L's sign

Lahore sore

LAK
    lymphokine-activated killer
        cell

lake
    venous l.

lakes of pus

LAMB
    lentigines, atrial myxoma,
        mucocutaneous
        myxomas, and blue
        nevi
    LAMB syndrome

lambda
    l. chain
    l. light chain

lame foliacée

mella *pl.* lamellae
   cornoid l.

lamellar
   l. calcification of the falx
     cerebri
   l. congenital ichthyosiform
     erythroderma
   l. desquamation of the
     newborn
   l. dominant
   l. dyshidrosis
   l. exfoliation of the
     newborn
   l. granule
   l. ichthyosis
   l. plates
   l. scale

lamelliform

lamin

lamina *pl.* laminae
   foliate l.
   l. lucida
   l. lucida deposit

laminar

laminated
   l. epithelial plug
   l. scales

lamination

Lamisil
   L. topical

lamp
   black light fluorescent l.
   black ray l.
   carbon arc l.
   cold quartz l.
   fluorescent sun l.
   germicidal l.
   heat l.
   high pressure mercury arc l.
   hot quartz l.
   Kromayer's l.
   low pressure mercury arc l.
   mercury arc l.

lamp (*continued*)
   mercury vapor l.
   quartz l.
   quartz-iodine l.
   sun l.
   ultraviolet l.
   Wood's l.
   xenon arc l.

Lamprene

Lanacort

Lanaphilic topical

lancet
   acne l.

lancinating

Landouzy
   L. disease
   L. purpura

Landry-Guillain-Barré syndrome

Landschutz tumor

Lane's disease

Langer's lines

Langerhans
   L's cell
   L's granules
   L's islets
   L's layer
   L's stria

Langhans'
   L's cell
   L's layer

langue au chat

lanolin, cetyl alcohol, glycerin,
   and petrolatum

lanosum
   Microsporum l.

lanuginosa
   acquired hypertrichosis l.
   hypertrichosis l.

lanuginous

lanugo
l. hair

Lanvisone topical

larbish

large
l. cell histiocytic lymphoma
l. cell lymphoma
l. vessel vasculitis
l. scars

large-plaque parapsoriasis

largish extravasation

larva *pl.* larvae
l. currens
cutaneous l. migrans
l. migrans
l. migrans cutanea
l. migrans, cutaneous
l. migrans profundus

larval

Larrea tridentata

laryngeal
l. edema
l. papillomatosis
l. webs

laryngospasm

Lasan

laser
l. ablation
l. beam
CO_2 l.
l. Doppler velocimetry
l. hair removal
l. therapy

Lassar
L. betanaphthol paste
L. plain zinc paste

lassitude

lata
condylomata l.
fascia l.

late
l. benign syphilis
l. latent syphilis
l. onset
l. onset neurofibromatosis
l. onset prurigo of
pregnancy
l. phase allergic reaction
l. reaction
l. reaction of Mitsuda

latency
l. period

latens
scarlatina l.

latent
l. allergy
l. infection
l. microbism
l. period
l. rat virus
l. stage
l. syphilis

lateral
l. margin
l. nail fold

lateralis
nevus unius l.
onychia l.

lateris
nevus unius l.

latex
l. agglutination test
l. particle agglutination

latrodectism

Latrodectus
L. mactans
L. mactans antivenom
L. mactans bite

lattice
l. fibers
l.-like pattern

latum

latum (*continued*)
    condyloma l.

Laugier-Hunziger syndrome

Launois-Bensaude
  lipomatosis

Lauth violet

law
    Jadassohn-Lewandowsky l.

lax

laxa
    cutis l.

layer
    basal l.
    basal l. of endometrium
    basal l. of epidermis
    basal cell l.
    clear l. of epidermis
    germinative l.
    germinative l. of epidermis
    germinative l. of nail
    granular cell l.
    granular l. of epidermis
    Henle's l.
    horny l.
    horny l. of epidermis
    horny l. of nail
    horny cell l.
    Huxley's l.
    Langhans l.
    malpighian l.
    membranous l. of
      subcutaneous tissue
    mucous l.
    palisade l.
    papillary l. of corium
    papillary l. of dermis
    prickle cell l.
    reticular l. of corium
    reticular l. of dermis
    spinous l.
    spinous l. of epidermis
    squamous cell l.
    surface l.

lazarine leprosy

lazy-S pattern

LBT
    lupus band test

LCD
    liquor carbonis detergens

LCV
    leukocytoclastic vasculitis

LDL
    low-density lipoprotein

LE
    lupus erythematosus
      LE cell
      discoid LE
      LE factor
      LE phenomenon

lead
    l. poisoning
    l. stomatitis

leaflike
    l. flakes
    l. scaling

leafy liverwort

leakage
    vascular l.

Ledderhose
    L's disease
    L's syndrome

Ledercillin VK Oral

leech
    American l.
    artificial l.
    horse l.
    land l.
    medicinal l.

leg
    Barbados l.
    elephant l.
    l. ulcer

Leiner
    L's dermatitis
    L's disease

leiodermia

leiomyoma *pl.* leiomyomas,
  leiomyomata
  l. cutis
  multiple cutaneous l's
  vascular l.

leiomyosarcoma

leiotrichous

Leishman
  L's cells
  L's stain
  L.-Donovan body

Leishmania
  L. aethiopica
  L. brasiliensis
  L. braziliensis
  L. braziliensis braziliensis
  L. braziliensis guyanensis
  L. braziliensis panamensis
  L. chagasi
  L. donovani
  L. donovani chagasi
  L. donovani donovani
  L. donovani infantum
  L. garnhami
  L. infantum
  L. major
  L. mexicana
  L. mexicana amazonensis
  L. mexicana mexicana
  L. mexicana pifanoi
  L. nilotica
  L. orientalis
  L. peruviana
  L. pifanoi
  L. tropica
  L. tropica aethiopica
  L. tropica major
  L. tropica minor
  L. tropica tropica
  L. viannia
  L. viannia braziliensis
  L. viannia guyanensis
  L. viannia peruviana

leishmania

leishmanial

leishmaniasis
  acute cutaneous l.
  l. aethiopica
  American l.
  l. Americana
  anergic l.
  anthroponotic cutaneous l.
  antimonial drug therapy for
    l.
  l. brasiliensis
  l. braziliensis
  l. braziliensis braziliensis
  l. braziliensis guyanensis
  l. braziliensis panamensis
  chronic cutaneous l.
  cutaneous l.
  diffuse cutaneous l.
  disseminated cutaneous l.
  l. donovani
  l. donovani chagasi
  l. donovani donovani
  dry cutaneous l.
  l. infantum
  lupoid l.
  l. major
  Mediterranean visceral l.
  mexicana l.
  mucocutaneous l.
  nasopharyngeal l.
  New World l.
  Old World l.
  post–kala-azar dermal l.
  pseudolepromatous l.
  l. recidivans
  rural cutaneous l.
  l. tegumentaria diffusa
  l. tropica
  urban cutaneous l.
  visceral l.
  visceral mucocutaneous l.
  wet cutaneous l.
  zoonotic cutaneous l.

leishmanicidal

leishmanid

leishmanin

leishmanin (*continued*)
l. intradermal test
l. test

leishmanoid
dermal l.
post–kala-azar dermal l.

Leishman-Montenegro-Donovan

Leiurus quinquestriatus

Leloir disease

lemic

lemon
l. oil
l. peel oil

LEN
linear epidermal nevus

Lennert lymphoma

lens opacities

lenticular
l. atrophia of the palmar creases
l. papules
l. syphilid

lenticulopapular

lentigines (*plural of* lentigo)
l., atrial myxoma, mucocutaneous myxomas, and blue nevi (LAMB)
solar l.

lentiginosis
centrofacial l.
l. endobuccalis
generalized l.
inherited patterned l.
l. profusa
l. syndrome

lentiginous
l. proliferation

lentigo *pl.* lentigines
genital l.

lentigo (*continued*)
l. maligna
l. maligna melanoma (LMM)
nevoid l.
nevus spilus l.
PUVA-induced l.
senile l.
l. senilis
simple l.
l. simplex
solar l.
Touraine centrofacial l.

lentil-shaped spot

Lenz' syndrome

Lenz-Majewski syndrome

leonine facies

leontiasis

LEOPARD
lentigines, electrocardiographic defects, ocular hypertelorism, pulmonary stenosis, abnormalities of genitalia, retardation of growth, deafness
LEOPARD syndrome

leopard
l. skin

leper

lepidic

Lepidoptera

lepidosis

lepothrix

lepra
l. alba
l. alphos
l. anaesthetica
l. arabum
l. bacillus
l. cells

lepra (*continued*)
    l. conjunctivae
    l. graecorum
    l. lepromatosa
    l. maculosa
    l. mutilans
    l. nervorum
    l. nervosa
    l. tuberculoides
    Willan l.

leprae
    Mycobacterium l.

leprechaunism syndrome

leprid

lepride

leprologist

leprology

leproma
    corneal l.

lepromatous
    l. forms
    l. infiltration
    l. leprosy
    l. macules
    l. nodule
    l. pole
    l. reaction

lepromin
    l. reaction
    l. skin test
    l. test

leprosarium

leprosary

leprose

leprosery

leprostatic

leprosum
    erythema nodosum l.

leprosus
    pemphigus l.

leprosy
    anesthetic l.
    articular l.
    Asturian l.
    l. bacillus
    borderline l.
    borderline lepromatous l.
    borderline tuberculoid l.
    cutaneous l.
    diffuse l. of Lucio
    dimorphous l.
    dry l.
    early l.
    histoid l.
    indeterminate l.
    intermediate l.
    lazarine l.
    lepromatous l.
    Lucio's l.
    macular l.
    macular lepromatous l.
    maculoanesthetic l.
    Malabar l.
    mixed l.
    multibacillary l.
    murine l.
    mutilating l.
    neural l.
    nodular l.
    l. of Lucio
    paucibacillary l.
    polar lepromatous l.
    pure neural l.
    rat l.
    reactional l.
    smooth l.
    spotted l.
    subclinical l.
    subpolar lepromatous l.
    trophoneurotic l.
    tuberculoid l.
    uncharacteristic l.
    virchowian l.
    water-buffalo l.

leprotic

leprotica
    alopecia l.

leprous

leptochroa

leptodermic

leptomeningeal
    l. component
    l. involvement
    l. melanoma
    l. melanosis

leptomeninges

leptomonad
    l. suspension

Leptopsylla segnis

Leptosphaeria
    L. senegalensis
    L. tompkinsii

Leptospira
    L. autumnalis
    L. icterohaemorrhagiae
    L. interrogans

leptospirosis
    anicteric l.
    icteric l.

Lesch-Nyhan syndrome

Leser
    L.-Trélat sign
    L.-Trélat syndrome

lesion
    acneform l.
    annular l.
    annular hyperpigmented l.
    l. arrangement
    atrophic l.
    basic l.
    blanchable red l.
    blue-gray l.
    blueberry muffin l.
    brown-black l.
    bullous l.
    bullous skin l.
    Bywaters l.
    cellulitic l.
    "classic" reticulate l.

lesion (*continued*)
    Cole herpetiform l.
    l. color
    l. configuration
    l. consistency
    cutaneous l.
    cystic l.
    dermal l.
    discoid l.
    l. distribution
    disseminated l.
    Division (I–IV) l.
    eczematous l.
    elementary l.
    eroded l.
    erysipelas-like skin l.
    l. evolution
    extragenital l.
    firm l.
    genital l.
    genital papulosquamous l.
    gross l.
    gummatous l.
    hemorrhagic l.
    herpetiform l. of Cole
    histologic l.
    indolent l.
    infarctive l.
    initial syphilitic l.
    Janeway l.
    kidney-shaped lesion
    lichenified l.
    linear l.
    l. margination
    medium l.
    l. morphology
    nickel and dime l.
    nonblanchable, abnormally
      colored l.
    nummular l.
    oil drop l.
    osseous l.
    papulopustular l.
    papulosquamous l.
    papulovesicular l.
    polypoid l.
    precancerous l.
    primary l.

lesion (*continued*)
    proliferative l.
    pruritic l.
    purpuric l.
    pustular l.
    pyodermatous skin l.
    reticular l.
    reticulate l.
    ringed l.
    rolled shoulder l.
    rupioid l.
    satellite l.
    scaling l.
    scaling skin-colored l.
    scarring scalp l.
    secondary l.
    sesslle l.
    shagreen l.
    l. size
    skin l.
    skin-colored l.
    slope shouldered l.
    smooth l.
    smooth skin-colored l.
    soft l.
    special l.
    square shouldered l.
    suppurating cystic l.
    l. surface characteristic
    target l.
    traumatic l.
    tuberculoid l.
    typical reticulate l.
    ulcer l.
    urticarial l.
    varicelliform l.
    vasculitic l.
    venular l.
    vesicobullous l.
    violaceous papulonodular,
      hyperkeratotic lesions
    vulvar l.
    warty lichenoid l.
    weeping l.
    white l.
    yellow l.
Lester iris

lethal
    l. midline granuloma
    l. midline granulomatosis

lethalis
    epidermolysis bullosa l.
    ichthyosis l.

lethargy

Letterer-Siwe disease

leukasmus

leukemia
    l. cutis
    non-mast-cell l.

leukemic
    l. erythroderma
    l. infiltration
    l. phase

leukemid

leukocyte
    l. adhesion molecule
      deficiency
    l. count
    l. function antigen-3 (LFA-3)
    l. migration
    polymorphonuclear l.

leukocytic elements

leukocytoclastic
    l. angiitis
    l. vasculitis (LCV)

leukocytosis

leukoderma
    acquired l.
    l. acquisitum centrifugum
    chemical l.
    l. colli
    contact l.
    genital l.
    occupational l.
    patterned l.
    postinflammatory l.
    syphilitic l.

leukodermatous

leukodermia

leukodermic

leukoedema
    oral l.

leukokeratosis
    l. nicotinica palati
    l. oris

leukokraurosis

leukonecrosis

leukonychia
    apparent l.
    l. partialis
    partial l.
    l. punctata
    l. striata
    total l.
    l. totalis
    l. trichophytica

leukopathia
    acquired l.
    congenital l.
    l. punctata reticularis
        symmetrica
    l. symmetrica progressiva
    l. unguium

leukopathy
    symmetric progressive l.

leukopenia

leukoplakia
    atrophic l.
    Candida l.
    candidal l.
    hairy l.
    oral hairy l.
    precancerous l.
    proliferative verrucous l.
    l. vulvae

leukoplakic vulvitis

leukoplasia

leukotrichia
    l. annularis

leukotrichous

leukotriene
    l. antagonist
    l. inhibition
    l. reduction
    l. regulation

leuprolide acetate

levamisole

level
    Clark l.

Lever 2000

levodopa therapy

levofloxacin

Lewandowski
    L. nevus elasticus
    nevus elasticus of L.
    rosacea-like tuberculid of L.
    L.-Lutz disease
    epidermodysplasia
        verruciformis of L.-Lutz

Leydig
    L. cells
    L. cylinders
    L. test

LGV
    lymphogranuloma
        venereum

Lhermitte-Duclos disease

l'homme rouge

lice (*plural of* louse)
    body l.
    End l.
    head l.
    pubic l.

Lice-Enz

lichen
    l. agrius
    l. albus
    l. amyloidosus
    l. annularis

lichen (*continued*)
- l. aureus
- l. chronicus simplex
- l. corneus hypertrophicus
- l. fibromucinoidosus
- l. frambesianus
- l. hemorrhagicus
- l. infantum
- l. iris
- l. leprosus
- l. myxedematosus
- l. myxedematous
- l. nitidus
- l. nitidus actinicus
- l. nitidus pinkus
- l. nuchae
- l. obtusus
- l. obtusus corneus
- l. pilaris
- l. pilaris seu spinulosus
- l. planopilaris
- l. planus
- l. planus, acute bullous
- l. planus, bullous
- l. planus, vesiculobullous
- l. planus actinicus
- l. planus acuminatus
- l. planus annularis
- l. planus atrophicans
- l. planus atrophicus
- l. planus et acuminatus atrophicans
- l. planus erythematosus
- l. planus exanthematicus
- l. planus follicularis
- l. planus generalisatus
- l. planus hypertrophicus
- l. planus mucosae erosivus
- l. planus of the mucosa
- l. planus of the mucosa, erosive
- l. planus of the oral mucosa
- l. planus pemphigoid
- l. planus pemphigoides
- l. planus pigmentosus
- l. planus planopilaris
- l. planus subtropicus
- l. planus tropicus

lichen (*continued*)
- l. planus verrucosus
- l. purpuricus
- l. ruber
- l. ruber acuminatus
- l. ruber follicularis decalvans capillitii
- l. ruber moniliformis
- l. ruber planus
- l. ruber verrucosus
- l. sclerosis et atrophicus (LS&A)
- l. sclerosus
- sclerosus l.
- l. sclerosus et atrophicus
- l. sclerosus scleroatrophy
- l. scrofulosorum
- l. scrofulosus
- l. simplex acutus
- l. simplex chronicus (LSC)
- l. simplex chronicus Vidal
- l. spinulosus
- l. striatus
- l. striatus epidermal nevus
- l. strophulosus
- l. syphiliticus
- l. trichophyticus
- tropical l.
- l. tropicus
- l. urticatus
- l. variegatus
- Wilson l.

lichen-type scale

lichenificatio
- l. gigantea

lichenification
- giant l.
- gigantean l.

lichenified
- l. dermatitis
- l. lesion
- l. plaque

licheniformis
- *Bacillus l.*

lichenization

lichenoid
l. acute pityriasis
l. amyloidosis
l. chronic dermatosis
l. dermatosis
l. distribution
l. drug eruption
l. eczema
l. eruption
l. interface inflammation
l. interface reaction
l. keratosis
l. melanodermatitis
l. papules
l. phase
l. photoeruption
l. purpura
l. reaction
l. syphilid
l. tissue reaction

lichenoides
chronica parapsoriasis l.
parapsoriasis l.
pityriasis l.
tuberculosis cutis l.

lid margins

Lida-Mantle HC topical

Lidex
L. topical

Lidex-E topical

lidocaine
bacitracin, neomycin,
polymyxin B, and l.
l. and epinephrine
l. hydrochloride
l. and hydrocortisone
l. prilocaine
l. solution

Lidoderm

LidoPen

lifelong infection

life-threatening reaction

ligament
Poupart's l.

ligand
l. binding region

light
actinic l.
l. amplification
l. chain
l. cryotherapy
l. dispersion
l. electrodesiccation
l. electrofulguration
l. electron microscopy
l. freezing
l. fulguration
infrared l.
ultraviolet l.
Wood's l.

lilac disease

limb
afferent l.
l. defects
efferent l.
l. paresthesia

limbus *pl.* limbi

lime
l. bergamot
slaked l.

limewater compresses

liminal

liminaris
alopecia l.

limited
l. joint mobility
l. progressive systemic
sclerosis
l. Wegener granulomatosis

limp skin

Lindane
L. dust

line

line (*continued*)
Aldrich-Mees l.
Beau's l.
cleavage l.
dynamic l.
Futcher's l.
Langer's l.
Mees' l.
Morgan's l.
l. of expression
l. of minimal tension
Pastia l's
relaxed skin tension l.
Voigt's l's
white l.

line of demarcation

linea *pl.* lineae
l. alba
l. alba buccalis
l. albicans
l. albicantes
l. atrophicae
l. nigra

linear
l. atrophic hypopigmented
hairless streaks
l. atrophoderma of Moulin
l. atrophy
l. circumscribed
scleroderma
l. closure
l. crusts
l. distribution
l. epidermal nevus
l. epidermal nevus
syndrome
l. fashion
l. focal elastosis
l. hyperkeratotic papules
l. hyperkeratotic plaques
l. IgA bullous dermatosis
l. IgA bullous disease
l. IgA dermatosis
l. IgA disease
l. IgM dermatosis of
pregnancy

linear (*continued*)
l. keratosis
l. keratotic streaks
l. lesion
l. lichen planus
l. melorheostotic
scleroderma
l. nevoid hypermelanosis
l. nevus
l. nevus sebaceus
syndrome
l. petechia
l. porokeratosis
l. progressive systemic
sclerosis
l. purpuric lesion
l. scleroderma
l. scleroderma variant
l. segmental lesion
l. streaking
l. telangiectases
l. verrucous epidermal
nevus
l. and whorled nevoid
hypermelanosis

linearis
morphea l.

lines
Blaschko's l.
l. of cleavage

lingua
l. Brocq-Pautrier
l. geographica
l. nigra
l. plicata
l. scrotalis
l. villosa nigra

linguae
exfoliatio areata l.
nigrities l.
pityriasis l.
tylosis l.

lingual artery

lingula

liniment

linoleate
ethyl l.

linoleic acid

a-linolenic acid

Linuche unguiculata

lip
l. cosmetic
l. pits
l. pomade
l. swelling

lipase determination

lipedema

lipedematous alopecia

lipid
l. deposition
l. disturbance
l. granulomatosis
l. vacuoles

lipidosis

lipoatrophia annularis

lipoatrophy
annular l.
l. insulin/corticoid-induced
partial l.
postinfection l.
semicircular l.
total l.

lipoblast

lipocyte

lipodermatosclerosis

lipodystrophia centrifugalis
abdominalis infantilis

lipodystrophy
congenital generalized l.
congenital progressive l.
generalized l.
intestinal l.
partial l.

lipodystrophy (*continued*)
progressive l.
progressive congenital l.
progressive partial l.
total l.

lipofibroma

lipofuscin

lipogranulomatosis
l. subcutanea

lipohypertrophy

lipoid
l. dermatoarthritis
l. granuloma
l. proteinosis

lipoidica
necrobiosis l.

lipoidosis
l. cutis et mucosa

lipoma
l. annulare colli
l. arborescens
atypical l.
l. cavernosum
l. fibrosum
l. of brown fat
pleomorphic l.
spindle cell l.
synovial l.
telangiectatic l.
l. telangiectodes

lipomatodes
nevus l.

lipomatosis
benign symmetric l.
mediastinal l.
multiple symmetric l.
l. neurotica

lipomatosus
nevus l.

lipomatous
nevus l.

lipomelanic reticulosis

lipomelanotic

lipomeningocele

Liponyssoides sanguineus

Liponyssus

lipophage

lipophagic
l. granuloma
l. panniculitis

lipophilic
l. organism

lipopolysaccharide

lipoprotein
l. lipase
l. lipase activator
l. lipase deficiency
l. metabolism

liposarcoma

liposuction
l. tumescent anesthesia

lipotrophy
semicircular l.

lips
cracked l.
dry l.
glowing red l.
large l.
pseudocolloid of l.

Lipschütz
L. bodies
L. cell
L. disease
L. erythema
L. ulcer

lipstick

liquefaction
l. degeneration
l. necrosis

Liquid Pred Oral

liquid nitrogen therapy

liquor carbonis detergens (LCD)

Lisch nodule

lisinopril

lissotrichic

Listeria monocytogenes

listeriosis
cutaneous l.
disseminated l.

lithium
l. carbonate
l. therapy

Little League elbow

Little's disease

live
measles virus vaccine l.
rubella virus vaccine l.
l. vaccine
varicella virus vaccine l.

livedo
l. annularis
l. pattern
l. patterned disease
l. racemosa
l. reticularis
l. reticularis, idiopathica
l. reticularis, symptomatic
l. reticularis-like lesion
l. reticularis with summer
ulceration
l. telangiectatica
l. vasculitis

livedoid
l. dermatitis
l. vasculitis
l. vasculopathy
l. violaceous patch

liver
l. dysfunction
l. fluke
l. spot

livid

lividity

livido
    lupus l.

livor

lizard
    l. bite
    l. skin

Loa loa

loaiasis

lobectomy

Loboa loboi

Lobo's disease

lobomycosis

Lobstein
    L's disease
    L's ganglion
    L's syndrome

lobular
    l. acanthosis
    l. necrosis of adipocytes
      with suppuration
    l. panniculitis

lobulated

lobule

local
    l. anaphylaxis
    l. immunity
    l. reaction
    l. skin flap
    l. urticaria
    l. wound care

localized
    l. acquired cutaneous
      pseudoxanthoma
      elasticum (PXE)
    l. acquired hypertrichosis
    l. albinism
    l. angiokeratoma
    l. argyria

localized (*continued*)
    l. congenital hypertrichosis
    l. cutaneous amyloidosis
    l. epidermolysis bullosa
      simplex
    l. granuloma annulare
    l. hypertrophy
    l. lipodystrophy
    l. mastocytoma
    l. morphea
    l. mucocutaneous
      candidiasis
    l. neurodermatitis
    l. pagetoid reticulosis
    l. pemphigoid of Brunsting-
      Perry
    l. progressive systemic
      sclerosis
    l. pustular psoriasis
    l. scleroderma
    l. vitiligo

loci (*plural of* locus)

Locoid

loculation

locus *pl.* loci

Löffler's syndrome

Loewenthal reaction

Lofgren's syndrome

logagraphia

logamnesia

logasthenia

loiasis

Loiasis filariasis

lomustine

Lone Star tick

long acting (LA)

long-acting
    l.-a. sulfonamides
    l.-a. vasoconstrictor

long-duration treatment

longitudinal
  l. axis
  l. black banding of the nail
  l. brown banding of the nail
  l. groove
  l. grooving
  l. hyperpigmented streaking
  l. melanonychia
  l. split
  l. splitting
  l. striae

long-term
  l.-t. complications
  l.-t. evaluation
  l.-t. psychologic
    consequences
  l.-t. sequelae
  l.-t. use

long-wave ultraviolet radiation

long-wavelength ultraviolet light
  (UVA)

loop
  amplification l.

looping

loose
  l. anagen hair syndrome
  l. anagen syndrome
  l. body
  l. skin

looseness of the skin

Loprox

loratadine
  l. and pseudoephedrine

Lortat-Jacobs
  L.-J. disease

loss
  eyebrow l.
  eyelash l.

lotion
  A/T/S l.

lotion (*continued*)
  calamine l.
  G-well l.
  Kwell l.
  Lotrimin AF l.
  Panscol l.
  phenolated calamine l.
  Scabene l.
  Tinver l.
  triamcinolone l. (TAL)

Lotrimin
  L. AF Cream
  L. AF Lotion
  L. AF Powder
  L. AF solution
  L. AF Spray Liquid
  L. AF Spray Powder

Lotrisone

Louis-Bar's syndrome

louse *pl.* lice
  body l.
  clothes l.
  crab l.
  head l.
  l. infestation
  pubic l.
  scalp l.
  sucking l.

louse-borne relapsing fever

lousiness

lousy

Lovibond
  L's angle
  L's file sign

low
  l.-dose radiation therapy
  l.-grade B-cell lymphoma
  l.-molecule-weight heparin
  l.-phenylalanine diet
  l.-risk tumor
  l.-strength corticosteroid
    creams
  l.-tyrosine diet

Löwenstein
  L.-Jensen agar
  L.-Jensen culture medium

lowest density chylomicrons

Loxosceles
  L. laeta
  L. reclusa
  L. reclusa bite

loxoscelism

LP
  lysylpyridinoline

LS&A
  lichen sclerosis et
    atrophicans

LSC
  lichen simplex chronicus

L-tryptophan

lubricant

lubricant/emollient
  Bag Balm l./e.
  Udder Butter l./e.

lubrication
  skin l

Lubriderm
  L. moisture recovery lotion
  L. moisturizer

lucida
  lamina l.

lucidum
  stratum l.

Lucio
  L's leprosy
  L's leprosy phenomenon
  L's phenomenon

lucotherapy

Ludwig's angina

Luer-Lok syringe

lues
  l. maligna

lues (*continued*)
  l. nervosa
  l. syphilitica
  l. tarda
  l. venerea

luetic mask

lumbar
  l. ganglionectomy
  l. puncture
  l. sympathectomy
  l. zoster

lumberman's itch

lumen

luminal
  l. amebicide
  l. border
  l. secretory cells

lump

lumpy
  l. jaw
  l. skin disease

Lund-Browder burn scale

lunula *pl.* lunulae
  diffusion of the l.
  l. of nail
  l. unguis

lupiform

lupinosa
  porrigo l.

lupoid
  l. leishmaniasis
  l. rosacea
  l. sycosis
  l. ulcer

luposa
  tuberculosis cutis l.

lupous

lupus
  l. anticoagulant (LA)
  l. band test (LBT)

lupus (*continued*)
l. carcinoma
Cazenave l.
chilblain l.
cutaneous l.
discoid l.
disseminated follicular l.
disseminated l.
  erythematosus
drug-induced l.
l. erythematodes
l. erythematosus (LE)
l. erythematosus cell
l. erythematosus cell test
l. erythematosus, chilblain
l. erythematosus, cutaneous
l. erythematosus, discoid
  (DLE)
l. erythematosus,
  hypertrophic
l. erythematosus, neonatal
l. erythematosus chronicus
  discoides
l. erythematosus chronicus
  disseminatus superficialis
l. erythematosus discoides
l. erythematosus
  disseminatus
l. erythematosus
  hypertrophicus
l. erythematosus–lichen
  planus overlap
l. erythematosus mucosae
  oris
l. erythematosus
  panniculitis
l. erythematosus profundus
l. erythematosus tumidus
l. erythematosus visceralis
l. erythematous–like rash
l. fibrosus
l. glomerulonephritis
l. hairs
l. hypertrophicus
l. livido
l. lymphaticus
l. miliaris disseminatus
  faciei

lupus (*continued*)
l. mutilans
neonatal l.
l. nephritis (LN)
l. panniculitis
l. papillomatosus
l. pernio
l. pernio besnier
photosensitive l.
  erythematosus
l. profundus
l. profundus/panniculitis
l. sebaceous
l. serpiginosus
l. superficialis
l. syndrome
systemic l. erythematosus
  (SLE)
transient neonatal systemic
  l. erythematosus
l. tuberculosus
tumid l.
l. tumidus
l. verrucosus
l. vorax
l. vulgaris
l. vulgaris verrucosus

lupuslike syndrome

luteoma

Lutz-Miescher
L.-M. disease

Lutz-Splendore-Almeida
L.-S.-A. disease

Lutzomyia
  L. flaviscutellata
  L. longipalpis
  L. noguchi
  L. olmeca
  L. peruensis
  L. sandflies
  L. trapidoi
  L. umbratilis
  L. verrucarum

LVG

LVG (*continued*)
    lymphogranuloma
      venereum

lycopene

lycopenemia

Lycopodium

Lyell
    L's disease
    L's syndrome

Lymantria
    L. dispar
    L. dispar sting

Lyme
    L. borreliosis
    L. disease

lymph
    l. node-based lymphoma
    l. node dissection
    l. node vessels

lymphadenitis
    necrotizing l.
    regional granulomatous l.

lymphadenoma

lymphadenomatosis

lymphadenopathy
    dermatopathic l.
    drug-induced l.
    regional l.

lymphadenosis
    benign l.
    l. benigna cutis
    l. cutis benigna

lymphangiectasia
    acquired l.

lymphangiectasis

lymphangiectatica
    pachyderma l.

lymphangiectodes

lymphangioleiomyomatosis

lymphangioma
    l. capillare varicosum
    cavernous l.
    l. cavernosum
    l. circumscriptum
    l. circumscriptum cysticum
    l. cysticum
    solitary simple l.
    l. superficium simplex
    l. tuberosum multiplex
    l. xanthelasmoideum

lymphangiomatosis

lymphangiomyomatosis

lymphangiosarcoma

lymphangiosis
    l. carcinomatosa cutis

lymphangitic
    l. sporotrichosis

lymphangitis
    bacterial l.
    l. carcinomatosa
    penile sclerosing l.
    sclerosing l.
    tuberculous l.

lymphatic
    l. blockage
    l. channels
    l. cisterns
    dermal l.
    l. drainage
    l. malformations
    l. microsurgery
    l. obstruction
    l. spread

lymphaticus
    lupus l.
    nevus l.

lymphedema
    chronic hereditary l.
    l.-distichiasis syndrome
    l. praecox
    primary l.
    secondary l.

lymphedema (*continued*)
l. tarda

lymphedematous keratoderma

lymphoblast

lymphoblastic

lymphoblastoma

lymphoblastosis

lymphocutaneous lesions

lymphocyte
l. activation
l. activation syndrome
B. l.
bystander l.
CD4 l.
effector l.
l. interaction
mature l.
myeloma tumor l.
peripheral blood l.
precursor B l.
recruited l.
l. stimulation
suppressor/cytotoxic l.
l. transformation test

lymphocytic
l. hypophysitis
l. infiltration
l. infiltration of Jessner
l. infiltration of Jessner-
Kanof
l. infiltration of the skin
l. inflammatory infiltration
l. lobular panniculitis
l. panniculitis
l. peribulbar infiltrate
l. perivascular infiltration

lymphocytoma
l. cutis

lymphoderma

lymphogranuloma
l. benignum
l. inguinale

lymphogranuloma (*continued*)
l. venereum (LGV)
l. venereum antigen
l. venereum conjunctivitis
l. venereum virus

lymphogranulomatosis
l. benigna
l. cutis
l. inguinalis
l. maligna

lymphohistiocytic infiltrate

lymphoid
l. cell
l. follicles
l. hyperplasia
l. markers

lymphokine
l.-activated killer cell (LAK)

lymphoma
l. cell disorder
cutaneous B-cell l.
cutaneous T-cell l. (CTCL)
l. cutis
immunoblastic l.
T-cell l., cutaneous

lymphomatoid
l. contact dermatitis
l. granulomatosis
l. papulosis
l. vasculitis

lymphomatosis
avian l.
fowl l.
ocular l.
visceral l.

lymphomatous

lymphopathia
l. venerea
l. venereum

lymphopenia

lymphoplasia
cutaneous l.

lymphoplasmacytoid
  immunocytoma

lymphoproliferative disease

lymphoreticular
  l. disorder
  l. malignancy
  l. system

lymphosarcomatosis

lymphostatic verrucosis

lymphotoxin

Lyngbya majuscula Gomont

LYOfoam dressing

lyonization

lyse

lysis
  endothelial l.

lysogenic
  l. bacterium

lysosomal
  l. membrane
  l. storage disease

lysosome

lysozyme

lysyl oxidase

lytic bone lesions

Lytta
  L. vesicatoria
  L. vesicatoria sting

lyze

M

Maalox

MAC
  membrane attack complex
  membranolytic attack
    complex
  Mycobacterium avium
    complex

Mace

macerate

macerated
  m. epidermis
  m. keratin

maceration
  interdigital m.
  moisture-induced m.
  plantar m.

McCusick's syndrome

macroaleuriospore

macrocephalia

macrocephalic

macrocephaly

macrocheilia

macrocheiria, macrochiria

macrochilia

macrocyclic

macrodactylia

macroglobulinemia

macroglossia

macrolabia

macrolide

macromelia

macromolecular
  bacterial m.
  m. protein

macronychia

macrophage
  m. activation syndrome
  activated m.
  cytokines m.
  Hansemann m.
  lipid-laden m.
  mature m.
  melanin-laden m.

macroscopic
  m. subepidermal
    vesicles
  m. vesicles

macrostomia

macula *pl.* maculae
  m. atrophicae
  cerebral m.
  m. ceruleae
  m. gonorrhoica
  mongolian m.
  m. retinae
  Saenger m.
  m. solaris

macular
  m. amyloidosis
  m. atrophy
  m. eruption
  m. erythema
  m. granuloma annulare
  m. hyperpigmentation
  m. leprosy
  m. lesion
  m. pigmentation
  m. purpura
  m. rash
  m. secondary syphilis
  m. syphilid

maculata
  pityriasis m.

maculate

maculation

maculatum
  atrophoderma m.

macule
    ash-leaf m.
    atrophic m.
    evanescent m.
    hypopigmented m.
    lance-ovate m.
    purpuric m.
    solitary m.
    subungual black m.

maculo-anesthetic leprosy

maculoerythematous

maculopapular
    m. rash
    m. scaly eruption
    m. syphilid

maculopapule

maculosa
    urticaria m.

maculosus

maculovesicular

MAD
    mandibuloacral dysplasia

mad itch

madarosis

Madelung's disease

madescent

madidans

Madura
    M. boil
    M. foot

Madurella
    M. grisea
    M. mycetomi

maduromycosis

mafenide
    m. acetate
    m. HCl

Maffucci's syndrome

magenta
    m. II
    basic m.

maggot
    Congo floor m.

MAGIC syndrome

magnesium
    m. carbonate
    m. sulfate

magnifying mirror

magnolia

mahogany hue

maintenance
    m. dose
    m. therapy

Majocchi
    M's disease
    M's granuloma
    M's purpura
    purpura annularis
        telangiectodes of M.

major
    aphthae m.
    m. aphthous ulcer
    erythema multiforme m.
    m. histocompatibility
        complex (MHC)
    variola m.

makeup
    Covermark corrective m.

mal
    m. de Cayenne
    m. de los pintos
    m. de Meleda
    m. de San Lazaro
    m. morado
    m. perforans
    m. perforant du pied

Malabar
    M. itch
    M. leprosy

malabsorption
    m. disorder
    m. syndrome

malachite green

malacoplakia

malaise

malakoplakia

malar
    m. butterfly rash
    m. erythema
    m. hypoplasia
    m. rash (MR)

malaria

Malassezia
    M. furfur
    M. ovalis

malathion
    m. emulsion
    m. powder

maldevelopment

male
    m. pattern alopecia
    m. pattern baldness
    m. pattern hair loss

malformation of extremities

malformed

Malherbe
    calcifying epithelioma
      of M.
    M's calcifying epithelioma
      and pilomatrixoma
    epithelioma of M.
    M's epithelioma

maligna
    lentigo m.
    lymphogranulomatosis m.
    onychia m.
    papulosis atrophicans m.
    scarlatina m.
    variola m.

malignancy
    myositis with m.
    systemic m.

malignant
    m. acanthosis nigricans
    m. angioendotheliomatosis
    m. atrophic papulosis
    m. blue nevus
    m. bubo
    m. chondroid syringoma
    m. clear cell acrospiroma
    m. clone
    m. degeneration
    m. down
    m. dyskeratosis
    m. eccrine poroma
    m. eccrine spiradenoma
    m. external otitis
    m. fibrous histiocytoma
    m. granulomatous angiitis
    m. hemangioendothelioma
    m. hemangiopericytoma
    m. histiocytoma
    m. histiocytosis
    m. lentigo melanoma
    m. lymphocyte
    m. lymphoma
    m. melanoma
    m. melanoma in situ
    m. melanoma precursor
      lesions
    m. metastatic melanoma
    m. mole syndrome
    m. neoplasia
    m. neoplasm
    m. neoplastic disease
    m. nodular hidradenoma
    m. pancreatic tumor
    m. papillomatosis
    m. papillomatosis of Degos
    m. pilomatricoma
    m. progression
    m. pustule
    m. pyoderma
    m. smallpox
    m. systemic mastocytosis
    m. transformation

malignant (*continued*)
    m. tumor

maligne
    papulose atrophicante m.

malignum
    keratoma m.

malingering

malleolar area

Malleomyces
    M. mallei
    M. pseudomallei

mallet toe

malleus *pl.* mallei

Mallorca acne

malnutrition
    episodic m.

malocclusion

malodor

malodorous
    m. exudate
    m. papillomatous growth
    m. sweating

malpighian
    m. cells
    m. layer

malpighii
    stratum m.

MALT
    mucosa-associated
      lymphoid tissue
    MALT lymphoma

Maltese cross

maltophilia
    Xanthomonas m.

malum
    m. perforans
    m. perforans pedis

mamanpian

mammary
    m. intraductal papilloma
    m. myxoid fibroma
    m. nipples

mammiform

mammilla *pl.* mammillae

mammillary muscle

mammillated

mammillation

mammilliform

mammillitis
    bovine herpes m.
    bovine ulcerative m.
    bovine vaccinia m.

mammose

mandibuloacral dysplasia

mandibulofacial dysostosis

mandrake

mange
    demodectic m.
    follicular m.
    sarcoptic m.

mango
    m. dermatitis
    m. fly

mangy

manicure

manifestation
    allergic m.
    clinical m.
    cutaneous m.
    mucocutaneous m.
    presenting clinical m.

Manson
    M. pyosis

Mansonella
    M. ozzardi
    M. streptocerca

Mantoux test

manus
　　tinea m.
　　tinea pedis et m.

manuum
　　keratolysis exfoliativa
　　　　areata m.

maple

marasmic kwashiorkor

marasmus

Marbaxin

marble skin

marbled mottling

marblelike

marbleization

Marcaine
　　M./Sensorcaine

Marcillin

Marfan's syndrome

marfanoid habitus

margarine disease

margin
　　free m. of nail
　　hidden m. of nail
　　lateral m. of nail
　　m. of nail, free
　　m. of nail, hidden
　　m. of nail, lateral

marginal
　　m. band
　　m. blepharitis
　　m. crusting
　　m. follicles
　　m. gingiva
　　m. keratitis
　　m. zone B-cell lymphoma

marginalis
　　alopecia m.
　　keratoelastoidosis m.

marginata
　　alopecia m.

margination
　　lesion m.
　　m. of lesions

marginatum
　　eczema m.
　　erythema m.

margo *pl.* margines
　　m. lateralis unguis
　　m. liber unguis
　　m. occultus unguis

Marie-Strümpell disease

marine
　　m. alga
　　m. animal sting
　　m. brown algae

Marinesco-Sjögren syndrome

Marjolin's ulcer

mark
　　beauty m.
　　birth m.
　　dhobie m.
　　ecchymotic m.
　　erythematous m.
　　pock m.
　　Pohl's m.
　　Pohl-Pinkus m.
　　port-wine m.
　　strawberry m.
　　Unna m.
　　washerman's m.

marked
　　m. dyspigmentation
　　m. localized reaction
　　m. propensity

marker
　　cell membrane m.
　　Gm m.

markings
　　skin m.

marks

marks (*continued*)
  stretch m.

marmorata
  cutis m.

marmorated

marmorization

Marshall
  M's syndrome
  M.-White syndrome

mask
  m. of pregnancy

marsupialization

mascara
  solvent-based m.
  water-based m.

maschalephidrosis

maschalyperidrosis

masculine
  m. habitus

masculinization

masculinize

masering phenomenon

mask
  Neutrogena acne m.
  m. of pregnancy
  Swiss Therapy eye m.
  tropical m.

masklike
  m. appearance
  m. expression

masochism

masochistic character traits

masoprocol
  m. cream

masque biliaire

MASS
  mitral valve prolapse, aortic anomalies, skeletal

MASS (*continued*)
  changes, and skin changes
  MASS syndrome

mass
  m. infection
  mushroomlike m.
  pendulous redundant m.

massive
  m. capillary proliferation
  m. lymphadenopathy
  m. subcutaneous swelling

massiveness

Masson
  M. intravascular endothelial proliferation
  M. pseudoangiosarcoma

mast cell
  m. c. degranulation
  m. c. growth factor
  m. c. mediator

Mastadenovirus

mastectomy
  radical m.

mastication

Mastigophora

mastigophoran

mastigophorous

mastigote

mastitis
  chronic m.

mastocyte

mastocytoma
  localized m.
  solitary m.

mastocytosis
  benign systemic m.
  cutaneous m.
  diffuse cutaneous m.
  malignant m.
  malignant systemic m.

mastocytosis (*continued*)
    papular m.
    systemic m.
    telangiectatic systemic m.

mat burn

material
    absorbent gelling m. (AGM)
    cross-reacting m.
    Epicel skin graft m.
    greenish purulent m.
    keratinous m.
    keratotic m.
    test m.
    yellowish purulent m.

maternal
    m. immunity
    m. varicella

matricectomy

matrix *pl.* matrices
    m. cell
    m. component
    distal nail m.
    extracellular m. (ECM)
    hair m.
    nail m.
    proximal nail m.
    m. unguis

mattress
    AkroTech m.
    convoluted foam m.
    m. itch
    vinyl-alternating air m.

maturation
    affinity m.

mature
    m. hyperkeratotic plaque
    m. lamellar bone
    m. lymphocytes
    m. myeloid cell
    m. secretory B lymphocyte

Mauriac
    M. syndrome

Max-Caro

Maxidex

Maxiflor
    M. topical

maxillaris

maxillary sinuses

Maximum Strength Desenex
    antifungal cream

Maxivate

May-Gruenwald stain

mayweed

mazamorra

Mazzotti
    M. test

MCI/MI
    methylchloroisothiazolinon
      e/methylisothiazolinone

M component immunoglobulin

MCTD
    mixed connective tissue
      disease

MCV
    molluscum contagiosum

MDS
    myelodysplastic syndrome

MDT
    multidrug therapy

meadow
    m. dermatitis
    m. grass dermatitis

measles
    atypical m.
    m. convalescent serum
    German m.
    m. immune globulin
      (human)
    m. immunoglobulin
    modified m.
    m., mumps, and rubella
      vaccine (MMR)

measles (*continued*)
    m., mumps and rubella
      vaccines, combined
    m. and rubella vaccines,
      combined
    three-day m.
    tropical m.
    m. virus
    m. virus vaccine
    m. virus vaccine live

Measurin

meatus

mebendazole

mechanica
    acne m.

mechanical
    m. abrasion
    m. cushion
    m. debridement and
      excision
    m. puncture
    m. treatment

mechanic's hands

mechanoblister

mechanobullous
    m. dermatosis
    m. disease
    m. eruption

mechanoreceptor

mechlorethamine hydrochloride

Mecholyl skin test

mecillinam

Meclan topical

meclocycline sulfosalicylate

MED
    minimal erythema dose

Mederma

media

medial thigh

median
    m. nail dystrophy
    m. raphe
    m. raphe cyst of the penis
    m. rhomboid glossitis

mediastinal
    m. disease
    m. lipomatosis

mediator
    cytolytic m.
    m. proteins
    secreted m.

Medical Research Council
   (MRC)
    M. R. C. Laboratories
      (MRCL)

medical therapy

medicamentosa
    acne m.
    alopecia m.
    dermatitis m.
    dermatosis m.
    rhinitis m.
    stomatitis m.
    urticaria m.

medicamentosus

medicaments

medicated
    m. baby oils
    m. creams

medication
    m. ingestion

medicinal eruption

medina worm

Mediplast Plaster

Medi-Quick Topical Ointment

Mediterranean
    M. exanthematous fever
    M. fever

medium

medium (*continued*)
  dermatophyte test m.
    (DTM)
  m. to deep chemical peel

Medlar bodies

Medralone injection

Medrol
  M. Dosepak
  M. oral

medulla *pl.* medullae
  m. of hair shaft
  thymic m.

medullary carcinoma

medullated

medullation

medulloblastoma

medusae
  caput m.

Mees
  M's lines
  M's stripes

mefenamic acid

mefloquine
  m. hydrochloride

megacolon

megadose corticosteroids

megaesophagus

megakaryocyte

megakaryocytic cell

megaloblastic anemia

megalobastoid

megalomania

megalonychia

megalonychosis

Megalopyge
  M. crispata

Megalopyge (*continued*)
  M. opercularis
  M. opercularis sting

megavitamin

meibomian
  m. gland
  m. gland dysfunction

meiotic
  m. recombination

Meirowsky phenomenon

Miescher's radial granulomas

Meissner corpuscle

Melaleuca oil

melanemia

melanidrosis

melanin
  m. deposits
  dermal m.
  hair m.
  m. synthesis
  white m.

melanism

melanization

melanoacanthoma
  oral m.

melanoblast

melanoblastoma

melanoblastosis neurocutanea
  touraine

melanocarcinoma

melanocomous

melanocyte
  m. dendrite
  dendritic m.
  m. differentiation
  m. dysplasia
  intradermal m.
  m. nevi

melanocytic
  m. activation
  m. infiltration
  m. lesion
  m. nevus
  m. oral lesion

melanocytoma
  compound m.
  dermal m.

melanocytosis
  oculodermal m.

melanoderma
  m. cachecticorum
  m. chloasma
  parasitic m.
  racial m.
  Riehl m.
  senile m.
  m. vegetative lesion

melanodermatitis
  m. toxica lichenoides

melanodermia

melanodermic

melanogenesis

melanogenic
  m. activity

melanohidrosis

melanoid

melanoleukoderma
  m. colli

melanoma
  acral-lentiginous m.
  acral-lentiginous malignant
    m.
  acrolentiginous m.
  amelanotic m.
  benign juvenile m.
  desmoplastic malignant m.
  halo m.
  m. in situ
  juvenile m.
  lentigo maligna m.

melanoma (*continued*)
  lentigo maligna malignant
    m.
  malignant m.
  malignant lentigo m.
  minimal deviation m.
  mucosal m.
  nevoid m.
  nodular m.
  nodular malignant m.
  nontumorigenic m.
  m. of the iris
  spindle cell m.
  subungual m.
  superficial malignant m.
  superficial spreading m.
  m. thickness
  tumorigenic m.
  m. warning signs

melanomatosis

melanomatous
  m. change

melanonychia
  longitudinal m.
  m. striata

melanopathy

melanophage

melanophore

melanoplakia

melanoprotein

melanosis
  m. ab igne
  addisonian m.
  m. cachecticorum
  m. circumscripta
    precancerosa
  m. circumscripta
    praecancerosa of
    Dubreuilh
  m. corii degenerativa
  m. cutis
  m. diffusa congenita
  generalized m.

melanosis (*continued*)
  m. lenticularis progressiva
  mucosal m.
  neonatal pustular m.
  m. neurocutanea
  neurocutaneous m.
  m. neviformis
  oculocutaneous m.
  oculodermal m.
  periorbital m.
  pustular m.
  Riehl's m.
  tar m.
  transient neonatal pustular
    m.

melanosity

melanosome

melanotic
  m. carcinoma
  m. freckle
  m. freckle of Hutchinson
  m. lesion
  m. precancerosis
  m. progonoma
  m. psammomatous type
  m. whitlow

melanotrichia

melanotrichous

melanuria

melarsoprol

melasma
  m. gravidarum
  m. medicamentosum
  m. universale

Meleda
  mal de M.
  M. disease

Meleney
  chronic undermining ulcer
    of M.
  M's gangrene
  M's ulcer

melioidosis

Melkersson
  M. syndrome
  M.-Rosenthal syndrome

Meloidae

Melophagus ovinus

melorheostosis

melphalan

MEM
  multiple eruptive milia

membrane
  basal cell m.
  basement m.
  cell m.
  glassy m.
  Huxley's m.
  hyaline m.
  keratogenous m.
  m. of epitrichium
  m. transport protein
  vitreous m.

membranous aplasia cutis

memory
  m. cell
  m. T helper cell

MEN
  multiple endocrine
    neoplasia
  multiple endocrine
    neoplasms
      MEN syndrome

mendelian
  m. dominant trait
  m. inheritance
  m. recessive mode of
    transmission

Mendes da Costa's syndrome

meninges

meningeal
  m. infiltration

meningioma
  cutaneous m.

meningitis *pl.* meningitides
  acute m.

meningocele

meningococcal sepsis

meningococcemia
  acute m.

meningoencephalitic
  m. phase

meningoencephalitis

meningomyelocele

meningo-oculofacial
  angiomatosis

meningovasculitis

Menkes
  M's disease
  M's kinky hair syndrome
  M's protein exports
    intracellular copper

menocelis

menopausal flushing

menopause

menstrual
  m. abnormalities
  m. acne

mentagra
  Alibert m.

mentagrophytes

mental
  m. confusion
  m. deficiency
  m. depression
  m. retardation

Mentax

menthol

menthyl
  m. anthranilate

MEP
  milia en plaque

mepacrine

meperidine HCl

mepivacaine
  m. hydrochloride

meradimate

meralgia paresthetica

merbromin

mercaptan

6-mercaptopurine (6-MP)

mercurial
  m. compound
  m. pigmentation

mercuric
  m. chloride

mercurochrome

mercury
  ammoniated m.
  m. granuloma
  m. poisoning

Merkel
  M. cell
  M. cell carcinoma
  M. cell tumor

Merlenate topical

merocrine
  m. gland

Mersol

Merthiolate

mesalamine

mesangial cells

mesangioproliferative
  glomerulonephritis

mesenchymal
  m. cell
  m. neoplasm

mesenchymal (*continued*)
 m. tissue
 m. tumor

mesentery

mesenteric
 m. vasculitis

meshed graft

mesoderm

mesodermal
 m. change
 m. dysplasia
 m. elements
 m. melanocytes
 m. nevus
 m. origin
 m. portion
 m. somite
 m. tissue

meta-analysis

metabolism
 baseline m.

metabolite

metacarpophalangeal
 m. joints

metacarpus

metachromasia

metachromatic
 m. granules
 m. leukodystrophy

metallic
 m. discoloration
 m. dysgeusia
 m. particle
 m. yarns

metalloid

metaplasia

metaplastic ossification

metaproterenol

Metasep

metastasis

metastatic
 m. breast carcinoma
 m. calcification
 m. calcinosis cutis
 m. carcinoma
 m. Crohn's disease
 m. deposits
 m. gastric adenocarcinoma
 m. granuloma
 m. liposarcoma
 m. osteoma cutis
 m. pancreatic carcinoma
 primary m.
 m. tuberculous ulceration

metatypic
 m. basal cell carcinoma

metatypical carcinoma

Metazoa

metazoal parasite

methacholine
 m. bromide
 m. chloride skin test
 m. sweat test

methantheline bromide

methdilazine

methemoglobinemia

methicillin-resistant
 Staphylococcus aureus
 (MRSA)

methimazole

methionine

methocarbamol

method
 prick-test m.

methotrexate (MTX)

methoxsalen

methoxycinnamate and
 oxybenzone

methoxypromazine maleate

8-methoxypsoralen (8-MOP)

methyl
  m. benzylidene camphor
  m. bromide
  m. bromide fumigation
  m. methacrylate monomer
  m. violet

methylbenzethonium chloride

methylchloroisothiazolinone

methyldopa

methylene blue

methylisothiazolinone

methylparaben

methylprednisolone
  m. acetate
  pulse m.

methylrosaniline chloride

methysergide
  m. maleate

Meticorten oral

metoprolol tartrate

metronidazole
  m. gel

metrorrhagia

metyrapone

MF
  mycosis fungoides

MFH
  malignant fibrous
    histiocytoma

MHC
  major histocompatibility
    complex

MI
  morphologic index
  myocardial
    infarction

Mibelli
  angiokeratoma of M.
  M's angiokeratoma
  M's disease
  porokeratosis of M.
  M's porokeratosis
  M's syndrome

MIC
  minimal inhibitory
    concentration
  minimum inhibitory
    concentration

micaceous
  m. balanitis
  m. scale

Micanol

Micatin
  M. cream
  M. topical

Michelin Tire baby syndrome

miconazole
  M. 7
  m. nitrate

microabscess
  intraepidermal m.
  Munro m.
  m. of Munro
  m. of mycosis fungoides
  neutrophilic intraepidermal
    m.
  Pautrier's m.
  m. of psoriasis

microadenoma

microaerophile

microaerophilic

microaleuriospore

microangiopathic
  m. anemia
  m. hemolytic anemia

microbe

microbial

microbial (*continued*)
    m. pathogens
    m. peptides

Microbilharzia variglandis

microcephaly

microcirculation

Micrococcus
    M. sedentarius

microconidia

microcornea

microcytic anemia

microemulsion
    m. formulation

microfilaria
    degenerated m.

microglial cells

microglossia

micrognathia

microhemagglutination
    m. assay for *T. pallidum*
    (MHA-TP)

microlesion

micronize

micronodular pattern

micronutrient

micronychia

microorganism

micropapular tuberculid

microphallus

microscopic
    m. adnexal carcinoma
    m. hypertrophy
    m. identification
    m. pattern
    m. polyangiitis

microscopy
    epiluminescent m.

Microspore Surgical Tape

microsporosis
    m. capitis
    m. nigra

Microsporum (Microsporon)
    M. audouinii
    M. canis
    M. canis var. *distortum*
    M. distortum
    M. ferrugineum
    M. gypseum
    M. nanum

microstomia

microthelia

microvascular abnormality

microvasculature

microvesicle

microvesiculation

microvivisection

microwave hyperthermia

midfoot

midline
    m. fissure
    m. granulomatosis
    m. hairy patch or pit
    m. lethal granuloma

midmetatarsal area

midpoint skin test

Miescher
    M's actinic granuloma
    M's cheilitis
    M's cheilitis granulomatosa
    M's elastoma
    M's granuloma
    M's granulomatous cheilitis

MIF
    migration-inhibitory
        factor
    microimmunofluorescence
        test

migrans
- annulus m.
- cutaneous larva m.
- erysipelas m.
- erythema m. (EM)
- erythema chronicum m.
- erythema nodosum m.
- larva m.
- ocular larva m.
- spiruroid larva m.
- ulcus m.
- visceral larva m.

migratory
- m. erythema
- m. thrombophlebitis

Mikulicz (von Mikulicz)
- M's aphthae
- M's cells
- M's disease
- M's syndrome
- M.-Sjögren syndrome

mild
- m. hypothyroidism
- m. irritant
- m. mononuclear cell infiltrate

milia (*plural of* milium)
- m. en plaque

Milian
- M's citrine skin
- M's disease
- M's erythema
- M's sign
- M's syndrome

miliaria
- m. alba
- apocrine m.
- m. crystallina
- m. papulosa
- m. profunda
- m. propria
- pustular m.
- m. pustulosa
- m. rubra
- m. vesiculosa

miliaris
- acne m.
- acne necrotica m.
- lupus m. disseminatus faciei
- tuberculosis cutis m.
- variola m.

miliary
- m. acne
- m. dissemination
- m. form
- m. lepromata
- m. papular syphilid
- m. sarcoid
- m. tuberculosis

milium *pl.* milia
- colloid m.
- milia cyst
- juvenile colloid m.
- multiple eruptive milia
- m. neonatorum
- pinhead-sized milia
- pinpoint-sized milia

milkers'
- m. node
- m. nodules
- m. nodule virus
- m. pox

milkpox

milky white fluid

Milleporina

millet

millijoule (mJ)

millipede
- m. burn
- m. sting

milphosis

Milroy's disease

Milton
- M. disease
- M. edema
- M. urticaria

mineral oil

minimal
m. deviation melanoma
m. pigment (MP)
m.-pigment
oculocutaneous albinism

minimum inhibitory
concentration (MIC)

Minipress

minocycline
m. hydrochloride
m. hyperpigmentation

minor
m. agglutinin
aphthae m.
erythema multiforme m.
variola m.

minoxidil solution plus

minutissimum
Corynebacterium m.

miracidia

miracidium

Mitchell
M. disease

mite
m. bite
m. control
dust m.
elevator grain dust m.
hair follicle m.
harvest m.
house dust m.
m. infestation
itch m.
pyroglyphid m.
scabietic m.
soybean grain dust m.
m. typhus
wheat grain dust m.

mithramycin

mitis

mitis (*continued*)
m. form
prurigo m.

mitochondria

mitogen
m. response
m.-driven lymphocyte
replication

mitoses

mitosis

mitotic
m. figure
m. inhibitor
m. rate

mitoxantrone hydrochloride

mitral
m. valve prolapse
m. valve prolapse, aortic
anomalies, skeletal
changes, and skin
changes (MASS)

Mitsuda
M. antigen
M. reaction
M. test

mittenlike deformity

mixed
m. aerobic/anaerobic
abscess
m. B-cell proliferation
m. cellular infiltrate
m. cellularity type
m. chancre
m. connective tissue
disease (MCTD)
m. cryoglobulinemia
m. hemangioma
m. hepatic porphyria
m. infection
m. leprosy
m. nail infection
m. papillary follicular
adenocarcinoma

mixed (*continued*)
    m. porphyria
    m. seborrheic-
      staphylococcal blepharitis
    m. tumor
    m. tumor of skin

mJ
    millijoule

MLNS
    mucocutaneous lymph
      node syndrome

MMR
    measles-mumps-rubella
      MMR vaccine
      MMR II

mnemic

mnemonic

moccasin
    m. foot
    m. snake bite
    m.-type tinea pedis

modification

modified
    m. measles
    m. smallpox
    m. varicella-like syndrome

modulation

modulator

Moeller
    M. hunter glossitis
    M. itch

Mohs
    M's chemosurgery
    M's fresh-tissue technique
    M's micrographic surgery
    M's microsurgery
    M's procedure
    M's surgery
    M's surgical removal
    M's technique

moiety

moist
    m. gangrene
    m. lesion
    m. papule
    m. tetter
    m. wart

Moisture ophthalmic drops

Moisturel moisturizer

moisturizer
    Aqua Care m.
    Betadine First Aid
      Antibiotics + m.
    body m.
    Eucerin m.
    Eucerin Plus m.
    facial m.
    Keri m.
    Lubriderm m.
    Moisturel m.
    Nivea m.
    occlusive m.
    RoEzIt skin m.
    topical m.
    Vaseline Intensive Care m.

moisturizing
    m. protective cream
    m. ointment

molar
    mulberry m.

mold
    nondermatophytic m.

mole
    atypical m.
    hairy m.
    pigmented m.
    spider m.

molecule
    class II storage m.
    histocompatibility m.
    integrin m.
    pentameric IgM m.
    reactive m.
    receptor m.

molle
 fibroma m.
 heloma m.
 papilloma m.

Moll's glands

mollusciformis
 verruca m.

molluscoid neurofibroma

molluscous

molluscum
 m. body
 cholesterinic m.
 m. contagiosum
 m. contagiosum
  cornuatum
 m. contagiosum virus
 m. corpuscle
 m. epitheliale
 m. fibrosum
 m. giganteum
 m. lipomatodes
 m. pendulum
 m. pseudocarcinomatosum
 m. pseudotumor
 m. sebaceum
 m. simplex
 m. varioliforme
 m. verrucosum

molt

mometasone furoate

Mondor's disease

mongolian
 m. macule
 m. facies
 m. spot

mongolism

monilated

monilethrix

Monilia
 M. albicans

Moniliaceae

monilial
 m. granuloma

moniliasis

moniliform
 m. hair

moniliformis
 lichen ruber m.

moniliid

Monistat
 M. cream
 M.-Derm topical
 M. lotion
 M. Vaginal

monkey
 m. B virus
 m. epithelium

monkeypox
 m. virus

monobenzone

monobenzyl ether of
 hydroquinone

monochroic

monochromasy

monochromat

monochromatic

monochromatism

monoclonal
 m. antibody (MAB, MoAb)
 m. antibody Ber H2
 m. antibody Ki-l
 m. B-cell neoplasm
 m. B- and T-cell cutaneous
  lymphoid hyperplasia
 m. cryoglobulinemia
 m. gammopathy
 m. IgG paraproteinemia
 m. plasmacytoma
 m. T-cell lymphoid
  hyperplasia

monocyte

monocyte-macrophage system

monocytic
    m. leukemia

monocytosis
    avian m.

Monodox oral

monoinfection

monomer

monomeric

monomer
    acrylic m.
    Actin m.
    methyl methacrylate m.
    vinyl m.

monomicrobic

monomorphous

mononeuritis
    m. multiplex

mononeuropathy

mononuclear
    m. cell
    m. phagocyte system
      (MPS)

monopolar current

monorecidive
    m. chancre

monosodium
    m. urate (MSU)
    m. urate crystal
    m. urate monohydrate

monosomy

monostotic lesion

monosymptomatic
  hypochondriasis psychosis

monotherapy
    dapsone m.

Monro
    M. abscess

Monsel's solution

Montenegro
    M. reaction
    M. test

Montgomery
    M's follicles
    M's glands
    M's tubercles

moon
    m. boot syndrome
    m. facies

5-MOP
    5-methoxypsoralen

8-MOP
    8-methoxypsoralen

Moraceae

morbid hair pulling

Morbihan's disease

morbilli

morbilliform
    m. basal cell carcinoma
    m. eruption
    m. reaction

Morbillivirus
    equine M.

morbus
    m. Darier
    m. majocchi
    m. moniliformis

MORFAN syndrome

morganii
    Morganella m.

Morgan's lines

morphe

morphea
    acroteric m.
    m. acroterica
    m. alba
    m. atrophica

Morgellons disease

morphea (*continued*)
    m. flammea
    generalized m.
    m. guttata
    guttate m.
    herpetiform m.
    m. herpetiformis
    linear m.
    m. linearis
    m. nigra
    m. pigmentosum
    m. profunda
    subcutaneous m.
    m. variant

morpheaform
    m. basal cell carcinoma
    m. sarcoid

morphologic
    m. category
    m. classification
    m. lesion type
    m. pattern
    m. units

morphology
    lesion m.

morpio, morpion *pl.* morpiones

Morquio
    M's disease
    M's sign
    M's syndrome

morsicatio buccarum

mortality

Mortierella
    M. wolfii

mortification

mortified

Mortimer
    M. disease
    M. malady

Morvan
    M's disease
    M's syndrome

mosaic
    m. fungus
    m. mutations
    m. skin
    m. wart

mosaicism

Moschcowitz
    M's disease

M's syndrome

mossy foot

moth
    brown-tail m.
    m. dermatitis
    flannel m.
    io m.
    m. patch
    tussock m.
    "moth-eaten"
    m.-e. alopecia
    m.-e. appearance
    m.-e. baldness

mother
    m. jaw
    m. lesion

motor and speech delay

Motrin

mottled
    m. bluish discoloration
    m. dyspigmentation
    m. pigmentation

mottling
    netlike m.

moulage

Moulin
    linear atrophoderma of M.

mountain disease

mouse
    m. flea
    house m.

mousepox

mousepox (*continued*)
  m. virus

mouth
  burning m.
  dry m.
  m. erythema multiforme
  painful m.
  scabby m.
  sore m.
  trench m.

Moynahan syndrome

moxibustion

mower's mite

moxa

M-Prednisol Injection

MPS
  mucopolysaccharidosis

MR
  malar rash

MRC
  Medical Research Council

MRCL
  Medical Research Council
    Laboratories

MRD
  minimal reacting dose

MRI
  magnetic resonance
    imaging

MSH
  melanocytic-stimulating
    hormone

Much granule

Mucha
  M. disease
  M. syndrome
  M.-Habermann disease
  M.-Habermann
    syndrome

mucicarmine stain

mucilage
  tragacanth m.

mucin
  m. deposition
  dermal m.

mucinoid

mucinosa
  alopecia m.

mucinosis *pl.* mucinoses
  cutaneous focal m.
  follicular m.
  m follicularis
  papular m.
  m. papulosa seu
    lichenoides
  plaquelike cutaneous m.
  reticular erythematous m.
    (REM)

mucinous
  m. cyst
  m. degeneration
  m. eccrine carcinoma

Muckle-Wells syndrome

mucocele

mucocutaneous
  m. borders
  m. candidiasis
  chronic m.
  m. disease
  m. fragility
  m. junction
  m. leishmaniasis
  m. lesion
  m. lymph node
    syndrome
  m. manifestation
  m. moniliasis
  m. sporotrichosis

mucoid
  m. degeneration

mucolytic

Mucomyst

mucophanerosis intrafollicularis
    et seboglandularis

mucopolysaccharide

mucopolysaccharidosis *pl.*
    mucopolysaccharidoses

mucopurulent
    m. sputum

Mucor

mucoraceous

Mucorales

mucormycosis
    cutaneous m.

mucosa *pl.* mucosae
    buccal m.
    hyalinosis cutis et m.
    lingual m.
    lipoidosis cutis et m.
    oral m.
    reddening of oropharyngeal
        m.
    ulceration of oral m.

mucosa-associated lymphoid
    tissue (MALT)

mucosal
    m. disease
    m. disease virus
    m. inflammation
    m. keratin pair K4 and K13
    m. lentigines
    m. melanoma
    m. melanosis
    m. neuroma
    m. pigmentation
    m. sarcoid

mucositis

mucosocutaneous

Mucosol

mucosum
    stratum m.

mucous

mucous (*continued*)
    m. cyst
    m. desiccation
    m. extravasation
        phenomenon
    m. granuloma
    m. membrane
    m. membrane disease
    m. membrane lesions
    m. membrane ulceration
    m. papule
    m. patch
    m. patches of syphilis
    m. plaque
    m. plug
    m. plugging
    m. retention cyst

mucous-membrane pemphigoid

Mucuna

mucus
    m. hypersecretion
    oyster mass of m.
    thick and sticky m.

mucus et mala pituita nasi

Muehrcke's line

Muir-Torre syndrome

mulberry
    m. cells
    m. lesion
    m. pattern
    m. rash
    m. spot

mule spinners' cancer of the
    scrotum

multiagent chemotherapy

multibacillary

multicentric
    m. basal cell carcinoma
    m. reticulohistiocytosis
        (MR)
    m. skin-limited disease

multicoloration

multidigit dactylitis

multifaceted syndrome

multifactorial
m. inheritance

multifidus

multifocal
m. extravasation
m. nature

multiforme
atypical erythema m.
bullous erythema m.
chronic erythema m.
drug-associated erythema m.
erythema m.
granuloma m.
mouth erythema m.
oral erythema m.
postherpetic erythema m.

multiformis
dermatitis m.

multigemini

multi-infection

multilating skin damage

multilocular
m. pustules

multinucleated
m. cell
m. cell angiohistiocytoma
m. epidermal giant cells
m. epithelioid cells
m. foam cell
m. foamy histiocytes
m. giant cell

multinucleation

multiorgan
m. disease
m. infarct
m. involvement

multiparous

multiple
m. benign cystic epithelioma
m. cerebrovascular ischemic event
m. chemical sensitivity
m. congenital defects
m. cutaneous leiomyoma
m. drug allergy syndrome
m. endocrine neoplasia (MEN)
m. endocrine neoplasms (MEN)
m. familial trichoepitheliomas
m. fibroepithelial tumor of Pinkus
m. fibrofolliculoma
m. hamartoma syndrome
m. hereditary hemorrhagic telangiectasis
m. idiopathic hemorrhagic sarcoma
m. keratoacanthoma
m. lentigines syndrome
m. minute digitate hyperkeratosis
m. minute keratotic papule
m. mucosal neuroma
m. mucosal neuroma syndrome
m. myeloma
m. myositis
m. neuroma
m. nevus cell nevi
m. plasmacytoma
m. puncture test (MPT)
m. puncture tuberculin test
m. reticulohistiocytoma
m. sclerosis
m. subcutaneous angiolipomas
m. sulfatase deficiency
m. sulfatase deficiency syndrome
m. symmetrical lipomatosis
m. trichoepithelioma

multiplex
  m. PCR
  osteitis tuberculosa cystica
    m.
  xanthoma m.

multisensitivity

multiseptate macroconidia

multisite involvement

multisystem
  m. ectodermal change
  m. disease
  m. sarcoidosis

multivariant analysis

mummification
  m. necrosis

mumps
  m. skin test antigen
  m. virus

Munchausen's syndrome

Munro
  M's abscess
  M's microabscess

mupirocin
  m. ointment

muriform
  m. fungal cells

muromonab-CD3

Mus
  M. alexandrinus
  M. decumanus
  M. musculus
  M. norvegicus
  M. rattus rattus

Muscidae

muscle
  arrector m. of hair
  cutaneous m.
  dermal m.
  m. origin

muscular

m. atrophy
m. dystrophy
m. weakness

musculus
  m. arrector pili

mustard
  nitrogen m.

Mustargen Hydrochloride

mutant

mutation of loricrin

mutational

mutilans
  arthritis m.
  keratoma
    hereditarium m.
  lupus m.
  psoriatic arthritis m.

mutilating
  m. keratoderma
  m. keratoderma of
    Vohwinkel
  m. leprosy

Mutilidae

muzzling

MVLS
  modified varicella-like
    syndrome

myasthenia gravis (MG)

Mycelex
  M. cream
  M.-G
  M. troche
  M.-7

mycelial
  m. form

mycelian

mycelioid

mycelium

mycete

mycethemia

mycetism

mycetoma
  actinomycotic m.
  Bouffardi black m.
  Bouffardi white m.
  Brumpt white m.
  Carter black m.
  eumycotic m.
  Nicolle white m.
  Vincent white m.

mycid

Mycifradin
  M. sulfate oral
  M. sulfate topical

Mycitracin topical

mycobacterial
  m. abscess
  m. DNA
  m. infection
  m. ulcer

mycobacteriosis
  environmental m.

Mycobacterium
  M. abscessus
  M. avium
  M. avium complex (MAC)
  M. avium-intracellulare
    (MAI)
  M. chelonae
  M. fortuitum
  M. gordonae
  M. haemophilum
  M. kansasii
  M. leprae
  M. leprae antigen
  M. malmoense
  M. marinum
  M. scrofulaceum
  M. simiae
  M. szulgai
  M. tuberculosis (MTB)
  M. ulcerans
  M. xenopei

mycodermatitis

Mycogen II topical

Mycolog-II topical

mycology

Myconel topical

mycophenolate mofetil

Mycoplasma
  M. pneumoniae

mycoplasmal infection

mycosis *pl.* mycoses
  cutaneous m.
  m. cutis chronica
  deep m.
  m. favosa
  m. framboesioides
  m. fungoides
  m. fungoides d'emblée
  m. fungoides palmaris et
    plantaris
  m. interdigitalis
  m. intestinalis
  opportunistic systemic m.
  rare m.
  subcutaneous m.

mycostatic

Mycostatin
  M. oral
  M. topical

mycotic
  m. endophthalmitis
  m. infections

myelin
  m. basic protein
  m. metabolic products
  m. protein

myelitis

myelocytic
  m. leukemia

myelodysplastic syndrome
  (MDS)

myelofibrosis

myelogenous
    m. leukemia

myeloid
    m. form
    m. metaplasia

myeloma
    m. tumor lymphocyte

myelomonocytic
    m. leukemia

myeloperoxidase (MPO)
    m. deficiency

myeloproliferative
    m. disease
    m. disorder

myelosuppression

myelosuppressive
    m. therapy

Myerson's nevi

myiasis
    botfly facultative m.
    botfly obligate m.
    creeping m.
    cutaneous m.
    dermal m.
    facultative m.
    furuncular m.
    m. linearis
    obligate m.
    m. oestruosa
    subcutaneous m.
    wound m.

Myliobatidae

myoblastoma
    granular cell m.

myocardial
    m. infarction
    m. sarcoidosis

myocarditis

myocardium

Myochrysine

myoclonus

myocutaneous

myoepithelial
    m. cells
    m. contraction

myoepithelioid cell
  reduplication

myoepithelioma

myoepithelium

myofibroblast

myofibromatosis
    infantile m.

myoma

myonecrosis

myopathy

myopia

myosclerosis

myosin

myositis
    nodular m.
    nonclostridial m.

myotonia atrophica

myotonic muscular dystrophy

myriad microfilariae

Myriapoda

myringitis
    m. bulbosa
    bullous m.

myringodermatitis

myrmecia
    m. type
    m. wart

Myroxilon

myrtle

Mytrex
  M. F topical

myxedema
  circumscribed m.
  generalized m.
  papular m.
  pretibial m.

myxedematosus
  lichen m.

myxedematous
  m. arthropathy
  m. lichen

myxoderma papulosum

myxoedema
  m. circumscriptum
    symmetricum praetibiale
  pretibial m.

myxofibroma

myxoid
  m. cyst
  m. finger cyst
  m. neurofibroma
  m. pseudocyst
  m. stroma

myxoma *pl.* myxomas,
  myxomata
    lipomatous m.

myxomatous
  m. degeneration
  m. material

myxosarcoma

myxovirus

N

NAAF
  National Alopecia Areata
    Foundation

nabumetone

NACDG
  North American Contact
    Dermatitis Group

nacreous ichthyosis

NADPH oxidase

Naegeli's syndrome

Naegleria

naeslundii
  Actinomyces n.

naevoid (*variant of* nevoid)

naevus (*variant of* nevus)

nafarelin
  n. acetate

Nafcil injection

nafcillin
  n. sodium

naftifine
  n. hydrochloride

Naftin
  N. cream
  N. topical

Naga sore

nail
  azure lunula of n.
  n. biting
  brittle n.
  n. change
  clubbing of n.
  n. clubbing
  convex n.
  n. discoloration
  double-edge n.
  n. dystrophy
  eggshell n.

nail (*continued*)
  n. en raquette
  n. fold
  n. fold capillaroscopy
  n. fold capillary loop
    abnormality
  n. fold inflammation
  n. fragility
  geographic stippling of n.
  n. groove
  half-and-half n.
  hang n. (*hangnail is
    preferred*)
  n. hardeners
  hippocratic n.
  n. horn
  ingrown n.
  n. keratin
  n. lacquers
  n. matrix
  n. matrix melanoma
  n. matrix nevus
  Ony-Clear N.
  parrot beak n.
  pigmented changes of the
    nails
  pincer n.
  n. pit
  pitted n.
  n. pitting
  pitting of n.
  n. plate
  n. plate staining
  n. plate thinning
  n. polish
  n. polish base coat
  n. polish removers
  racket n.
  racquet n.
  ram horn n.
  reedy n.
  ringworm of n.
  n. root
  shell n.
  splitting n.
  spoon n.

nail (*continued*)
    stippled n.
    Terry's n.
    turtleback n.
    n. wall
    watch-crystal n.
    whole n.
    yellow n.

nailbed
    n. hyperkeratosis
    n. nevus

nailbiting

nail fold
    n. f. capillary microscopy
    proximal n. f.

naillike shape

nail nipper
    Amico n. n.

nail-patella-elbow syndrome

naked
    n. granulomas
    n. papillary epithelioma
    n. tubercle

nalidixic acid

Nallpen injection

naloxone
    n. HCl
    n. hydrochloride

naltrexone
    n. HCl

NAME
    nevi, atrial myxoma,
      myxoid neurofibromas,
      and ephelides
        NAME syndrome

nape
    n. nevus
    n. of the neck

naphtha

naphthalene

napkin
    n. dermatitis
    n. rash

naproxen
    n. sodium

narcotic
    n. dermopathy

naris, narium
    folliculitis n. perforans

narrow
    n. band
    n. rim

narrowband
    n. UVB
    n. UVB phototherapy

nasal
    n. glioma
    n. hypoplasia
    n. packing
    n. papillomata
    n. septal cartilage

nasi
    granulosis rubra n.

nasociliary
    n. branch

nasolabial
    n. angle
    n. crease
    n. fold (NLF)
    n. grooves

nasopharyngeal
    n. leishmaniasis
    n. ulcer

natal teeth

native

natural killer (NK)
    n. k. cell
    n. k. cytotoxic factor
      (NKCF)
    n. k. cell stimulating factor
      (NKSF)

Naxos disease

NBT
   nitroblue tetrazolium

NebuPent inhalation

Necator americanus

necatoriasis

neck
   n. dermatitis
   fiddler n.
   Madelung's n.
   n. of hair follicle
   n. sign

necklace
   Casal's n.
   n. of pearls
   n. of Venus

necrobiosis
   n. lipoidica
   n. lipoidica diabeticorum
   n. lipoidica-granuloma
      annulare
   n. lipoidica-like lesions

necrobiotic
   n. connective tissue
   n. xanthogranuloma

necrogenic
   n. tubercle
   n. wart

necrogenica
   verruca n.

necrolysis
   toxic epidermal n. (TEN)

necrolytic migratory erythema

necrosis *pl.* necroses
   cold-induced n.
   pressure n.
   n. progrediens
   radiation n.
   radium n.
   stellate n.
   subcutaneous fat n.
   traumatic fat n.

necrotic
   n. arachnidism
   n. center
   n. connective tissue
   n. crust
   n. cutaneous loxoscelism
   n. detritus
   n. grayish substance
   n. papule
   n. pocket
   n. scab
   n. slough
   n. tissue
   n. ulcer

necrotica
   acne n.
   dermatitis nodularis n.

necrotisans
   sycosis nuchae n.

necrotization

necrotizing
   n. angiitides
   n. angiitis
   n. arteritis
   n. fasciitis
   n. glomerulitis
   n. glomerulonephritis
   n. granuloma
   n. infection
   n. livedo reticularis
   n. livedo vasculitis
   n. panarteritis
   n. vasculitis

needle
   n. biopsy

negative
   n. nevus
   n. patch test
   n. reaction
   n. Schick test

NEH
   neutrophilic eccrine
      hidradenitis

neighboring skin

Neisseria
  N. gonorrhoeae
  N. meningitidis
  N. meningitidis B

Nelson's syndrome

nemathelminth

Nemathelminthes

nemathelminthiasis

nematization

Nematocera

nematocyst
  venom-bathed n.

Nematoda

nematode
  n. dermatitis

nematodiasis

neoangiogenesis

Neo-Cortef topical

neodymium (Nd)
  n.:yttrium-aluminum-garnet
    (Nd:YAG) laser

neoformans
  Cryptococcus n.
  Saccharomyces n.

Neoloid

Neomixin topical

neomycin
  n. dermatitis
  n. and polymyxin B
  n., polymyxin B, and
    dexamethasone
  n., polymyxin B, and
    gramicidin
  n., polymyxin B, and
    hydrocortisone
  n., polymyxin B, and
    prednisolone
  n. sulfate

neonatal

neonatal (*continued*)
  n. acne
  n. candidiasis
  n. citrullinemia
  n. hemochromatosis
  n. herpes
  n. herpes simplex virus
  n. icterus
  n. lupus
  n. lupus erythematosus
    (NLE)
  lupus erythematosus, n.
  n. pustular melanosis
  n. systemic candidiasis

neonate

neonatorum
  acne n.
  dermatitis exfoliativa n.
  edema n.
  erythema toxicum n.
  ichthyosis congenita n.
  impetigo n.
  pemphigus n.
  sclerema n.
  seborrhea squamosa n.

neoplasia

neoplasm

neoplastic
  n. angioendo
    theliomatosis
  n. B cell
  n. cell
  n. disease
  n. infiltrate
  n. mass
  n. process
  n. proliferation
  n. transformation

neoplastica
  acrokeratosis n.
  alopecia n.

Neoral
  N. oral

Neosar injection

Neosporin
  N. Cream
  N. solution
  N. Topical Ointment

neostibosan

NeoSynalar

Neotestudina rosatii

Neotrombicula autumnalis

neovascularization

nephelometry

nephritic syndrome

nephritogenic
  n. streptococcus

nephroerysipelas

nephrolithiasis

nephropathy

nephrotic syndrome

nephrotoxic

nephrotoxicity

NERDS
  nodules, eosinophilia,
    rheumatism, dermatitis,
    and swelling
      NERDS syndrome

nerve
  n. deafness
  n. sheath myxoma

Nervocaine

nervosa
  purpura n.

Nesacaine
  N.-MPF

nest
  junctional n.
  n's of nevus cells

Netherton's syndrome

netlike

netlike (*continued*)
  n. distribution
  n. mottling

netted pattern

nettle
  n. rash

Nettleship's disease

nettling hair

network
  idiotype n.

Neucalm

Neumann
  N's disease
  N's type

neural
  n. crest
  n. fibrolipoma
  n. leprosy
  n. nevus
  n. tissue

neural-mediated flushing

neuralgia
  postherpetic n. (PHN)
  red n.

neurilemmoma

neurinoma

neuritic

neuritis

neuriticum
  atrophoderma n.

neuritis
  optic n.

neuroblast

neuroblastoma

neurocutaneous
  n. disorder
  n. melanocytosis
  n. melanosis
  n. syndrome

neurodermatitic

neurodermatitis
  n. atopica
  circumscribed n.
  n. circumscripta
  n. disseminata
  disseminated n.
  exudative n.
  genital n.
  localized n.
  nodular n.
  nummular n.

neurodermatosis

neurodermite disseminée

neuroectodermal
  n. defect
  n. structures

neuroendocrine
  n. carcinoma of the skin
  n. cell
  n. tumor

neuroepidermal

neurofibroma

neurofibromatosis (*types–8*)
  abortive n.
  central type n.
  classic n.
  n. generalisata (of von
    Recklinghausen)
  incomplete n.
  late onset n.
  segmental n.
  variant n.

neurofibrosarcoma

neurohumoral

neurolemmoma (*variant of*
  neurilemmoma)

neuroleprosy

neuroleptic
  n. drug

neurolipomatosis
  n. dolorosa

neurologic
  n. abnormality
  n. alopecia
  n. degeneration
  n. genodermatosis

neuroma
  n. cutis
  false n.
  nevoid n.
  n. telangiectodes

neuromatosa
  elephantiasis n.

neuromatosis

neuromatous

neuron

neuronevus

Neurontin

neuropathic pain

neuropathy

neuropeptide

neurosensory deafness

neurosyphilis
  asymptomatic n.
  late n.
  meningeal n.
  meningovascular n.
  parenchymatous n.

neurothekeoma

neurotic
  n. excoriation

neurotica
  alopecia n.

neurotoxic poison

neurotoxicity

neurotrophic
  n. origin
  n. ulcer
  n. ulcerations

neurotropic forms

neurovascular
  n. junction
  n. structure

neutral
  n. lipid
  n. lipid storage
  n. lipid storage disease

neutralization

Neutrogena
  N. Acne Mask
  N. Healthy Skin
  M. Moisture SPF 15
  N. T/Derm
  N. Sensitive Skin Sunscreen
    SPF 17
  N. soap
  N. Sunblock SPF 30

neutropenia

neutrophil
  n. chemotaxis
  n. migration
  n. superoxide generation

neutrophilia

neutrophilic
  n. dermatosis
  n. eccrine hidradenitis
  n. exocytosis
  n. inflammation
  n. intraepidermal IgA
    dermatosis
  n. leukocytoclastic
    vasculitis
  n. microabscess
  n. necrosis
  n. vessel-based dermal
    inflammation

nevi (*plural of* nevus)
  compound, benign
    acquired n.
  intradermal, benign
    acquired n.
  junctional, benign acquired
    n.

nevoblast

nevocellular

nevocyte

nevocytic nevus

nevoid (*variant* naevoid)
  n. anomaly
  n. basal cell carcinoma
  n. basal cell carcinoma
    syndrome
  n. basalioma syndrome
  n. distribution
  n. elephantiasis
  n. hyperkeratosis of nipple
    and areola
  n. hypermelanosis
  n. hypertrichosis
  n. lentigo
  n. process
  n. telangiectasia

nevolipoma

nevoxanthoendothelioma

nevus *pl.* nevi (*variant* naevus)
  achromic n.
  n. acneiformis unilateris
  acquired n.
  acquired melanocytic n.
  amelanotic n.
  n. anemicus
  n. angiectodes
  n. angiomatodes
  angiomatous n.
  n. arachnoideus
  n. araneosus
  n. araneus
  nevi, atrial myxoma,
    myxoid neurofibromas,
    and ephelides (NAME)
  n. avasculosus
  balloon cell n.
  basal cell n.
  bathing trunk n.
  Becker's n.
  n. Bleu
  blue n.

nevus (*continued*)
  blue rubber bleb nevi
  capillary n.
  n. cavernosus
  n. cell
  n. cell, A-type
  n. cell, B-type
  n. cell, C-type
  cellular n.
  cellular blue n.
  n. cell nevus
  n. cerebelliformis
  n. ceruleus
  chromatophore n. of
    Naegeli
  comedo n.
  comedones epidermal n.
  n. comedonicus
  n. comedonicus
    syndrome
  common n.
  compound n.
  congenital n.
  connective tissue n.
  n. depigmentosus
  dermal n.
  dermoepidermal n.
  dysplastic n.
  n. elasticus
  n. elasticus of
    Lewandowski
  epidermal n.
  epidermic-dermic n.
  epithelial n.
  epithelioid cell n.
  n. epitheliomatocylindro-
    matosus
  erectile n.
  fatty n.
  faun tail n.
  n. fibrosus
  flame n.
  n. flammeus
  n. flammeus nuchae
  n. flammeus phakomatosis
    pigmentovascularis
  n. follicularis
  n. follicularis keratosis

nevus (*continued*)
  n. fragarius
  n. fuscoceruleus
  n. fuscoceruleus
    acromiodeltoideus
  n. fuscoceruleus
    ophthalmomaxillaris
  garment n.
  giant congenital n.
  giant congenital pigmented
    n.
  giant hairy n.
  giant pigmented n.
  n. giganteus
  hair follicle n.
  hairy n.
  halo n.
  hard n.
  hepatic n.
  honeycomb n.
  inflamed linear verrucous
    epidermal n. (ILVEN)
  intracutaneous n.
  intradermal n.
  intraepidermal n.
  Ito n.
  n. of Ito
  Jadassohn's sebaceous n.
  Jadassohn-Tièche n.
  junction n.
  junctional n.
  lentigines, atrial myxoma,
    mucocutaneous
    myxomas, and blue nevi
    (LAMB)
  lichen striatus epidermal n.
  linear n.
  linear epidermal n.
  n. lipomatodes
  n. lipomatodes superficialis
  n. lipomatosis
  n. lipomatosus
  n. lipomatosus cutaneus
    superficialis
  lymphatic n.
  n. lymphaticus
  n. maculosus
  malignant blue n.

nevus (*continued*)

marginal n.
m. maternus
melanocytic n.
mesodermal n.
mixed n.
n. mollusciformis
n. molluscum
n. morus
multiplex n.
nape n.
negative n.
n. nervosus
neural n.
neuroid n.
nevocellular n.
n. nevocellularis
nevocytic n.
nevus cell n.
nodular connective tissue n.
nonpigmented n.
nuchal n.
n. of Ota
n. oligemicus
n. ophthalmomaxillaris
oral epithelial n.
organoid n.
Ota's n.
n. of Ota
n. papillaris
n. papillomatosus
pigmented n.
pigmented hair epidermal n.
n. pigmentosus
n. pigmentosus et pilosus
n. pilosus
plane n.
polyploid n.
port-wine n.
n. profundus
raspberry n.
n. sanguineus
scarf n.
n. sebaceous
sebaceous n.
n. sebaceus of Jadassohn
sebaceus n. of Jadassohn

nevus (*continued*)

segmental n.
n. simplex
soft n.
speckled lentiginous n.
spider n.
n. spilus
n. spilus lentigo
n. spilus tardus
spindle cell n.
spindle and epithelioid cell n.
Spitz n.
n. spongiosus albus mucosae
stellar n.
stocking n.
straight hair n.
strawberry n.
subcutaneous n.
n. sudoriferous
Sutton's n.
n. syringocystadenosus papilliferus
systematized n.
n. tardus
n. telangiectaticus
n. unilateralis comedonicus
n. unius lateralis
n. unius lateris
Unna's n.
n. varicosus osteohypertrophicus
vascular n.
n. vascularis
n. vascularis fungosus
n. vasculosus
n. venosus
venous n.
n. verrucosus
verrucous n.
n. vinosus
vulvar n.
Werther n.
white sponge n.
white sponge n.
woolly-hair n.
zoniform n.

nevus-cell nevus

newborn
    bullous impetigo of n.
    n. erythroderma
    spontaneous gangrene of n.
    subcutaneous fat necrosis
        of n.

Newcastle
    N. disease (ND)
    N. disease virus

New World leishmaniasis

Nezelof
    N. syndrome

NF
    neurofibromatosis

NGT topical

Niacels

niacin
    n. deficiency

niacinamide

NIAMS
    National Institute of
        Arthritis, Musculoskeletal
        and Skin Disorders

nicardipine hydrochloride

nickel
    n. allergy
    n. dermatitis
    n. oxides
    n. sensitivity

Nicobid

Nicolar

Nicolas
    N.-Durant-Favre disease
    N.-Favre disease

Nicolau syndrome

Nicolle-Novy-MacNeal medium

nicotinamide

nicotine
    n. gum
    n. picrate

Nicotinex

nicotinic acid

Niemann-Pick disease

nifedipine

nifurtimox

night blindness

nigra
    dermatosis papulosa n.
    linea n.
    lingua n.
    pityriasis n.
    seborrhea n.
    tinea n.

nigricans
    acanthosis n. (AN)
    drug-induced acanthosis n.
    keratosis n.
    malignant acanthosis n.
    pseudoacanthosis n.
    Rhizopus n.
    type A acanthosis n.
    type B acanthosis n.
    type C acanthosis n.

NIH
    National Institutes of Health

Nikolsky's sign

Nilstat topical

ninth-day erythema

NIP
    National Immunization
        Program

nipple, accessory

nisoldipine

nit

nitidus
    lichen n.

Nitro-Bid ointment

nitrofurantoin

nitrofurazone

nitrogen (N)
    liquid n.
    n. mustard
    n. spray

Nitrostat ointment

nitrosurea

nitrous oxide

Nix
    N. Creme Rinse

Nizoral
    N. oral
    N. topical

NK
    natural killer
        NK cell

NKCF
    natural killer cytotoxic
        factor

NLE
    neonatal lupus
        erythematosus

NMSC
    National Comprehensive
        Cancer Network
    nonmelanoma skin cancer

No Pain-HP

Nocardia
    N. asteroides
    N. brasiliensis
    N. caviae
    N. farcinica
    N. madurae
    N. tenuis
    N. transvalensis

nocardiosis

nociceptor stimulation

nocturnal itching

nodal
    n. involvement

node
    Heberden n.
    milkers' n.

nodi (*plural of* nodus)

nodosa
    n. ball-and-socket deformity
    cutaneous polyarteritis n.
    dermatitis n.
    periarteritis n.
    tinea n.
    trichomycosis n.
    trichomycosis axillaries n.
    trichorrhexis n.

nodose
    n. condition
    n. lesions

nodosity

nodosum
    erythema n. (EN)

nodous

nodular
    n. basal cell carcinoma
    n. elastosis with cysts and
        comedones
    n. fasciitis
    n. hidradenoma
    n. fasciitis
    n. fat necrosis
    n. histology
    n. intraoral herpes
    n. leprosy
    n. malignant melanoma
    n. melanoma (NM)
    n. neurodermatitis
    n. pattern
    n. process
    n. prurigo
    n. pseudosarcomatous
        fasciitis
    n. scabies

nodular (*continued*)
   n. skin eruption
   n. skin lesion
   n. subcutaneous fasciitis
   n. vasculitis
   n. xanthomas

nodularis
   prurigo n.
   trichomycosis axillaris n.

nodularity

nodulated

nodulation

nodule
   apple jelly n.
   athlete's n.
   Bohn n.
   cutaneous n.
   cutaneous-subcutaneous n.
   dark-staining n.
   interconnecting pustular n.
   Jeanselme n.
   juxta-articular n.
   lepromatous n.
   Lisch n.
   milkers' n.
   paraumbilical n.
   picker's n.
   red n.
   red papule and n.
   rheumatic n.
   rheumatoid n.
   sharply circumscribed n.
   Sister Mary Joseph n.
   Stockman n.
   subcutaneous n.
   subcutaneous
     granulomatous n.
   subcutaneous rheumatoid
     n.
   surfers' n.

nodules, eosinophilia,
  rheumatism, dermatitis, and
  swelling (NERDS)

noduli (*plural of* nodulus)

nodulocystic
   n. acne
   n. lesion

nodulosis
   rheumatoid n.

nodulo-ulcerative lesions

nodulous

nodulus *pl.* noduli
   n. cutaneus

nodus *pl.* nodi

noire
   tache n.

Nolahist

noma

nomenclature

nonacnegenic

nonallergenic foods

nonallergic inflammatory
  reaction

nonblanchable
   n., abnormally colored
     lesion

nonbullous
   n. congenital erythrodermic
     ichthyosis
   n. congenital ichthyosiform
     erythroderma
   n. ichthyosiform
     erythroderma
   n. impetigo

noncaseating
   n. granuloma
   n. granulomatous
     inflammatory lesion
   n. tuberculoid granuloma

noncomedogenic

nondermatophyte fungal
  infection

nondiagnostic
   n. lesions

nonencapsulated

nonepidermolytic palmoplantar
  keratoderma

nonerosive arthritis

nongonococcal bacterial
  arthritis

nonhealing sore

nonhereditary
  n. bullous disease
  n. disease
  n. mesodermal dysplasia
    disorder

non-Hodgkin's lymphoma
  (NHL)

noniatrogenic

nonimmunologic
  n. complication
  n. drug reaction
  n. mechanism

noninfectious

noninflammatory
  n. edema
  n. thrombosis

noninvasive melanoma

nonisomerizable
  n. class
  n. retinoid

nonlipidized histiocytic cell

nonmelanoma
  n. cutaneous malignancy
  n. skin cancer

Nonne-Milroy-Meige syndrome

nonneoplastic
  n. disease
  n. infiltrating cell

nonnucleoside

nonocclusive dressing

nonpalpable purpura

nonpathogenic fungus

nonpharmacologic measure of
  treatment

nonphotochromogen

nonpigmented nevus

nonpitting
  n. edema

nonpoisonous

nonproteinous

nonscarring
  n. alopecia
  n. blister

nonsedating antihistamine

nonspecific
  n. dermatitis
  n. serologic test

nonspiny skin

nonsteroidal
  n. antiinflammatory
  n. antiinflammatory drug
    (NSAID)

nonstick gauze

nonsyphilitic
  n. interstitial keratitis
  n. treponematosis

nonthrombocytopenic purpura

nonvenereal
  n. contagiosity
  n. sclerosing lymphangitis
    of the penis
  n. syphilis

Noonan's syndrome

Norape cretata

Nordryl
  N. injection
  N. Oral

norepinephrine bitartrate

norgestimate

normal
n. acral skin
n. cholesteremic
xanthomatosis
n. hair follicle
n. oral mucosa
n. skin

normolipemic xanthomatosis

normolipoproteinemic
n. mucocutaneous
xanthomatosis
n. xanthomatosis

Norplant contraceptive system

Norpramin

Nor-tet oral

North American
N. A. blastomycosis
N. A. Contact Dermatitis
Group (NACDG)

northern
n. rat flea
n. rat flea bite

Norway itch

Norwegian scabies

nosocomial infection

nosologic

nostras
elephantiasis n.
piedra n.

notalgia paresthetica

notched incisors

notochord

Nova Scotia Niemann-Pick
disease

Novacet
N. topical

Novocain
N. injection

NP-27

NSAID
nonsteroidal
antiinflammatory drug

NSHD
nodular sclerosing Hodgkin
disease

nuchae
acne keloidalis n.
cutis rhomboidalis n.
erythema n.
lichen n.
ligamentum n.
nevus flammeus n.
sycosis n.

nuchal
n. area
n. comedones
n. rigidity

nuclear
n. antigens
n. chromatin
n. dust
n. IgG deposition
n. membrane
n. pleomorphism
n. vacuolization

nuclear/cytoplasmic ratio

nucleated blood cells

nuclei (*plural of* nucleus)

nucleic acid

nucleolar protein

nucleolus

nucleoside
n. reverse transcriptase
inhibitors

nucleotide
n. excision repair process

Nu-Hope skin barrier strip

nummular

nummular (*continued*)
  n. dermatitis
  n. eczema
  n. eruptions
  n. lesion
  n. neurodermatitis
  n. pattern
  n. syphilid

nummulare
  eczema n.

nummularis
  psoriasis n.

Nupercainal

Nutracort

Nutramigen

Nutraplus topical

nutritional
  n. deficiency
  n. development
  n. disorder

NVAC
  National Vaccine Advisory
    Committee

nyctalopia

Nygmia phaeorrhoea

nylon

nystagmus

nystatin
  n. and triamcinolone

Nystat-Rx

Nystex topical

Nyst-Olone II topical

O

oak
> poison o.
> o. tree
> western poison o.

oasthouse disease

oat cell
> o. c. carcinoma

oatmeal
> colloidal o.

obesity
> morbid o.

obligate
> o. aerobe
> o. myiasis

obligatory
> o. intracellular parasites
> o. pathogenicity

obliterans
> balanitis xerotica o.

obliterative arteritis
syndrome

obsessive-compulsive disorder
(OCD)

obsolescent

obstipation

obstructive
> o. jaundice
> o. liver disease
> o. purpura

obtusus
> lichen o.

OCA
> oculocutaneous albinism

occipital
> o. forelock
> o. horn syndrome
> o. scalp

occlude

Occlusal-HP

occlusion
> o. miliaria
> portal o.

occlusive
> o. arterial disease
> o. dressing
> o. moisturizer
> o. patch test
> o. permeable biosynthetic
> wound dressing
> o. therapy

occult primary melanoma

occupational
> o. acne
> o. allergic alveolitis
> o. contact dermatitis
> o. dermatosis
> o. exposure
> o. vitiligo

occupation-related syndrome

ochrodermia

ochronosis
> endogenous o.
> exogenous o.
> ocular o.

ochronotic arthropathy

octinoxate

octisalate

Octocaine
> O. injection

octreotide acetate

octyl
> o. methoxycinnamate
> o. salicylate

ocular
> o. abnormality
> o. albinism
> o. atopic dermatitis

ocular (*continued*)
    o. canthus
    o. dysplasia
    o. hypertelorism
    o. larva migrans
    o. lesion
    o. pemphigus
    o. rosacea

oculocerebral syndrome of
  Cross and McKusick

oculocerebral-
  hypopigmentation syndrome

oculocutaneous
    o. albinism
    o. telangiectasias

oculodermal
    o. melanocytosis
    o. melanosis

oculoglandular syndrome of
  Parinaud

oculo-oral-genital syndrome

Ocutricin
    O. HC otic
    O. topical ointment

odaxetic

ODD
  once-daily dosing

Odland body

odonto-tricho-ungual-digital-
  palmar syndrome

odontogenic
    o. cyst
    o. etiology
    o. infection

odontogenous sinus

odor
    volatile o.

odoriferous

Oedemeridae

Oesophagostomum

oestruosa
    myiasis o.

OET
  open epicutaneous test

Off!

ofloxacin

Ofuji's disease

Ohara's disease

OHL
  oral hairy leukoplakia

OI
  osteogenesis imperfecta

oidiomycin

Oidiomycetes

oidiomycosis

oidiomycotic
  "oid-oid" disease

oil
    o. acne
    bergamot o.
    bhilawanol o.
    birch tar o.
    cade o.
    castor o.
    citronella o.
    coal tar, lanolin, and
      mineral o.
    Derma-Smoothe o.
    o. drop lesion
    o. gland
    jojoba o.
    light mineral o.
    mineral o.
    o. of argemone
    o. of bergamot
    o. of cade
    olive o.
    ricinus o.
    o. spots
    sweet o.

oil (*continued*)
    theobroma o.
    trypsin, balsam peru, and
       castor o.
    white mineral o.

Oil of Olay

oilated colloidal oatmeal bath

oil-based facial foundation

oiliness

oily
    o. areas of the skin
    o. granuloma
    o. yellow fluid

ointment
    benzoic and salicylic acid
       o.
    coal tar o.
    compound resorcinol o.
    Hebra o.
    Jarisch o.
    Medi-Quick Topical O.
    Neosporin Topical O.
    rose water o.
    triamcinolone o. (TAO)
    Whitfield's O.

olamine
    ciclopirox o.

old burn scars

old man's pemphigus

Old World
    O. W. disease
    O. W. leishmaniasis

Olea

olefin

oleic acid

oleoresin
    plant o.

oleosa
    hyperhidrosis o.
    seborrhea o.

oleosus

olfactory acuity

olighidria

oligoarthritis

oligoclonal
    o. stage
    o. T-cell proliferation

oligocystic

oligodactyly

oligohidria

oligohidrosis

oligotrichia

oligotrichosis

olive

Ollendorf
    O's sign
    O's syndrome

Ollier
    O's disease
    O's layer

Olmsted
    O. syndrome

olsalazine sodium

omega
    o.-3 fatty acids
    o.-6 fatty acids

Omenn's syndrome

omental patch

Omnipen

Omnipen-N

omphalocele

once-daily dosing (ODD)

Onchocerca
    O. caecutiens
    O. volvulus

onchocercal dermatitis

onchocerciasis

onchocercoma *pl.*
    onchocertomas,
    onchocertomata

onchocercosis

oncogenic

oncology

oncosphere

oncovirus

ondansetron hydrochloride

one hand-two foot
    syndrome

ongles en raquette

onion
    o. skin surface

onion-mite dermatitis

onset
    insidious o.

onychalgia
    o. nervosa

onychatrophia

onychatrophy

onychauxis

onychectomy

onychia
    Candida o.
    o. craquelé
    o. lateralis
    o. maligna
    monilial o.
    o. parasitica
    o. periungualis
    o. piannic
    o. punctata
    o. sicca
    syphilitic o.

onychitis

onychoclasis

onychocryptosis

onychodystrophia mediana
    canaliformis

onychodystrophy

onychogenic

onychogryphosis,
    onychogryposis

onychoheterotopia

onychoid

onychology

onycholysis
    distal o.
    o. partialis
    proximal o.
    o. semilunaris

onycholytic

onychoma

onychomadesis

onychomalacia

onychomycosis
    Candida o.
    dermatophytic o.

onychonosus

onycho-osteodysplasia

onychopathic

onychopathology

onychopathy

onychophagia

onychophagy

onychophosis

onychophyma

onychoptosis

onychorrhexis

onychoschizia

onychosis

onychotillomania

onychotomy

onychotrophy

Ony-Clear Nail

onyx

onyxis

onyxitis

oophorectomy

oozing
 o. dermatitis

opacifier

opalescent

open
 o. comedo
 o. epicutaneous test (OET)
 o. patch test

open-angle glaucoma

operation
 Cotting's o.

ophiasis

ophritis

ophryitis

ophryogenes
 ulerythema o.

ophthalmic
 o. zoster

ophthalmica
 zona o.

ophthalmicus
 herpes zoster o.

ophthalmomaxillaris
 nevus o.
 nevus fuscoceruleus o.

ophthalmomyiasis

ophthalmoplegia

opiate
 o. analgesia

opioid

Opisocrostis hirsutus

oppilation

opportunistic
 o. infection
 o. organism
 o. pathogen
 o. systemic fungal infection
 o. systemic mycosis

opsonin

opsonization
 o./phagocytosis

opsonize

optic
 o. disk
 o. glioma
 o. neuritis

Optimine

optimum temperature

optomechanical scanner

Orabase
 O. HCA
 Kenalog in O.
 O. with benzocaine

Oracit

oral
 o. aphthous ulcer
 o. birth control pills
 o. candidiasis
 o. Crohn's disease
 o. commissure
 o. condyloma planus
 o. contraceptives
 o. epithelial nevus
 o. (erosive) lichen planus
 o. erythema multiforme
 o. florid papillomatosis
 o. frenula and clefts
 o. gold
 o. hairy leukoplakia
 o. hyposensitization

oral (*continued*)
    o. keratosis
    o. leukoplakia
    o. lichen planus
    o. melanoacanthoma
    o. melanosis
    o. methoxsalen
      photochemotherapy
    o. mucosa
    o. mucosa lesion
    o. mucosal papules
    o. nevus
    o.-ocular-genital syndrome
    o. papillomatosis
    o. postinflammatory
      hyperpigmentation
    o. psoriasis
    o. retinoids
    o. squamous cell
      carcinoma
    o. submucous fibrosis
    o. tattoo
    o. thrush
    o. ulceration
    o. zinc

oral lesion
    atrophic o. l's
    erosive o. l's
    reticulate o. l's
    ulcerative o. l's

orange-bronze color

Orap

Orasone oral

orbicular
    o. eczema

orbiculare
    Pityrosporon o. (*former
    name for Malassezia
    furfur*)

orbicularis
    o. oculi
    psoriasis o.

orbital
    o. inflammatory disease

orbital (*continued*)
    o. myositis
    o. pseudotumor

ordinal designation of the
    exanthemata

orf
    human o. virus
    o. virus

organ
    o.-specific autoantigen
    o. transplantation rejection
      prophylaxis

organ of Corti

organelle

organism
    prokaryotic extracellular o.

organoid nevus

oriental
    o. boil
    o. button
    o. rat flea
    o. rat flea bite
    o. ringworm
    o. sore
    o. ulcer

orientalis
    furunculosis o.
    Leishmania o.

orifice
    follicular o.
    pilosebaceous o.

orificial

orificialis
    tuberculosis cutis o.

oris
    cancrum o.
    leukokeratosis o.

ornidazole

ornithodoriasis

Ornithodoros

Ornithodoros (*continued*)
  O. tholozani

Ornithonyssus
  O. bacoti
  O. bursa
  O. sylviarum

ornithosis virus

orofacial
  o. edema
  o. granulomatosis
  o. infections

orogenital sexual contact

orolabial herpes simplex

oropharyngeal candidiasis

oropharynx

Oroya fever

orris

Orthoclone OKT3

orthographists

orthokeratinization

orthokeratosis

orthokeratotic cell

Orthomyxoviridae

orthomyxovirus

Orthopoxvirus
  O. vaccinia

orthostatic
  o. hypotension
  o. purpura

Osler
  O's disease
  O's hemangiomatosis
  O's nodes
  O's sign
  O's syndrome II
  O's triad
  O.-Vaquez disease
  O-Weber-Rendu disease
  O.-Weber-Rendu syndrome

osmidrosis

osseous
  o. anomalies
  o. choristoma
  o. heteroplasia
  o. lesion
  o. syphilis
  o. yaws

ossificans
  myositis o.

ossification
  para-articular o.

osteitis fibrosa cystica
  disseminata

osteoarthritic disfigurements

osteoarthritis (OA)

osteoarthropathy
  idiopathic hypertrophic o.
  primary hypertrophic o.

osteoblast

osteoblastic

osteochondritis dissecans

osteochondrodysplasia

osteoclast
  o.-activating factor (OAF)
  o.-type cell

osteoclastic activity

osteocope

osteocopic

osteodermatopoikilosis

osteodermatous

osteodermia

osteogenesis
  o. imperfecta
  o. imperfecta tarda

osteogenic sarcoma

osteohypertrophic nevus
  flammeus

osteolysis

osteolytic bone lesion

osteoma
    o. cutis

osteomalacia

osteomatoid

osteomatosis

osteomyelitis

osteopenia

osteoperiostitis

osteopoikilosis

osteosis
    o. cutis

osteotelangiectasia

ostia

ostium
    pilosebaceous o.

ostracea
    parakeratosis o.

ostraceous
    o. scale

ostreacea
    psoriasis o.

Ota
    nevus of O.
    O's nevus

oticus
    herpes zoster o.

otitis
    external o.
    o. externa

otomycosis

otosclerosis

outbreak

outermost
    o. envelope
    o. membrane

ova

ova and parasites (O&P)

oval
    o. areas
    o. nuclei

ovale
    Pityrosporum o. (former
        name for Malassezia
        ovaliss)
    Plasmodium o.

ovalis
    Malassezia o.

ovarian
    o. dysgenesis
    o. neoplasm
    o. teratoma

overdosage

overdose
    drug o.

overgrowth
    fungal o.

overlap
    o. disease
    o. myositis (OVLP)
    o. syndrome

overlapping
    o. metabolic pathway
    o. morphologies

overuse syndrome

overwintering

oviducal

ovinia

oviposition

ovipositor

OVLP
    overlap myositis

ovoid
    o. configuration
    o. nuclei

oxacillin
    o. sodium

oxalate crystal occlusion

oxalosis

oxaprozin

oxiconazole
    o. nitrate

oxidized cellulose

oxidizing agent

Oxistat
    O. topical

Oxsoralen
    O. topical
    O.-Ultra oral

oxybenzene

oxychlorosene

Oxy-5
    O. Tinted

oxybenzone
    methoxycinnamate and o.

Oxycel

oxychlorosene sodium

oxygen
    hyperbaric o. (HBO)
    o. saturation

oxyhemoglobin

oxymetholone

oxytetracycline
    o. hydrochloride
    o. and hydrocortisone
    o. and polymyxin B

oxyuriasis

Oxyuris vermicularis

oyster
    o. mass of mucus

ozochrotia

P

P
    P gene
    P gene codes
    P selectin activation

PAB
    para-aminobenzoate

PABA
    para-aminobenzoic acid

PAC
    papular acrodermatitis of
        childhood

pachonychia

pachycheilia

pachyderma
    p. lymphangiectatica
    p. verrucosa
    p. vesicae

pachydermatocele

pachydermatosis

pachydermatous

pachydermia

pachydermic

pachydermie vorticelle

pachydermoperiostosis
    p. plicata

pachyglossia

pachyhymenia

pachyhymenic

pachylosis

pachymenia

pachymenic

pachyonychia
    p. congenita
    p. congenital tarda
    p. congenital
        hereditaria

pachyotia

pad
    knuckle p.

padimate
    p. A
    p. O

Paecilomyces

Paederus
    P. gemellus
    P. gemellus sting
    P. limnophilus
    P. limnophilus sting

PAFD
    percutaneous abscess and
        fluid drainage

Paget
    P's abscess
    P's abscess syndrome
    P's cells
    P's disease
    P's disease, extramammary
    P's disease, mammary

pagetoid
    p. basal cell carcinoma
    p. cells
    p. melanoma
    p. reticulosis

pagoplexia

pain
    limb p.

painful
    p. adiposity
    p. auricular nodule
    p. bruising syndrome
    p. ear nodule
    p. piezogenic pedal papule

paint
    Castellani's p.

Pak
    Shingles Relief P.

palatal
    p. mucosa
    p. rugae

palate
    p. cross of espundia
    hard p.
    itchy soft p.
    soft p.

pale
    p. cell acanthoma
    p. cell walls
    p. color
    p. eosinophilic
    p. irides

palisaded
    p. collection
    p. granulomatous
        dermatoses
    p. granulomatous
        inflammation

palisading
    p. granuloma
    p. parallel rows

pallescense

palliative

pallida
    Spirochaeta p.

pallidum
    Treponema p.

Pallister mosaic aneuploid
    syndrome

pallor
    circumoral p.

palm
    reddening of p.

palmar
    p. aponeurosis
    p. crease
    p. erythema
    p. fascia
    p. fasciitis and polyarthritis
        syndrome

palmar (*continued*)
    p. hyperhidrosis
    p. keratoses
    p. pits
    p. seed dermatoses
    p. pustulosis
    p. syphilid
    p. xanthomas

palmare
    erythema p.
    xanthoma striatum p.

palmaris
    pyosis p.
    xanthochromia striata p.
    xanthoma striata p.

palmellina
    trichomycosis p.

palmitoleic acid

palmoplantar
    p. erythrodysesthesia
        syndrome
    p. fibromatosis
    p. hyperhidrosis
    p. hyperkeratosis
    p. keratoderma (PPK)
    p. pigmentation
    p. pustular psoriasis
    p. pustulosis

palmoplantaris
    pustulosis p.

palm-sole involvement

palpable purpura

palpebral
    p. antimongoloid fissures
    p. edema

palpebrarum
    pediculosis p.
    xanthelasma p.
    xanthoma p.
    p. xanthoma

pamidronate

PAN

PAN (*continued*)
    polyarteritis nodosa

Panafil

panaritium

panarteritis
    p. nodosa

Panasol II home phototherapy
    system

Panasol-S

panatrophy
    Gowers p.
    p. of Gower

P-ANCA
    positive peripheral
        antineutrophil cytoplasmic
        autoantibody

Pancoast
    P's syndrome
    P's tumor

pancreatic
    p. carcinoma
    p. disease
    p. neoplasm
    p. pseudocyst
    p. sprue

pancreatitis

pancytopenia

pandemic

pandemicity

panhidrosis

panhypopituitarism
    autoimmune p.
    idiopathic p.
    secondary p.

panidrosis

panimmunity

panleukopenia

Panmycin Oral

panniculalgia

panniculitides (*plural of*
    panniculitis)
    inflammatory p.
    lobular p.

panniculitis *pl.* panniculitides
    antitrypsin deficiency p.
    chemical p.
    cold p.
    cytophagic histiocytic p.
    cytophagic lobular p.
    enzyme-related p.
    histiocytic cytophagic p.
    inflammatory p.
    idiopathic p.
    idiopathic lobular p.
    lobular p.
    lupus erythematosus p.
    nodular migratory p.
    nodular nonsuppurative p.
    pancreatic p.
    pancreatic lobular p.
    physical p.
    physical lobular p.
    popsicle p.
    poststeroid p.
    prototypical septal p.
    relapsing febrile nodular
        nonsuppurative p.
    scleroderma septal p.
    sclerosing p.
    septal p.
    subacute migratory p.
    subacute nodular migratory
        p.
    traumatic p.
    vessel-based lobular p.
    Weber-Christian p.

panniculus *pl.* panniculi
    p. adiposus

pannus
    p.-cartilage junction
    p. formation

panophthalmitis

PanOxyl

PanOxyl-AQ

Panretin

pansclerotic
p. morphea of children
p. forms

Panscol
P. lotion
P. ointment

panthenol

pantothenol

Pap test

PAPA syndrome
pyogenic sterile arthritis,
    pyoderma gangrenosum
    and acne

papain

Papanicolaou test (Pap test)

papaverine

paper-white patch

papilla *pl.* papillae
anogenital vestibular p.
p. corii
dermal papillae
p. dermatis
p. dermis
hair p.
hypertrophy of tongue
    papillae
nerve p.
p. of corium
p. pili
skin p.
tactile papillae
vestibular p.

papillaris
pars p.

papillary
p. adenocarcinoma
p. adenoma
p. atrophy
p. base

papillary (*continued*)
p. connective tissue
p. dermal blood vessels
p. dermal edema
p. dermal fibrosis
p. dermal vessels
p. dermis
p. eccrine adenoma
p. ectasia
p. elements
p. hidradenoma
p. necrosis
p. part
p. tumor

papillate

papillation

papilliferous

papilliferum
hidradenoma p.
syringocystadenoma p.

papilliferus
nervus
    syringocystadenomatosus
    p.

papilliform

papillitis

papilloadenocystoma

papillocarcinoma

papilloma
p. acuminatum
basal cell p.
p. colli
cutaneous p.
p. diffusum
p. durum
hard p.
inguinale tropicum
intracanalicular p.
p. lineare
p. molle
soft p.
p. venereum
p. virus infection

papilloma (*continued*)
    warty p.
    zymotic p.

papillomatosis
    confluent and reticulate p.
    p. cutis carcinoides
    florid cutaneous p. (FCP)
    florid oral p.
    p. of Gougerot-Carteaud
    juvenile p.
    malignant p. of Degos
    oral florid p.
    palatal p.
    recurrent respiratory p.
    reticulated p.
    verrucous p.

papillomatosus
    lupus p.
    nevus p.

papillomatous
    p. epidermal hyperplasia

Papillomavirus

papillomavirus
    human p. (HPV)

Papillon-Lefèvre syndrome

Papineau graft

Papovaviridae

papovavirus
    p. group

pappose

pappus

papula

papular
    p. acantholysis
    p. acne
    p. acne scars
    p. acne vulgaris
    p. acrodermatitis
    p. acrodermatitis of
      childhood
    p. center

papular (*continued*)
    p. dermatitis
    p. dermatitis of pregnancy
    p. eruption
    p. fever
    p. fibroplasia
    p. histiocytosis of the head
    p. mastocytosis
    p. mucinosis
    p. pityriasis rosea
    p. pruritic dermatosis
    p. purpuric stocking and
      glove syndrome
    p. sarcoid
    p. scrofuloderma
    p. syphilid
    p. urticaria
    p. xanthoma

papulation
    granular p.
    perifollicular p.

papulatum
    erythema p.

papule
    Celsus p.
    discrete p.
    discrete umbilicated p.
    fibrous p.
    follicular p.
    follicular erythematous p.
    follicular spinous p.
    Gottron's p.
    indolent p.
    indurated p.
    keratotic p.
    moist p.
    mucous p.
    painful piezogenic pedal p.
    penile pearly p.
    perifollicular erythematous
      p.
    peripheral violaceous p.
    persistent pearly penile p.
    piezogenic pedal p.
    primary p.
    prurigo p.

papule (*continued*)
   pruritic p.
   purple-red p.
   red p.
   scaly p.
   split p.

papuliferous

papuloerythematous

papuloerythroderma
   p. of Ofuji

papuloid

papulonecrotic
   p. lesions
   p. tuberculid

papulonecrotica
   tuberculosis p.
   tuberculosis cutis p.

papulonodular deposition

papulopustular
   p. lesion
   p. secondary syphilis

papulopustule

papulosa
   acne p.
   dermatitis p. nigra
   p. nigra dermatosis
   stomatitis p.
   urticaria p.

papulose atrophicante maligne

papulosis
   atrophic p.
   p. atrophicans maligna
   bowenoid p.
   lymphomatoid p.
   malignant atrophic p.
   p. of the face

papulosquamous
   p. dermatitis
   p. disease
   p. disorder
   p. eruption

papulosquamous (*continued*)
   p. lesion
   p. syphilid

papulosum
   eczema p.

papulovesicle

papulovesicular
   p. acrolocated syndrome
   p. lesion
   p. rash
   p. satellite lesion

papyraceous
   p. scar

para
   p.-aminobenzoate (PAB)
   p.-aminobenzoic acid (PABA)

parachlorometaxylenol

parachlorophenylalanine

parachroma

parachromatosis

paracoccidioidal granuloma

Paracoccidioides brasiliensis

paracoccidioidin
   p. skin test

paracoccidioidomycosis

paraffin
   p.-fixed tissue
   liquid p.
   white soft p.
   yellow soft p.

paraffinoma

parafollicularis
   hyperkeratosis follicularis et p.

parafrenal abscess

parahidrosis

parainfluenza

parainfluenza (*continued*)
  p. virus

parakeratosis (*compare*
    porokeratosis)
  focal p.
  p. Mibelli
  p. ostracea
  p. papulosa
  p. psoriasiformis
  p. pustulosa
  p. scutularis
  p. variegata

parakeratotic
  p. cell
  p. crust
  p. hair cast
  p. horny layer
  p. nuclei
  p. scale

parallel linear scratch marks

parallergic

paralytic
  p. ileus

paramedian lines

parameter

paramethasone acetate

Paramyxoviridae

Paramyxovirus

paraneoplastic
  p. acrokeratosis
  p. pemphigus
  p. syndrome

paraneoplastica
  acrokeratosis p.

parangi

paranoia

paranuclear inclusion body–like
    aggregate

paraphenylenediamine
  p. dermatitis

paraphimosis

paraprotein

paraproteinemia

parapsoriasis
  p. acuta
  p. acuta et varioliformis
  acute p.
  atrophic p.
  p. atrophicans
  chronic p.
  p. digitiformis
  p. en gouttes
  p. en grandes plaques
  p. en plaque
  p. en plaque Brocq, benign
    small-plaque type
  p. en plaque Brocq, large
    focal type
  p. en plaque Brocq, large
    plaque type
  p. en plaque Brocq, small
    focal type
  p. guttata
  guttate p.
  large plaque p.
  p. lichenoid
  p. lichenoides
  p. lichenoides chronica
  p. lichenoides et
    varioliformis acuta
  p. maculata
  poikilodermatous p.
  poikilodermic p.
  retiform p.
  small plaque p.
  p. variegata
  p. varioliformis
  p. varioliformis acuta
  p. varioliformis chronica

pararama

parascarlatina

Paraschoengastia nunezi

parasitaria
  achromia p.

parasite
  metazoal p.
  ova and p's (O&P)

parasitemia

parasitic
  p. cyst
  p. disease
  p. granuloma
  p. invasion
  p. melanoderma

parasitica
  achromia p.
  onychia p.

parasiticidal

parasiticum
  eczema p.

parasitization

parasitosis
  delusion of p.

parasyphilis

parathyroid
  p. disease
  p. metabolism
  p. neoplasm

parathyroidectomy

paratrichosis

paratrimma
  erythema p.

paratripsis

paratriptic

paraumbilical nodule

paraungual

paravaccinia
  p. virus
  p. virus infection

paravertebral
  p. ossification

parchment skin

parchmentlike membrane

paregoric

pareleidin

parenchyma

parenchymal organs

parenchymatous

parental
  p. consanguinity
  p. gold therapy

parenteral antibiotic

paresis
  generalized p.

paresthesia

paresthetica
  meralgia p.
  notalgia p.

paridrosis

Parkes
  P.-Weber hemangiomatosis
  P.-Weber syndrome

Parkinson's disease

paromomycin
  p. sulfate

paronychia
  acute p.
  Candida p.
  candidal p.
  chronic p.
  herpetic p.
  suppurative p.
  p. tendinosa

paronychial
  p. infection
  p. wart

paronychomycosis

paronychosis

parotid duct cyst

parotitis

paroxetine
    p. HCl
    p. hydrochloride

paroxysm

paroxysmal
    p. flushing
    p. hand hematoma
    p. hemoglobinuria
    p. nocturnal
        hemoglobinuria (PNH)
    p. vasodilation

parrot-beak nail

Parry-Romberg syndrome

pars
    p. papillaris
    p. reticularis

parsley

parson spider

Parsonage-Turner syndrome

Parthenium hysterophorus

parti-colored

partial
    p. albinism
    p. anonychia
    p. combined
        immunodeficiency
        disorder
    p. dermal thickness
    p. nail ablation
    p. thromboplastin time
    p. unilateral lentiginosis

partial-thickness
    p.-t. burn
    p.-t. graft

partialis
    hypertrichosis p.

particle
    latex p's

parturition

parvilocular cyst

Parvoviridae

Parvovirus

parvovirus
    human p. (HPV)
    human p. B19

PAS
    periodic acid–Schiff
        PAS stain
        PAS technique
    positive basement
        membrane

Paschen bodies

PASI
    psoriasis area severity index

Pasini
    P. epidermolysis bullosa
    P.-Pierini idiopathic
        atrophoderma

passage
    percutaneous p.

passion purpura

passive
    p. cutaneous anaphylactic
        reaction
    p. cutaneous anaphylaxis
        (PCA)
    p. cutaneous anaphylaxis
        test
    p. immunization

paste
    Ihle's p.
    Lassar's p.
    Lassar's plain zinc p.
    Veiel's p.
    zinc oxide p.
    zinc oxide and salicylic acid
        p.

Pasteurella
    P. haemolytica
    P. multocida
    P. pestis
    P. tularensis

Pasteurellaceae

pasteurellosis

Pastia
    P's line
    P's sign

pasty content

patch
    ash-leaf p.
    bandlike p.
    butterfly p.
    circinate p.
    eczematous p.
    herald p.
    isolated p.
    lance-ovate p.
    moth p.
    mucous p.
    opaline p.
    oval p.
    pruritic erythematous p.
    salmon p.
    scaling p.
    shagreen p.
    sharply marginated p.
    soldier p.
    p. stage
    p. test
    p. test positive
    p. testing
    p. test interpretation
    p. test scarring
    Trans-Ver-Sal transdermal
        p.

patchy hyperpigmentation

patent
    p. ductus arteriosus
    p. extrahepatic bile
        ducts

pathergy

pathobiology

Pathocil

pathogen
    opportunistic p.

pathogenic
    p. bacteria
    p. blastomycetes
    p. species
    p. staphylococci

pathogenesis

pathogenetic
    p. mechanism

pathogenicity

pathognomic

pathognomonic
    p. feature

pathologic
    p. diagnosis
    p. feature
    p. tissue

pathologically confirmed
    complete remission (PCR)

pathomechanism

pathophysiology

pathway
    endogenous p.
    exogenous p.
    p. of heme

patient
    p. education

pattern
    annular p.
    circular p.
    p. of distribution
    irregular reticulated p.
    lacelike p.
    lichenoid histologic p.
    linear p.
    livedo p.
    nodular p.
    psoriasiform histologic p.
    serpiginous p.
    sporotrichoid p.
    stellate p.
    webbed p.
    zosteriform p.

patterned
p. acquired hypertrichosis
p. alopecia
p. leukoderma

patterning
linear p.
zosteriform p.

patulous
p. opening

paucibacillary
p. disease
p. leprosy

pauci-inflammatory

paucilesional primary
cutaneous plasmacytoma

Pautrier
P's abscess
P's microabscess

PAUVA
phenylalanine/UVA

Paxton disease

PBG
porphobilinogen

PBZ
Pyribenzamine
PBZ-SR

PCA
passive cutaneous
anaphylaxis

PCE oral

PCMX
para-chlorometaxylenol

PCR
polymerase chain reaction

PCT
porphyria cutanea tarda

PCV
polycythemia vera

PDT
photodynamic therapy

peanut agglutinin

pearl
epidermic p.
epithelial p.

pearly penile papules

peau
p. de chagrin
p. d'orange

pectinate
p. bodies
p. hyphae

pectus deformity

pederin

PediaPatch transdermal patch

Pediapred oral

pediatric
American Academy of P's
(AAP)
p. scleroderma

pedicle

Pedi-Cort V topical

pedicular

pediculation

pediculi

Pediculoides ventricosus

pediculosis
p. capillitii
p. capitis
p. corporis
p. corporis vel
vestimentorum
p. inguinalis
p. palpebrarum
p. pubis
p. vestimenti
p. vestimentorum

pediculous

Pediculus
P. capitis

Pediculus (*continued*)
    P. corporis
    P. humanus
    P. humanus capitis
    P. humanus capitis
      infestation
    P. humanus corporis

pedicure

Pedi-Dri

Pedi-Pro topical

pedis
    dermatomycosis p.
    tinea p.

peduncle

peduncular

pedunculated
    p. fibromas
    p. lesion
    p. papilloma
    p. tumor

peel
    chemical p.
    facial p.
    familial continuous skin p.
    skin p.

peeling-skin syndrome

PEG
    polyethylene glycol

peg
    rete p.

pelade

pelage

Pelea anisata

pelidnoma

pelioma

peliosis

pellagra
    p.-associated dermatitis
    p.-like eruption

pellagrin

pellagroid
    p. changes
    p. dermatitis
    p. drug eruption

pellagrosis

pellagrous skin

pellicle
    acquired p.

pellitory
    wall p.

Pelodera strongyloides

pelt

pelvic ultrasonography

pemphigoid
    benign mucosal p.
    benign mucous membrane
      p.
    bullous p. (BP)
    bullous p., localized
    cicatricial p.
    p. gestationis
    lichen planus p.
    localized chronic p.
    mucous-membrane p.
    p. nodularis
    p. syphilid

pemphigoides

pemphigosa
    variola p.

pemphigus
    p. acutus
    benign familial chronic p.
    p. benignus chronicus
      familiaris
    Brazilian p.
    p. contagiosus
    p. erythematosus
    p. erythematous
    familial benign chronic p.
    foliaceous p.
    p. foliaceus

pemphigus (*continued*)
    p. gangrenosus
    p. gravidarum
    p. hemorrhagicus
    p. IC antibodies
    p. leprosus
    p. malignus
    p. mucosae
    p. neonatorum
    ocular p.
    old man's p.
    p. seborrheicus
    South American p.
    syphilitic p.
    p. syphiliticus
    p. vegetans
    p. vegetans, benign
    p. vulgaris
    p. vulgaris antigen
    wildfire p.

pemphigus-like eruption

penciclovir

pendulous
    p. abdomen
    p. breasts

pendulum
    fibroma p.

Penecare cream

Penecort

penetrans
    hyperkeratosis follicularis et
      parafollicularis in cutem
      p.
    Tunga p.

penetrant

penetrating wound virus

penicillamine

penicillin
    benzathine p. G
    p.-induced anaphylaxis
    p. G crystalline
    p. G, parenteral, aqueous

penicillin (*continued*)
    p. G procaine
    penicillinase-resistant
      penicillin
    p. v potassium
    procaine p. G
    p. therapy
    p. type I allergy

penicillin-induced anaphylaxis

Penicillium marneffei

penile
    p. melanosis
    p. pearly papule
    p. sclerosing lymphangitis
    p. squamous cell
      carcinoma

penis
    p. cancer, squamous cell
      carcinoma
    glans p.
    median raphe cyst of the p.

penoscrotal fold

Pentacarinat injection

Pentacef

pentad

pentaerythritol
    p. tetranitrate

Pentam-300 injection

pentamer

pentamidine
    p. in aerosol form
    p. isethionate

pentapeptide

Pentasa oral

pentavalent
    p. antimony

pentazocine

pentostatin

pentoxifylline

Pentrax

Pen-Vee K oral

penultimate toes

Pepcid
P. IV
P. oral

pepper-dot

peppermint oil

peptic ulcer disease

peptide
antigenic p.
immunogenic p.

Peptostreptococcus
P. anaerobius
P. asaccharolyticus
P. magnus
P. prevotii
P. productus
P. saccharolyticus

peracute

perambulating ulcer

percussion and postural
drainage (P and PD)

percutaneous
p. absorption
p. passage
p. test

perforans
folliculitis nares p.
folliculitis narium p.

perforated ulcer

perforating
p. calcific elastosis
p. collagenosis
p. disease
p. disease of hemodialysis
p. disorder of uremia
p. folliculitis
p. granuloma annulare
p. pseudoxanthoma
  elasticum

perforating (*continued*)
p. ulcer of foot

perfrigeration

perfume
p. dermatitis

Periactin

periadenitis
p. mucosa necrotica
  recurrens

periadnexal
p. dermis

perianal
p. Bowen's disease
p. candidiasis
p. itching
p. pruritus
p. streptococcal cellulitis

periarteriolar lymph sheath

periarteritis
p. gummosa
p. nodosa

periarticular
p. region
p. site

periauricular

péribuccale
erythrose pigmentaire p.

peribulbar
p. area of anagen
p. infiltrate

pericapillary fibrin

pericardial effusion

pericarditis

pericardiotomy

pericardium

perichondritis
infectious p.

pericyte

periderm

peridermal

perifollicular
  p. accentuation
  p. fibroma
  p. granulomatous
    inflammation
  p. hyperkeratosis
  p. hypopigmentation
  p. infiltrate
  p. inflammation
  p. lymphocytic infiltrate
  p. papulation
  p. pattern
  p. petechiae
  p. pigment retention

perifolliculitis
  p. abscendens et suffodiens
  p. capitis abscedens et
    suffodiens
  dissecting p.
  pustular p.
  superficial pustular p.

perilesional skin

perimeatal balanitis

perinatal
  p. gangrene
  p. hypothermia
  p. lethal

perineal
  p. erythema
  p. lesions
  p. pruritus
  p. skin lesion

perineural
  p. infiltration
  p. invasion

perinevoid vitiligo

perinuclear
  p. clear space
  p. halo

periocular area

period
  incubation p.

periodic edema

periodic acid–Schiff (PAS)
  p. a.–S. stain
  p. a.–S. technique

periodontal bone

periodontia

perionychia

perionychium

perionyx

perioral
  p. area
  p. dermatitis
  p. hypertrophic granulation
    tissue

periorbital
  p. area
  p. dermatitis
  p. hemangioma
  p. hyperpigmentation
  p. purpura

periorificial
  p. keratoses
  p. keratotic plaques
  p. lentiginosis
  p. skin

periosteum

periostia

periostitis
  idiopathic p.

periostosis

peripheral
  p. ameloblastoma
  p. areola
  p. arthritis
  p. blood eosinophilia
  p. eosinophilia
  p. extension
  p. gangrene

peripheral (*continued*)
p. giant cell granuloma
p. nerves
p. nerve block
p. nerve sarcomas
p. nerve section
p. neuritis
p. neuropathy
p. neurotransmission
p. ossifying fibroma
p. palisading
p. pattern
p. rings of scales
p. seventh-nerve palsy
p. splaying
p. tissue
p. type
p. ulcerative keratitis
p. vascular disease
p. vesiculation

peripheral

peripheralis

periphery

periporate

periporitis

periporoma

perisynovitis

perisyringitis

peritoneal
p. dialysis
p. effusion

peritoneum

periumbilical
p. ecchymosis
p. lesions
p. perforating PXE

periungual
p. erythema
p. fibroma
p. telangiectasia
p. wart

periungualis
onychia p.

perivascular
p. dermal component
p. dermal infiltrate
p. hemorrhage
p. inflammation
p. inflammatory cells
p. invasion
p. lymphocyte inflammatory
infiltrate
p. lymphocytic infiltrate
p. lymphohistiocytic
infiltrate
p. macrophages
p. mantle
p. mixed cell inflammatory
infiltrate
p. pattern

perivasculitis

perlèche

permanent
p. alopecia
p. epilation
p. macrocheilia

Permapen injection

permeability

permeable

permethrin
p. cream

pernicious anemia

pernio *pl.* perniones
p. cyanosis
erythema p.
lupus p.

perniosis

Pernox

peroxidase

peroxide
benzoyl p.

peroxide (*continued*)
   erythromycin and benzoyl
      p.

Peroxin
   P. A5
   P. A10

perpendicular groove

Persa-Gel

Persantine

persistent
   p. acantholytic dermatosis
   p. bleeding
   p. edema
   p. light reaction
   p. pearly penile papules
   p. pyoderma
   p. ulceration

persister

Persoonia elliptica

perspiratio
   p. insensibilis

perspiration
   insensible p.
   sensible p.

perspire

perstans
   acrodermatitis p.
   erythema p.
   erythema dyschromicum p.
   erythema figuratum p.
   erythema gyratum p.
   hyperkeratosis lenticularis
      p.
   telangiectasia macularis
      eruptiva p. (TMEP)
   urticaria p.

pertenue
   Treponema p.

Pertofrane

pertussis

Peru
   balsam of P.

peruana
   verruca p.

Peruvian wart

peruviana
   verruca p.

pes
   p. cavus
   p. planus

pesticide

petechia *pl.* petechiae
   calcaneal p.
   linear p.
   Tardieu p.

petechial
   p. eruption
   p. hemorrhage

petechiasis

petrolatum
   p. gauze dressing
   heavy liquid p.
   hydrophilic p.
   lanolin, cetyl alcohol,
      glycerin, and p.
   light liquid p.
   liquid p.
   white p.

petroleum
   p. jelly
   p. oil

Peutz-Jeghers syndrome

Peyer patch

Peyronie's disease

PF
   pemphigus foliaceus

PFAPA
   periodic fever, aphthous
      stomatitis, pharyngitis,
      adenitis

Pfizerpen
    P.-AS injection
    P. injection
PG
    pyoderma gangrenosum
P/G
    Fulvicin P.
PGL-1
    phenolic glycolipid-1
PH
    pseudohypoparathyroidism
PHA
    phytohemagglutinin
PHACE
    *p*osterior fossa brain
      malformation,
      *h*emangiomas, *a*rterial
      anomalies, *c*oarctation of
      the aorta and cardiac
      defects, and *e*ye
      abnormalities
    PHACE syndrome
Phacelia
    P. campanularia
    P. crenulata
phacomatosis
Phaeoannellomyces werneckii
phaeohyphomycosis
    systemic p.
phagedena
    p. gangrenosa
    p. nosocomialis
    sloughing p.
    tropical p.
    tropical sloughing p.
phagedenic
    p. ulcer
    p. ulceration
phagocyte
phagocytic cells

phagocytosis
phagolysosome
phakoma
phakomatosis
    p. pigmenti keratotica
    p. pigmenti vascularis
phaneroscope
phantom
    p. limb syndrome
    p. tumor
pharmaceutical agent
pharmacokinetic
    Dapsone p's
pharmacologic
    p. effects
    p. mediators of anaphylaxis
    p. therapy
pharmacopeial
pharyngeal pouch syndrome
pharyngitid
pharyngitis vesicularis
phase
    convalescent p.
    efferent p.
phenacetin
Phenameth Oral
Phendry Oral
Phenergan
    P. injection
    P. Oral
Phenetron Oral
phenformin
    p. HCl
phenindamine tartrate
phenobarbital
    p. hypersensitivity
      syndrome

phenobarbital (*continued*)
theophylline, ephedrine, and p.

phenol
camphor and p.
camphor, menthol and p.
liquefied p.
p.-preserved extract

phenolated disinfectant

phenolic
p. antiseptic detergent
p. compounds

phenolization

phenolphthalein

phenomenon *pl.* phenomena
p. of Arthus
Chase-Sulzberger p.
coagulation p.
hemorrhagic p.
Koebner's p.
Lucio's p.
Meirowsky p.
"prozone" p.
Raynaud's p.
Sulzberger-Chase p.

phenothiazine

phenotype
p. classification

phenotypic
p. dimorphism
p. expression

phenotypical forms

phenoxybenzamine hydrochloride

phenoxymethyl penicillin

phentolamine
p. HCl

phenyl
p. hydrate

phenylalanine
p. hydroxylase

phenylalanine (*continued*)
p. metabolism

phenylbenzimidazole sulfonic acid

phenylbutazone

phenylketonuria

phenylmercuric
p. acetate
p. propionate
p. salts

phenylpyruvic
p. acid
p. oligophrenia

phenytoin

pheochromocytoma

pheomelanin

pheromone

Phialophora
P. parasitica
P. verrucosa

Philodendron
P. crystallinum

"philosopher's nooks"

philtrum

phimosis
acquired p.

pHisoderm

pHisoHex

phlebectasia
congenital generalized p.

phlebectasis

phlebothrombosis

Phlebotomus
P. argentipes
P. ariasi
P. chinensis
P. longipes
P. major

Phlebotomus (*continued*)
    P. martini
    P. noguchi
    P. orientalis
    P. papatasi
    P. pedifer
    P. perniciosus
    P. sandflies
    P. sergenti
    P. verrucarum

phlebotomy

phlegmasia
    p. alba
    p. alba dolens
    p. malabarica

phlegmon
    diffuse p.

phlegmonous
    p. cellulitis
    p. erysipelas
    p. ulcer

phlogosin

phlogotherapy

phlycten

phlyctena *pl.* phlyctenae

phlyctenar

phlyctenoid

phlyctenosis

phlyctenous

phlyctenular

phlyctenule

PHN
    postherpetic neuralgia

phobia

Phormia
    P. regina

phosphatides

phosphatidyl

phosphatidylinositol

phospholipid
    p. cholesterol

phosphorescence

phosphorus

phosphorylase

photoaccentuated

photoaccentuation

photoactivatable drug

photoaging

photoallergen

photoallergic
    p. contact dermatitis
    p. drug reaction
    p. reaction
    p. sensitivity

photoallergy

photochemotherapy
    extracorporeal p.

photochromogen

photocontact
    p. dermatitis

photocutaneous

photodermatitis

photodermatosis

photodistributed
    p. bullous reaction
    p. lichenoid reaction
    p. pattern

photodistribution

photodrug
    p. reaction

photodynamic
    p. sensitization
    p. therapy

photoerythema

photoexposed area

Photofrin

photographic developer

photoinactivation

photoingestant dermatitis

photolichenoid reaction

photomedicine

photoncia

photonosus

photo-onycholysis

photo-patch, photopatch
    p.-p. test

photopathy

photopheresis

photophobia

photophoresis
    extracorporeal p.

photophytodermatitis

photoprotection

photosensitive
    p. nonscarring dermatitis

photosensitivity
    p. dermatitis
    drug-induced bullous p.
    p., ichthyosis, brittle hair,
      intellectual
      impairment
    p., ichthyosis, brittle hair,
      intellectual impairment,
      decreased fertility, and
      short stature (PIBIDS)
    p. reaction

photosensitive

photosensitivity

photosensitization
    contact p.

photosensitize

photosensitizing
    p. disease
    p. drugs
    p. substance
    p. weed

phototherapy
    ultraviolet
    UVA/UVB p.

photothermolysis
    selective p.

phototoxic
    p. contact dermatitis
    p. drug reaction
    p. events
    p. injury
    p. reaction
    p. sensitivity

phototoxicity

phototoxis

PHP
    pseudohypoparathyroidism

phrynoderma

phthiriasis
    p. capitis
    p. corporis
    p. inguinalis
    pubic p.

Phthirus pubis

phycomycosis
    subcutaneous p.

phyla

phylaxis

phylum
    p. Annelida
    p. Arthropoda
    p. Chordata
    p. Cnidaria
    p. Nemathelminthes
    p. Protozoa
    p. Platyhelminthes

phyma *pl.* phymata

phymatorhusin

phymatorrhysin

phymatosis

Physalia

physical
  p. allergy
  p. barrier
  p. change
  p. dimensions of the skin
  p. lobular panniculitis
  p. stimulus
  p. sunscreen
  p. urticaria

physiognomy

physiologic mottling

phytanic
  p. acid
  p. acid storage
  p. acid storage disease

phytodermatitis

phytohemagglutinin (PHA)

phytophlyctodermatitis

phytophotodermatitis

phytosterolemia

phytotoxic

phytotoxin

pian
  p. bois
  hemorrhagic p.

piannic
  onychia p.

PIBIDS
  photosensitivity, ichthyosis,
    brittle hair, intellectual
    impairment, decreased
    fertility, and short stature
  PIBIDS syndrome

Picker nodule

picker
  p's acne
  p's nodule

Picornaviridae

picornavirus

picric acid

piebald
  p. skin

piebaldism

piebaldness

piedra
  black p.
  p. nostras
  white p.

Piedraia
  P. hortae

piercing manner

Pierini
  atrophoderma of Pasini and
    P.
  idiopathic atrophoderma of
    Pasini and P.

piezogenic
  p. nodule
  p. pedal papule

piezogenous

pig
  p. skin

pigeon breast

pigment
  abnutzung p.
  age p.
  p. cell transplantation
  p. change
  p.-free zones
  p. granule
  incontinence of p.
  p. incontinence
  melanotic p.
  minimal p. (MP)

pigment (*continued*)
    p. spot polyposis

pigmentary
    p. abnormality
    p. anomaly
    p. atopic dermatitis
    p. changes
    p. demarcation boundaries
    p. demarcation line
    p. dermatosis of Gougerot
      and Blum
    p. dilution
    p. incontinence
    p. purpuric eruption
    p. syphilid

pigmentation
    abnormal p.
    addisonian dermal p.
    amiodarone p.
    arsenic p.
    Atabrine p.
    exogenous p.
    postinflammatory p.

pigmented
    p. basal cell carcinoma
    p. basal cell epithelioma
    p. dendritic melanocyte
    p. follicular cyst
    p. hair epidermal nevus
    p. hairy epidermal nevus
      syndrome
    p. lesion
    p. nevi
    p. patches
    p. purpura
    p. purpuric lichenoid
      dermatitis
    p. purpuric lichenoid
      dermatitis of Gougerot
    p. purpuric lichenoid
      dermatosis
    p. seborrheic keratosis
    p. spindle cell tumor of
      Reed
    p. villonodular synovitis
      (PVNS)

pigmenti
    incontinentia p.

pigmentolysin

pigmentophage

pigmentosa
    urticaria p.

pigmentosum
    morphea p.
    urticaria p.
    xeroderma p.

pigmentosus
    nevus p.

pilar
    p. cyst
    p. differentiation
    p. sheath acanthoma
    p. tumor of scalp

pilaris
    juvenile pityriasis rubra p.
    keratosis p.
    lichen p.
    pityriasis rubra p.

pilary
    p. apparatus
    p. complex
    p. elements

pileous

pili (*genitive and plural of* pilus)
    p. annulati
    p. annulatus
    arrector p.
    p. bifurcati
    p. canaliculi
    p. incarnati
    p. multigemini
    p. pseudoannulatus
    p. recurvati
    p. torti
    p. triangulati et canaliculi

pilial

piliferous
    p. cyst

piliform

pilocarpine
    p. iontophoresis sweat test

piloerection

piloid

piloleiomyoma

pilomatricoma

pilomatrixoma
    p. carcinoma

pilomotor
    p. reflex

pilonidal
    p. cyst
    p. fistula
    p. sinus

pilorum
    arrectores p.
    atrophia p. propria

pilose

pilosebaceous
    p. apparatus
    p. duct
    p. follicle
    p. gland hyperplasia
    p. orifice
    p. ostium
    p. structure
    p. unit

pilosis

pilosus
    nevus p.
    nevus pigmentosus et p.

pilus *pl.* pili
    p. annulati
    p. annulatus
    arrector p.
    pili bifurcates
    pili canaliculi
    pili cuniculati
    pili incarnati
    pili incarnati recurvati

pilus (*continued*)
    p. incarnatus
    pili multigemini
    F p.
    I p.
    R p.
    pili torti
    p. tortus
    p. triangulati et canaliculi

pimeloma

pimozide

Pimpinella anisum

pimple

pincer nail

pinch
    p. graft
    p. purpura

pinching

pine

pineal gland

pinealoma

pinealopathy

pinhead
    p. size
    p.-sized milia
    p.-sized papule

pink
    p. disease
    p. seeds

Pinkus' tumor

pinna

pinocyte

pinocytosis
    active p.

pinosome

pinpoint
    p. electrocoagulation
    p. papules

pinpoint (*continued*)
p. pustules
p. milia

Pin-Rid

pinta
tertiary p.

pintids

pintoid

pintos
mal de los p.

pinworm
p. infection

Pin-X

PIP
proximal interphalangeal

piperacillin
p. sodium
p. sodium and tazobactam sodium

piperazine
p. citrate
p. derivative

piperonyl butoxide

piroxicam photosensitivity

pit
palmar p.
plantar p.

pitch wart

pitches

pitlike depression

pitted
p. acneform scar
p. keratolysis
p. nails
p. scar

pitting
p. edema
nail p.
p. of nail

pituitary
p. basophilic tumors
p. basophilism
p. cachexia
p. disorder
p. growth hormone–secreting tumor
p. MSH-producing tumor

pityriasic

pityriasiform scaling

pityriasis
p. alba
p. alba atrophicans
p. amiantacea
p. capitis
p. circinata
p. circinata et marginata
p. folliculorum
p. furfuracea
Gibert p.
Hebra p.
p. lichenoid
lichenoid p., acute
lichenoid p., chronic
lichenoid acute p.
p. lichenoides
p. lichenoides acuta
p. lichenoides chronica
p. lichenoides et varioliformis acuta (PLEVA)
p. linguae
p. maculata
p. nigra
p. pilaris
p. rosea
p. rosea–like eruption
p. rotunda
p. rubra (Hebra)
p. rubra pilaris
p. rubra pilaris Devergie
p. sicca
p. sicca faciei
p. simplex
p. steatoides
p. streptogenes
p. versicolor

pityriasis-type scale

pityrodes
    alopecia p.

pityroid

*Pityrosporon (former name for
    Malassezia)*
        P. orbiculare
        P. ovale

*Pityrosporum (former name for
    Malassezia)*
        P. folliculitis
        P. orbiculare
        P. ovale

pizotifen

placebo

placenta

placental infiltration

pladaroma

plaited

plana
    verruca p.

planar
    p. xanthoma

plane
    p. of sectioning
    p. wart
    p. xanthoma

planing

planopilaris
    lichen p.

plant
    p. dermatitis
    p. sterols

planta *pl.* plantae
    verruca p.

plantar, plantare
    p. bromidrosis
    p. dermatitis
    p. dermatosis, juvenile

plantar (*continued*)
    p. desquamation
    p. fascia
    p. fasciitis
    p. fibromatosis
    p. hyperhidrosis
    p. hyperkeratosis
    p. inoculum
    keratoderma palmare et p.
    p. maceration
    p. nerve syndrome
    p. nevi
    p. pits
    p. pitting
    p. psoriasis
    p. pustulosis
    p. seed dermatoses
    p. syphilid
    p. verrucous cyst
    p. wart

plantaris
    epidermolytic keratosis
        palmaris et p.
    ichthyosis palmaris et p.
    keratoderma palmaris et p.
    keratosis palmaris et p.
    pustulosis palmaris et p.
    tylosis palmaris et p.
    verruca p.

planum
    xanthoma p.

planus
    annular lichen p.
    atrophic lichen p.
    bullous lichen p.
    condyloma p.
    erosive lichen p.
    follicular lichen p.
    genital erosive lichen p.
    hypertrophic lichen p.
    lichen p.
    lichen ruber p.
    linear lichen p.
    oral condyloma p.
    oral (erosive) lichen p.
    pes p.
    ulcerative lichen p.

plaque
annular erythematous p.
atrophic p.
attachment p.
bacterial p.
cytoplasmic p.
degenerative collagenous p.
discrete p.
disseminées parapsoriasis
en p's
eczematoid pruritic p's
erythematous p.
herald p.
Hutchinson's p's
inflammatory p.
lichenified p.
mucous p.
p. of pregnancy
palm-sized p.
parapsoriasis en p.
pneumonic p.
p. psoriasis
psoriatic p.
red-purple p.
septicemia p.
shagreen p.
shiny p.
p. stage
p. stage mycosis
fungoides
submucosal p.
ulcerovegetating p.
urticarial p.
violaceous p.
warty keratotic p's

plaquelike
p. cutaneous mucinosis
p. mucinosis

plaque-type psoriasis

Plaquenil

plasma
p. cell
p. cell cheilitis
p. cell dyscrasia with
polyneuropathy,
organomegaly,

plasma (*continued*)
endocrinopathy,
monoclonal protein
p. cell infiltration
p. cell orificial mucositis
p. dopamine level
p. coproporphyrins
p. cortisol
p. exchange
p. heparin level
p. lipoprotein
p. membrane
p. norepinephrine level
p. protoporphyrins

plasmacytoid immunoblasts

plasmacytoma
extramedullary p.
monoclonal p.
paucilesional primary
cutaneous p.
polyclonal p.
primary p.
secondary p.
secondary cutaneous p.
solitary p.

plasmacytosis circumorificialis

plasmapheresis
exchange p.

plasminogen
p. activator
p. activator inhibitor-1 level
p. factor

plasmocytoma penis

Plasmodium
P. malariae

plaster

plastic
p. adhesive dressing
p. surgery

plasticizers

plastics

plate
nail p.

platelet
p. aggregation
p. count
p.-fibrin thrombus
p. thromboxane B3 generation

plateaulike

Platinol
P.-AQ

platyhelminth

Platyhelminthes

platyonychia

pledgets

pleocytosis

pleomorphic
p. cellular elements
p. cellular infiltrate
p. lipoma
p. sweat gland adenoma
p. T-cell lymphoma
p. T-cell lymphoma (large cell)
p. T-cell lymphoma (medium-sized)
p. T-cell lymphoma (small cell)

pleomorphism

plessigraph

plessimeter

plessimetric

plethora

plethoric

plethysmograph

plethysmography

pleura

pleural effusion

pleurodynia
epidermic p.

PLEVA
pityriasis lichenoides et varioliformis acuta

plexiform
p. capillary pattern
p. neurofibroma
p. neuroma

pleximeter

pleximetric

pleximetry

plexometer

plexus
superficial vascular p.
upper reticular dermal p.

pliable scar

plica
p. neuropathica
p. polonica

plicated tongue

PLSI
Psoriasis Life Stress Inventory

plucked chicken-skin appearance

plucking

plug
central horny p.
follicular p.
keratinous p.
laminated epithelial p.
mucous p.

plugging
eccrine p.
follicular p.
hyperkeratosis p.
mucous p.

plum-colored papules

Plummer
P's nails
P.-Vinson syndrome

pluriorificialis
    ectodermosis erosiva p.

pluripotent

pluripotential
    p. adnexal cells
    p. cells

pluriresistant

PM
    polymyositis

PMLE
    polymorphous light
    eruption
        eczematous PMLE
        familial PMLE

pneumatic
    p. hammer operation
    p. pumps

pneumatophore

pneumococcal
    p. pneumonia
    p. sepsis

Pneumocystis carinii

pneumoderma

pneumonitis

pneumothorax *pl.*
    pneumothoraces
        iatrogenic p.

pock
    p. marks

pocket
    necrotic p.

pockmark

podagra

Pod-Ben-25

podobromidrosis

Podocon-25

Podofilox

podofilox

Podofin

podophyllin

podophyllotoxin

podophyllum
    p. resin

PodoSpray nail drill system

POEMS
    polyneuropathy,
        organomegaly,
        endocrinopathy,
        monoclonal gammopathy,
        and skin changes
    POEMS syndrome

pogoniasis

Pohl-Pinkus constriction

poikilocarynosis

poikiloderma
    p. atrophicans and cataract
    p. atrophicans vasculare
    Civatte p.
    p. of Civatte
    p. congenitale
    reticulated pigmented p.
    p. vasculare atrophicans
    p. vascularis atrophicans

poikilodermatomyositis

poikilodermatous
    p. condition
    p. parapsoriasis

poikilodermia (*variant of*
    poikiloderma)
        p. congenitalis

point
    Kienböck-Adamson p's

pointed
    p. condyloma
    p. wart

pointing

poison
  contact p.
  corrosive p.
  p. ivy
  p. ivy dermatitis
  p. oak
  p. oak dermatitis
  p. sumac
  p. sumac dermatitis

poisonwood tree

Poladex

polar
  p. lepromatous form
  p. tuberculoid form

Polaramine

polarization

polarized light

polarizing electron microscopy

polaroscopy

poliosis
  p. circumscripta
  p. eccentrica

polish
  nail p.

Polistes
  P. sting

pollinosis

Polocaine injection

polyamine

polyangular flecks

polyarteritis
  p. nodosa

polyarthralgia

polyarthritis (PA)
  asymmetric p.
  epidemic p.
  erosive p.
  juvenile chronic p.

polyarticular
  p. arthritis
  p. gonococcal arthritis
  p. juvenile rheumatoid
    arthritis

polychemotherapy

polychondritis
  relapsing p.

polychromatic

polychrome toluidine blue

Polycillin
  P.-N
  P.-PRB

polyclonal
  p. hypergammaglobulinemia
  p. hyperglobulinemia
  p. plasmacytoma

polycyclic
  p. annular lesions
  p. aromatic hydrocarbons
  p. border
  p. configuration
  p. patches
  p. serpiginous
    eruption
  p. shape

polycystic
  p. ovary
  p. ovary disease
  p. ovary syndrome

polycythemia vera

polydactylia

polydactylism

polydactyly

polyenes (*class of drugs*)

polyester
  p. fibers
  p. film
  p. plasticizers
  p. resins

polyethylene
    p. film (*Saran Wrap*)
    p. glove
    p. occlusive dressing
    p. sheet bath PUVA

Polygam S/D

polygenic

polyglandular
    p. autoimmune disease

polyglucosan
    p. inclusions

polygonal
    p. cell
    p. fragments
    p. papules

polyhedral
    p. balloon cell
    p. body
    p. cells
    p. spores

polyhidrosis

polyidrosis

polymastia

polymer
    p. film dressing
    p. foam dressing

polymerase
    p. chain reaction (PCR)

polymerization

polymerized

polymorphe
    erythema p.

polymorphic
    p. eruption of pregnancy
    p. exanthemata-purpuric
    p. leukocytes
    p. light eruption
    p. neutrophils
    p. reticulosis

polymorphism

polymorphonuclear
    p. cells
    p. infiltrate
    p. leukocyte (PML)

polymorphous
    p. cellular infiltrate
    p. exanthema
    p. light eruption (PMLE)
    p. skin lesion

Polymox

polymyalgia
    p. rheumatica

polymyositis
    juvenile dermato/p.
        (JDMS/PM)

polymyxin
    p. B
    p. B and hydrocortisone
    p. B sulfate
    p. B sulfate and bacitracin
        zinc
    p. B sulfate, bacitracin zinc,
        and neomycin sulfate
    p. B sulfate, gramicidin, and
        neomycin sulfate
    p. B sulfate, neomycin
        sulfate, dexamethasone
    p. B sulfate and
        trimethoprim sulfate

polynesic

polyonychia

polyostotic
    p. fibrous dysplasia
    p. lesion

polyoxyethylene

polyp
    fibroepithelial p.
    lipomatous p.

polypapilloma

polypectomy

polypeptide
    p. chain

polyphasic

polypi (*plural of* polypus)

polypoid
    p. lesion
    p. melanoma

polyposis

polypus *pl.* polypi

polyradiculomyopathy

polysaccharide

polyserositis

Polysporin
    P. ophthalmic
    P. topical

polystichia

Polytar

polythelia

polytrichia

polytrichosis

polyunguia

polyunsaturated fatty acids

polyurethane
    p. fiber

polyvinyl
    p. chloride (PVC)
    p. resins

POMA
    postoperative margin
      assessment

pomade
    p. acne

pomphoid

pompholyx

pomphus

Poncet-Spiegler tumor

Pontocaine

poor
    p. circumscription
    p. mouth hygiene
    p. muscle tone

poorly
    p. demarcated malar
      erythema
    p. designed flap

popliteal
    p. artery pulse
    p. cyst
    p. fossa
    p. pterygium syndrome
    p. space
    p. web

popsicle panniculitis

poral occlusion disease

porcupine
    p. boy
    p. disease
    p. man
    p. skin

pore
    dilated p. of Winer
    sweat p.

porencephalia

porencephalic

porencephalitis

porencephalous

porencephaly

porfimer sodium

Porges-Meier test

pori (*genitive and plural of* porus)

porocarcinoma
    eccrine p.

poroid hidradenoma

porokeratosis
    actinic p.

porokeratosis (*continued*)
disseminated superficial actinic p.
p. excentrica
linear p.
p. linearis unilateralis
Mibelli p.
p. of Mibelli
p. neviformis
p. palmaris et plantaris disseminata
p. plantaris discreta
plaque-type p.
p. punctata
punctate p.
p. superficialis disseminata actinica

porokeratotic
p. eccrine ostial

poroma
eccrine p.
follicular p.

porphobilinogen
p. deaminase
urinary p.

porphyria
p. cutanea tarda (PCT)
p. cutanea tarda hereditaria
erythropoietic p.
p. hepatica chronica
symptomatic p.
p. variegata
variegate p. (VP)

porphyric

porphyrin
p. gallstones
p. metabolism
p. precursor
X p.

porphyrinogen

porphyrinuria

porrigo
p. decalvans

porrigo (*continued*)
p. favosa
p. furfurans
p. larvalis
p. lupinosa
p. scutulate

porta
p. hepatis

portal
p. fibrosis
p. hypertension
p. of entry

Portuguese
P. man-of-war dermatitis
P. man-of-war
P. man-of-war sting

port-wine
p.-w. malformation
p.-w. mark
p.-w. nevus
p.-w. stain

porus *pl.* pori
p. sudoriferus

Posada mycosis

positive
p. nontreponemal condition
p. nontreponemal test
p. reaction

postacne
p. anetoderma-like scars
p. osteoma cutis

postadolescent

postauricular
p. fissures
p. fold
p. sulcus

postcapillary
p. venule walls

postcardiotomy syndrome

postcryosurgical pigmentary changes

postdermabrasion

postdysenteric form of Reiter's syndrome

postencephalitic trophic ulcer

posterior
  p. auricular fold
  p. iliac horns
  p. root ganglia
  p. tibial pulse

posterolateral

posteromedial

postherpetic
  p. erythema multiforme
  p. neuralgia (PHN)

posthitis

postictal purpura

postinfection

postinflammatory
  p. dermal melanosis
  p. elastolysis
  p. epidermal cytokines
  p. hyperpigmentation
  p. hypopigmentation
  p. leukoderma
  p. variant

post–kala azar dermal leishmanoid

postmastectomy lymphedema

postmiliarial hypohidrosis

postmenopausal
  p. women

postmortem
  p. pustule
  p. tubercle
  p. wart

postnatal
  p. life
  p. telogen effluvium

postoperative hematoma

postpartum
  p. alopecia
  p. period
  p. telogen effluvium

postphlebitic syndrome

postpubertal

postpuberty

postpubescence

postpubescent

postradiation therapy

poststeroid panniculitis

postsynaptic terminal

postthrombotic leg ulcer

posttransfusion isoantibody

posttransplantation plasma cell dyscrasia

posttraumatic
  p. hemorrhage
  p. pustular eruption

postural
  p. drainage
  p. hypotension

posturethritic form of Reiter's syndrome

postvaccinial
  p. retinitis

postvenereal reactive arthritis

postzygotic
  p. mutation
  p. somatic mutation

Potaba

potassium
  p. alum
  p. hydroxide (KOH)
  p. iodide
  p. permanganate
  p. titanyl phosphate laser

potatolike nodules

potential
    zoonotic p.

Pott
    P. gangrene
    P. puffy tumor

poultice

poultry handler's disease

poultryman's itch

Poupart
    P's ligament
    P's line

povidone-iodine

powder
    absorbable dusting p.
    dusting p.
    facial p.
    full-coverage facial p.
    Lotrimin AF P.
    Lotrimin AF Spray P.
    transparent facial p.
    Zeasorb-AF P.

pox
    chicken p.
    Kaffir p.

Poxviridae

poxvirus
    p. officinalis

PPD
    purified protein derivative
        of tuberculin

PPDA
    paraphenylenediamine

PPH
    pseudopseudohypopara-
        thyroidism

PPHP
    pseudopseudohypopara-
        thyroidism

PPK
    palmoplantar keratoderma

Prader-Willi syndrome

prairie itch

PrameGel

Pramosone
    P. cream

pramoxine
    p. HCl
    p. hydrochloride

pratensis
    dermatitis p. striata

Pratt procedure

Prausnitz
    P.-Küstner (PK) antibody
    P.-Küstner (PK) reaction
    P.-Küstner (PK) test

Prax lotion

praziquantel

prazosin hydrochloride

preadolescent acne
    childhood p. a.
    infantile p. a.
    neonatal p. a.

preandrogen

preauricular
    p. cyst
    p. nodes
    p. sinus

prebetalipoproteinemia

precancer

precancerosa
    melanosis circumscripta p.

precancerous
    p. lesion

precipitate
    p. in gel
    p. in solution

precipitation
    p. assays
    agar p.

precocious
 p. growth
 p. puberty

precursor
 p. B cells
 myeloid p.

Predaject injection

Predalone injection

Predcor injection

Predicort-50 injection

predictive
 p. patch test
 p. testing

predilection
 genetic p.

predispose

predisposition

prednicarbate

Prednicen-M Oral

Prednisol TBA injection

prednisolone
 chloramphenicol and p.
 p. and gentamicin
 neomycin, polymyxin b,
   and p.
 sodium sulfacetamide and
   p.
 p. tebutate

prednisone

preengraftment

preeruptive

preexisting
 p. bulla

Pregestimil

pregnancy
 papular dermatitis of p.
 pruritic urticarial papules
   and plaques of p. (PUPPP)

pregnancy (*continued*)
 p.-related dermatoses
 p. striae
 p. tumor

Prelone Oral

premalignant
 p. condition
 p. fibroepithelial tumor of
   Pinkus
 p. form of parapsoriasis en
   plaque
 p. tumor

prematura
 alopecia p.

premature
 p. aging
 p. alopecia
 p. alveolar bone loss
 p. cataract formation
 p. gray
 p. sebaceous hyperplasia
 p. thinning

premenstrual acne

premorbid

premunition

premunitive

premycotic

prenatal
 p. metastatic lesion
 p. skin

preoperative anesthetic

preparation
 KOH p.
 scabies p.
 Tzanck p.

Pre-Pen

prepolypoid

prepubertal

prepuce

preputial orifice

preputiale
  sebum p.

presenile spontaneous
  gangrene

presenilis
  alopecia p.

presenting clinical manifestation

preservative

pressure
  p. alopecia
  p. blister
  p. dressing
  p. gangrene
  light p.
  p. sore
  p. urticaria

pressure ring
  Walsh p. r.

PreSun
  P. lotion and gel

presymptomatic phase

presynaptic
  p. neuromuscular blockade
  p. terminal

pretibial
  p. hyperpigmentation
  p. myxedema

prevention
  Centers for Disease Control
    and P. (CDC)

preventive
  p. treatment

prick
  p. puncture test
  p. skin testing
  p. test
  p. test concentration
  p. testing
  p. wounds

Pricker needle

prickle cell
  p. c. carcinoma
  p. c. epithelioma
  p. c. layer

prickle layer

prickly heat

prilocaine

primary
  p. amyloidosis
  p. anetoderma
  p. antiphospholipid
    syndrome
  p. atrophy
  p. biliary cirrhosis
  p. cold urticaria
  p. complex
  p. cutaneous adenoid cystic
  p. cutaneous B-cell
    lymphoma
  p. cutaneous follicular
    center cell lymphoma
  p. cutaneous
    histoplasmosis
  p. cutaneous Hodgkin's
    disease
  p. cutaneous
    immunocytoma
  p. cutaneous
    (ulceroglandular)
    infection
  p. cutaneous lymphoma
  p. cutaneous meningioma
  p. cutaneous
    plasmacytoma
  p. cutaneous T-cell
    lymphoma
  p. effusion lymphoma
  p. facial basal cell
    carcinoma
  p. function
  p. genital herpes simplex
    virus
  p. herpes simplex infection
  p. herpetic stomatitis

primary (*continued*)
  p. hypercoagulable state
  p. hyperhidrosis
  p. hyperlipoproteinemia
  p. immune response
  p. immunodeficiency
    syndrome
  p. infection
  p. irritant
  p. irritant dermatitis
  p. lesion
  p. lues
  p. lymphedema
  p. lymphocytic perifollicular
    inflammatory infiltrate
  p. lymphocytic perivascular
    inflammatory infiltrate
  p. macular atrophy of skin
  p. milia
  p. neuroendocrine
    carcinoma of the skin
  p. nodular malignant
    melanoma
  p. pigmented nodular
    adrenocortical disease
  p. pyoderma
  p. reaction
  p. rejection
  p. squamous cell
    carcinoma
  p. sensitization reaction
  p. Sjögren's syndrome
  p. syphilis
  p. tuberculous complex
  p. tufted hairs
  p. vasculopathy

primigravid

primigravida

Primula obconica

Principen

prion

prior drug exposure

Priscoline HCl

Pro-Banthine

probenecid
  ampicillin and p.
  colchicines and p.

probiosis

probiotic

problem-oriented
  p.-o. diagnosis

procainamide

procaine
  p. hydrochloride
  penicillin g p.

Procardia

procedure
  Mohs p.
  Z-plasty p.

process
  generalized systemic p.

processionary caterpillar

procoagulant synthesis

procoagulation defect

Procort

proctitis

proctocolitis
  ulcerative p.

Proctocort

Pro-Depo Injection

prodromal
  p. stage
  p. symptom

prodromata

prodrome

prodromic

product
  Exact skin p.
  home cleaning p.

professor angle

profile
  angioedema p.

profunda
  miliaria p.
  tinea p.

profundus
  lupus p.
  lupus erythematosus p.

profundus/panniculitis
  lupus p./p.

profusa
  lentiginosis p.
  p. scaling

progenitalis
  herpes p.

progeria
  p. adultorum
  Hutchinson-Gilford p.
  true p.

progeroid factors

progesterone
  p. binding
  p. receptor

proglottid

proglottis

prognathia

prognathic

prognathism

prognathous

prognosis *pl.* prognoses

prognostic

progonoma
  melanotic p.

progression
  malignant p.

progressiva
  granulomatous disciformis
    chronica et p.

progressive
  p. bacterial synergistic
    gangrene
  p. cerebellar ataxia
  p. deforming
  p. disseminated
    histoplasmosis
  p. facial hemiatrophy
  p. fatal encephalitis
  p. glomerular disease
  p. idiopathic atrophoderma
  p. kyphoscoliosis
  p. lipodystrophy
  p. muscular atrophy
  p. neuromyopathy
  p. nodular histiocytoma
  p. paresis
  p. pigmentary dermatosis
  p. pigmentary disease of
    Schamberg
  p. pigmented purpura
  p. postoperative gangrene
  p. systemic scleroderma
  p. systemic sclerosis

proinflammatory
  p. effects

prolactin
  p.-secreting adenoma
  p.-secreting microadenoma
  p.-secreting tumor

prolapsed uterus

prolidase deficiency

proliferated

proliferating
  p. angioendotheliomatosis
  p. basaloid cells
  p. epidermoid cyst
  p. epithelial cyst
  p. pilar cyst
  p. systematized
    angioendotheliomatosis
  p. trichilemmal cyst

proliferation
  acanthotic epidermal p.

proliferation (*continued*)
    B-cell p.
    clonal p.

proliferative
    p. dermatitis
    p. fasciitis
    p. lesion
    p. synovitis
    p. synovium
    p. verrucous leukoplakia-
      associated carcinoma

prolonged
    p. febrile illness
    p. intravenous
      supplementation
    p. remission

promastigote

promethazine (*Phenergan*)
    p. HCl
    p. hydrochloride

prominent
    p. ears
    p. inferior labial artery

promyelocyte

promyelocytic
    p. leukemia

pronounced
    p. scars
    p. swelling

propagation

propagative

propantheline bromide

properdin
    p. factor A
    p. factor B
    p. factor D
    p. factor E
    p. system

prophylactic
    p. antibody
    p. measures

prophylactic (*continued*)
    p. systemic antivirals
    p. treatment

prophylaxis
    active p.
    p. agent
    chemical p.
    malaria p.
    passive p.

Prophyllin

porphyrin
    p. intermediates
    p. production

Propionibacterium
    P. acnes
    P. propionicus

propionicus
    Propionibacterium p.

propofol

propoxyphene HCl

propranolol hydrochloride

propria
    atrophia pilorum p.
    lamina p.

proptosis

propylene glycol

propylthiouracil

proquazone

Proscar

prosecutor
    p's tubercle
    p's wart

prosodemic

prosopitis granulomatosa

prostaglandin (PG)
    p. D (PGD)
    p. D_2 (PGD_2)
    p. E (PGE)

prostaglandin (*continued*)
    p. E_1 (PGE$_1$)
    p. E_2 (PGE$_2$)
    p. H_2 (PGH$_2$)
    p. synthesis inhibition

Prostaphlin
    P. injection
    P. oral

prostate-specific antigen

prostatitis

prosthetic

prostration

protease
    p. inhibitor

protection
    photo p.
    p. test

protective
    p. barrier cream
    p. factor
    p. protein

protector
    Heelbo decubitus p.

protein
    autologous heat shock p.
    p. C
    p. C deficiency
    p. C replacement
    p. deposition
    p. electrophoresis
    p. filaggrin
    p. fragment
    human heat shock p.
    p. hydrolysate
    p. kinase C
    mediator p.
    milk p.
    nonantibody plasma p.
    p.-purified derivative
    p. S
    p. synthesis

proteinuria

proteoglycan
    95-kD membrane-bound p.

proteolysis

Proteus
    P. mirabilis
    P. syndrome
    P. vulgaris

Prothazine
    P. injection
    P. oral

prothrombin time

protionamide

protopianoma

Protopic

protoplasmic
    p. cylinder
    p. poison

protoporphyria
    erythropoietic p.
    p. erythropoietica

protoporphyrin IX

protoporphyrinogen oxidase

Prototheca
    P. wickerhamii
    P. zopfii

protothecosis

prototype
    p. antigen-presenting cell

prototypic lesion

prototypical septal panniculitis

Protozoa

protozoacide

protozoal parasitic disease

protozoan

protozoiasis

protracted

protuberans
dermatofibrosarcoma p.

protuberant abdomen

proud flesh

Provatene

provocative
p. skin test
p. test

prowazekii
Rickettsia p.

proximal
p. fingernail folds
p. interphalangeal (PIP)
p. nailfold
p. nail matrix
p. phalanges
p. subungual
onychomycosis
p. symphalangism
p. trichorrhexis nodosa

Prozac

PRP
pityriasis rubra pilaris

pruriginosus
strophulus p.

pruriginous
p. dermatoses
p. papule

prurigo
actinic p.
acute childhood prurigo
p. aestivalis
p. agria
p. annularis
Besnier's p.
p. of Besnier
p. of Borda
p. chronica multiformis
p. diathsique
p. estivalis
p. ferox
p. gestationis

prurigo (*continued*)
p. gestationis of Besnier
p. gravidarum
Hebra p.
p. of Hebra
p. hiemalis
Hutchinson summer p.
p. infantilis
melanotic p.
p. mitis
nodular p.
p. nodularis
p. nodularis of Hyde
p. papule
p. of Pierini
p. pigmentosa
polymorphic p.
p. simplex
p. simplex acuta infantum
(Brocq)
p. simplex chronica
p. simplex subacuta
summer p.
summer p. of Hutchinson
p. universalis
p. vulgaris
winter p.

pruritic
p. autoimmune vesicular
bullous disease
p. dermatosis
p. erythematous patch
p. folliculitis of pregnancy
p. inflammatory
dermatoses of pregnancy
p. lesion
p. papule
p. urticarial papules and
plaques of pregnancy
(PUPPP)
p. vesiculopustular eruption
p. wheals

pruritogenic

pruritus
p. aestivalis
p. ani

pruritus (*continued*)
    aquagenic p.
    p. balnea
    bath p.
    central p.
    Duhring p.
    essential p.
    p. estivalis
    genital p.
    p. gravidarum
    p. hiemalis
    perianal p.
    psychogenic p.
    p. scroti
    senile p.
    p. senilis
    symptomatic p.
    uremic p.
    p. vulvae

psammoma bodies

psammous

Pseudallescheria
    P. boydii

pseudoacanthosis
    p. nigricans

pseudoainhum

pseudoalopecia areata

pseudoanaphylactic
    p. shock

pseudoanaphylaxis

pseudoangiosarcoma
    Masson p.

pseudoarthrosis

pseudoatrophoderma colli

pseudochancre redux

pseudochromidrosis

pseudocolloid
    p. of lips

pseudocomedones

pseudocowpox

pseudocowpox (*continued*)
    p. virus

pseudocyst

pseudocystic rheumatoid
   arthritis

pseudoedema

pseudoephedrine
   hydrochloride

pseudoepicanthic fold

pseudoepitheliomatous
    p. hyperplasia
    p. keratotic
    p. nodule
    p. reaction

pseudoerysipelas

pseudoexfoliation

pseudofolliculitis
    p. barbae
    p. of the beard

pseudoform

pseudoglandular squamous cell
   carcinoma

pseudohorn cyst

pseudo-Hutchinson's sign

pseudoicterus

pseudoinfection

pseudojaundice

pseudo-Kaposi's sarcoma

pseudokeloidal nodules

pseudolepromatous
   leishmaniasis

pseudoleukoderma
   angiospasticum

pseudolymphoma
    p. reaction
    Spiegler-Fendt p.

pseudomalignant

pseudomalignant (*continued*)
  p. epitheliomatous
    hyperplasia
  p. lymphoma

pseudomelanoma

pseudomembrane

pseudomembranous
  p. colitis
  p. patches

Pseudomonas
  P. aeruginosa
  P. aeruginosa bacteremia
  P. elastase
  P. mallei
  P. mesophilica
  P. pseudomallei
  P. septicemia

pseudomonilethrix

pseudomycelium

pseudonit

pseudoobstruction

pseudopalsy

pseudopapilledema

pseudoparalysis
  Parrot's p.
  syphilitic p.

pseudopelade
  p. of Brocq

pseudophlegmon
  Hamilton p.

pseudopodagra

pseudoporphyria
  p. uremica

pseudopseudohypopara-
  thyroidism (PPHP)

pseudoreaction

pseudorheumatoid
  p. nodule

pseudorubella

pseudosarcoma Kaposi

pseudosarcomatous fasciitis

pseudoscar
  spontaneous p.
  stellate p.

pseudoscarlatina

pseudosclerodermatous
  reaction

pseudoseptic

pseudosmallpox

pseudosyndactylism

pseudosyndactyly

pseudotrichinosis

pseudotumor
  p. cerebri

pseudo-Turner syndrome

pseudovariola

pseudoverrucous papules

pseudovesicle

pseudoxanthoma
  p. elasticum (PXE)

pseudoxanthomatous
  p. mastocytosis
  p. variant

psilate

psilosis

psilothin

psilotic

psittacosis

psora

psoralens (*class of drugs*)
  p.-311 nm UVB therapy
  p. plus UVA light (PUVA)
  p. and ultraviolet A (PUVA)

Psorcon
    P. topical
    P. topical steroid

psorelcosis

psoriasic

psoriasiform
    p. acanthosis
    p. dermatitis
    p. epidermal hyperplasia
    p. eruption
    p. histologic pattern
    p. hyperkeratosis
    p. lesion
    p. patch
    p. plaque
    p. syphilis

psoriasiformis
    parakeratosis p.

psoriasis
    annular p.
    p. annularis
    p. annulata
    arthritic p.
    p. arthropathica
    p. arthropica
    Barber's p.
    p. buccalis
    p. circinata
    circinate p.
    p. diffusa
    discoid p.
    p. discoidea
    p. discoides
    droplike p.
    erythrodermic p.
    exfoliative p.
    p. figurata
    figurate p.
    flexural p.
    follicular p.
    p. follicularis
    generalized pustular p.
    genital p.
    p. geographica
    p. guttata

psoriasis (*continued*)
    guttate p.
    p. gyrata
    gyrate p.
    intertriginous p.
    intraepidermal
      microabscess of p.
    p. inversa
    inverse p.
    p. inveterata
    p. linguae
    p.-linked alloantigens
    localized acral-pustular p.
    localized pustular p.
    microabscess of p.
    napkin p.
    nummular p.
    p. nummularis
    p. of palms and soles
    p. orbicularis
    p. ostracea
    ostraceous p.
    palmar p.
    p. palmaris et plantaris
    p. palmoplantaris
    plaque p.
    plaque-type p.
    p. punctata
    pustular p.
    pustular p., generalized
    pustular p., localized
    p. pustulosa generalisata
    p. pustulosa hypocalcemica
    p. pustulosa palmaris et
      plantaris (Barber-
      Konigsbeck type)
    recalcitrant p.
    rupial p.
    rupioid p.
    p. rupioides
    seborrheic p.
    seborrheic-like p.
    p. spondylitica
    p. universalis
    volar p.
    von Zumbusch's pustular p.
    p. vulgaris

psoriasis (*continued*)
    p. vulgaris, chronic
        stationary type
    p. vulgaris, guttate type
    p. vulgaris, nail changes
    Zumbusch's p.

Psoriasis Area Severity Index
    (PASI)

Psoriasis Life Stress Inventory
    (PLSI)

psoriatic
    p. arthritis
    p. arthritis mutilans
    p. arthritis with spinal
        involvement
    p. arthropathy
    p. dermal papillae
    p. erythroderma
    p. keratinocytes
    p. nail changes
    p. nails
    p. plaque
    p. sacroiliitis
    p. scale
    p. spondylitis

psoriatica
    arthropathia p.

psoriaticum
    erythroderma p.

psoric

psoriGel

Psorion Cream

psoroid

Psorophora

psorophthalmia

psoroptic acariasis

Psoroptes
    P. bovis
    P. cuniculi
    P. equi
    P. ovis

psoroptid carpet mite

psorous

P&S Shampoo

PSS
    progressive systemic
        sclerosis

psychiatric disease

psychocutaneous

psychodermatology

Psychodidae

psychogalvanic

psychogalvanometer

psychogenic
    p. factor
    p. pain syndrome
    p. pruritus
    p. purpura
    p. reaction

psychological stimuli

psychomotor

psychopathologic condition

psychopathology

psychopharmacology

psychopharmacologic
    p. intervention
    p. medication

psychophysical

psychophysiologic
    p. disorder

psychosis

psychotherapy

PT
    prothrombin time

PTEN
    pentaerythritol tetranitrate

pteridine

pteronyssinus
    Dermatophagoides p.

pterygium *pl.* pterygia
    p. colli
    p. formation
    p. inversum unguis
    p. unguis

pthiriasis
    p. capitis
    p. corporis
    p. pubis

Pthirus
    P. pubis
    P. pubis infestation

PTK
    protein tyrosine kinase

ptosis

PTT
    partial thromboplastin time

puberty
    precocious p.

pubes

pubescence

pubic
    p. baldness
    p. lice
    p. louse
    p. phthiriasis
    p. trichomycosis

pubis
    pediculosis p.
    pthiriasis p.
    Pthirus p.

pubomadesis

pudenda (*plural of* pudendum)

pudendal ulcer

pudendi (*genitive of* pudendum)
    granuloma p.

pudendum *pl.* pudenda
    ulcerating granuloma of p.

pudoris
    erythema p.

Puente disease

puerperium

puffiness

Pulex
    P. irritans

pulicans
    purpura p.

pulicicide

pulicide

pulicosis

pull test

"pulling boat" hand

pulmonary
    p. artery stenosis
    p. aspergillosis
    p. carcinoma
    p. fibrosis
    p. hypoplasia
    p. infiltration
    p. lymphangiolei-
      omyoma
    p. metastasis
    p. osteoarthropathy
    p. sarcoidosis
    p. stenosis

pulpitis sicca

pulse
    p. chlorambucil
    p. methylprednisolone

pulsed dye laser (PDL)

pulseless disease

pultaceous

punch
    p. biopsy
    Dyonics suction p.
    p. grafts
    skin p.
    upcurved p.

punched-out
   p.-o. cyst
   p.-o. ulceration

puncta
   p. pruritica

punctata
   acne p.
   chondrodysplasia p.
   keratodermia p.
   keratosis p.
   keratosis palmoplantaris p.
   onychia p.
   porokeratosis p.
   psoriasis p.

punctate
   p. brown scabs
   p. erosion
   erythema p.
   p. erythematous papule
   p. hemorrhage
   p. keratitis
   p. keratoderma
   p. keratoses
   p. keratosis of the palmar
      creases
   p. leukonychia
   p. palmoplantar
      keratoderma
   p. palmoplantar keratosis
   p. porokeratotic
      keratoderma
   p. superficial necrosis
   p. wheals

punctatum
   keratoderma p.

punctiform
   p. accentuation

punctum

puncture
   p. technique
   p. wound

pupate

pupil
   Argyll Robertson p.

PUPPP
   pruritic urticarial papules
      and plaques of pregnancy

pura (plural of pus)

purified calf thymus DNA

purine nucleotides
   phosphorylase deficiency

PURPLE
   painful purpuric ulcers with
      reticular pattern of the
      lower extremities

purple
   p. patches
   p.-red papule

purplish discoloration

Purpose
   P. Alpha Hydroxy Moisture
   P. Dry Skin
   P. soap

purpura
   actinic p.
   acute idiopathic
      thrombocytopenic p.
   acute vascular p.
   allergic p.
   allergic
      nonthrombocytopenic p.
   anaphylactoid p.
   p. angioneurotica
   p. annularis telangiectodes
   p. annularis telangiectodes
      of Majocchi
   p.-associated disease
   autoimmune p.
   autoimmune
      thrombocytopenia p.
   p. bullosa
   p. cachectica
   chronic idiopathic
      thrombocytopenic p.
   p. cryoglobulinemia
   cutaneous p.
   drug p.
   drug-induced p.

purpura (*continued*)
    eczematid-like (Doucas-
      Kapetanakis) p.
    essential p.
    essential thrombocytopenic
      p.
    factitious p.
    fibrinolytic p.
    p. fulminans
    p. gangrenosa
    Gardner-Diamond p.
    p. hemorrhagica
    Henoch's p.
    Henoch-Schönlein p. (HSP)
    hypergammaglobulinemic
      p.
    hyperglobulinemic p.
    p. iodica
    idiopathic p.
    idiopathic
      thrombocytopenic p. (ITP)
    itching p.
    Landouzy p.
    macular p.
    p. maculosa
    Majocchi's p.
    mechanical p.
    p. morphology
    p. nervosa
    nonpalpable p.
    nonthrombocytopenic p.
    orthostatic p.
    palpable p.
    passion p.
    periorbital p.
    pigmented p.
    p. pigmentosa chronica
    p. pigmentosa progressiva
    psychogenic p.
    p. pulicans
    p. pulicosa
    p. rheumatica
    Schamberg p.
    Schönlein p.
    Schönlein-Henoch p.
    senile p.
    p. senilis
    p. simplex

purpura (*continued*)
    skin p.
    solar p.
    steroid p.
    p. steroidica
    symptomatic p.
    p. symptomatica
    p. telangiectatic vascular
      papules
    thrombocytopenic p.
    thrombocytopenic p.,
      idiopathic
    thrombocytopenic p.,
      primary
    thrombocytopenic p.,
      secondary
    thrombopenic p.
    thrombotic
      thrombocytopenic p.
      (TTP)
    traumatic p.
    p. urticans
    p. variolosa
    Waldenström's p.
    Waldenström's benign
      hypergammaglobulinemic
      p.
    Waldenström's
      hyperglobulinemic p.
    Werlhof p.

purpureum

purpuric
    p. eruption
    p. halo
    p. lesion
    p. mottling
    p. phototherapy-induced
      eruption
    p. pityriasis rosea
    p. spots

pursed openings

purulent
    p. exudates
    p. otitis media
    p. synovitis

puruloid

pus
    glairy p.

pus-containing amebae

puss
    p. caterpillar
    p. caterpillar sting
    p. moth
    "pussy" *(slang for pustular, puslike)*

pustula *pl.* pustulae
    p. maligna

pustulant

pustular
    p. acne
    p. acrodermatitis
    p. bacterid
    p. bacterid Andrews
    p. blebs
    p. dermatosis
    p. drug eruption
    p. eruption
    p. folliculitis
    p. form
    p. lesion
    p. melanosis
    p. miliaria
    p. patch-test reaction
    p. perifolliculitis
    p. psoriasis
    p. psoriasis of the palms and soles
    p. psoriasis of Zumbusch
    p. syphilid

pustulation

pustule
    follicular p.
    Kogoj p.
    malignant p.
    multilocular p.
    postmortem p.
    simple p.
    spongiform p.
    spongiform p. of Kogoj

pustule *(continued)*
    sterile p.
    thin-walled p.
    unilocular p.

pustuliform

pustulocrustaceous

pustulosa
    acne p.
    acrodermatitis p.
    miliaria p.
    parakeratosis p.
    trichomycosis p.

pustulosis
    p. acuta varioliformis Juliusberg
    palmar p.
    p. palmaris
    p. palmaris et plantaris
    palmoplantar p.
    p. palmoplantaris
    plantar p.
    p. subcornealis
    p. vacciniformis acuta
    p. varioliformis acuta

pustulosum
    eczema p.
    erysipelas p.

pustulotic arthrosteitis

putrefaction

PUVA
    psoralen and ultraviolet A
        PUVA-associated nonmelanoma
        foil bath PUVA
        PUVA-induced squamous cell carcinoma
        PUVA-induced lentigo
        topical PUVA

PVNS
    pigmented villonodular synovitis

PXE

PXE (*continued*)
    pseudoxanthoma elasticum
    PXE-like papillary dermal
        elastolysis

pyarthrosis

pyemia

pyemic

Pyemotes
    P. boylei
    P. tritici
    P. ventricosus

pyknosis

pyknotic
    p. cell
    p. nucleus

pyloric atresia

pyocyanin

pyocyanolysin

pyoderma
    blastomycosis-like p.
    chancriform p.
    p. chancriforme faciei
    p. faciale
    p. facialis
    p. gangrenosa
    p. gangrenosum
    granulomatous p.
    intractable p.
    malignant p.
    persistent p.
    primary p.
    secondary p.
    streptococcal p.
    superficial follicular p.
    superficial granulomatous
        p.
    p. ulcerosum
    p. vegetans
    vegetating p.
    p. verrucosum

pyodermatitis

pyodermatosis

pyodermatous
    p. infection
    p. process
    p. skin lesion

pyodermia
    p. chancriformis
    p. faciale
    p. facialis
    p. gangrenosa
    p. gangrenosum
    p. vegetans

pyogenic
    p. abscess
    p. cocci
    p. folliculitis
    p. granuloma
    p. granuloma formation
    p. granuloma-like
        proliferation
    p. infection
    p. liver abscess
    p. organism
    p. paronychia
    p. sterile arthritis
    p. superficial infection

pyogenicum
    granuloma p.

pyohemia

pyomyositis

pyorrhea

pyosis
    Corlett p.
    p. of Corlett
    Manson p.
    p. palmaris
    p. tropica

pyostomatitis
    p. vegetans

pyrazinamide (PZA)
    rifampin, isoniazid, and p.

pyrazolone

Pyrenochaeta romeroi

pyrethrins

pyrethroid
   synthetic p.

pyrethrum spray

pyrexia
   tick p.

pyridostigmine bromide

pyridoxine
   p. deficiency
   p. excess

pyriform
   p. flagellate

pyriform (*continued*)
   p. sinuses

pyrimethamine
   sulfadoxine and p.

Pyrinyl II

pyrithione
   zinc p.

pyrithyldione

pyruvate kinase deficiency

pythiosis

pyuria

Q

Q
  Q fever
  Q-switched alexandrite laser
  Q-switched mode
  Q-switched Nd:YAG laser
  Q-switched neodymium:YAG laser
  Q-switched ruby laser
  Q-switching

qualitative
  q. platelet function abnormality

quarantine

quarter
  q.-evil
  q.-ill

quartz light

quaternary
  q. ammonium
  q. syphilis

quaternium
  q.-15
  q.-18 bentonite

Questran

Queyrat
  erythroplasia of Q.

quicklime

quiescence

quiescent stage

Quiess

quinacrine
  q. anhidrosis

Quincke
  Q's angioedema
  Q's disease
  Q's edema
  Q's I syndrome

quinidine

quinine sulfate

quinolones

quinone

Quinquaud
  Q's disease

Quinsana Plus topical

R

R
    roentgen

rabbit botfly

Rabson-Mendenhall syndrome

raccoon eyes

racemosa
    livedo r.

Racet topical

racial
    r. background
    r. melanoderma

racket nails

rad

radial
    r. head abnormality
    r. scar

radiation
    r. burn
    r. dermatitis
    r. dermatitis, chronic
    r. dermatosis
    electromagnetic r.
    r. erythema
    r.-induced EM
    r. spectrum
    r. therapy
    r. ulcer
    ultraviolet r.

radical
    r. mastectomy

radices (plural of radix)

radiciform

radicis (genitive of radix)

radiculoneuritis

radioactive
    r. gold
    r. isotope

radioallergosorbent test (RAST)

radiocontrast material

radiodense

radiodensity

radiodermatitis
    chronic r.

radioepidermitis

radioepithelitis

radiofrequency

radioimmunoassay (RIA)

radiolabeled
    r. highly purified SAP
    r. octreotide scans

radiolabeling

radiolucency

radiolucent

radionuclide
    r. ventriculography

radiosensitivity

radiotherapist

radium ulcers

radix *pl.* radices
    r. pili
    r. unguis

radon

ragweed
    r. dermatitis

raised border

ram horn nail

Ramsay Hunt syndrome

random
    r. distribution

randomized double-blind
    prospective study

ranitidine hydrochloride

ranula

raphe
  median r.

rapid
  r. growers
  r. growth rate

Rapp-Hodgkin ectodermal
  dysplasia syndrome

rare
  r. mycosis
  r. recurrence
  r. plasma cell leukemia
  r. system reaction

rash
  ammonia r.
  antitoxin r.
  astacoid r.
  atopic dermatitis r.
  black currant r.
  brown-tail r.
  butterfly r.
  cable r.
  caterpillar r.
  crystal r.
  diaper r.
  drug r.
  ecchymotic r.
  generalized maculopapular
    r.
  gum r.
  heat r.
  heliotrope r.
  hemorrhagic r.
  hydatid r.
  JRA r.
  lupus erythematous-like r.
  macular r.
  maculopapular r.
  malar r. (MR)
  malar butterfly r.
  mulberry r.
  Murray Valley r.
  napkin r.
  nettle r.
  papulovesicular r.

rash (*continued*)
  red r.
  rose r.
  serum r.
  skin r.
  "slapped cheek" r.
  summer r.
  sunburn-like r.
  tooth r.
  wandering r.
  wildfire r.

Rasmussen's syndrome

raspberry
  r. tongue

RAST
  radioallergosorbent test
  RAST test

rat
  r.-bite fevers
  r. flea bite
  r. mite dermatitis
  r. mite itch
  r. tapeworm

rate
  erythrocyte sedimentation
    r. (ESR)

ratio
  risk (RR)

rattlesnake
  r. bite

RAV
  Rous-associated virus

raw base

Rayer disease

Raynaud
  R's disease
  R's gangrene
  R's phenomenon
  R's syndrome

razor blade

RBC fluorescence

RD
    rhabdomyosarcoma
    human RD

RDEB
    recessive dystrophic
      epidermolysis bullosa
      (Hallopeau-Siemens)

reaction
    accelerated r.
    acute anaphylactic r.
    acute phase r.
    adverse drug r.
    allergic r.
    anaphylactic r.
    anaphylactic
      hypersensitivity r.
    anaphylactoid r.
    antigen-antibody r.
    angry back r.
    Bloch r.
    cell-mediated r.
    cutaneous r.
    cutaneous basophil
      hypersensitivity r.
    cutaneous graft versus host
      r.
    delayed hypersensitivity r.
    demarcated r.
    dermatophytid r.
    dermotuberculin r.
    dopa r.
    downgrading r.
    drug r.
    early r.
    eczematous r.
    epicutaneous r.
    foreign body r.
    fungal id r.
    Goetsch skin r.
    granulomatous
      inflammatory r.
    Herxheimer r.
    hypersensitivity r.
    id r.
    inflammation r.
    intradermal r.
    irritant patch-test r.

reaction (*continued*)
    Jarisch-Herxheimer r.
    Jones-Mote r.
    Lepra r.
    lepromatous r.
    lepromin r.
    local r.
    marked localized r.
    miscellaneous r.
    Mitsuda r.
    non-drug-related r.
    photoallergic r.
    photoallergic drug r.
    photosensitivity r.
    polymerase chain r. (PCR)
    primary sensitization r.
    pustular patch-test r.
    reversal r.
    skin r.
    specific r.
    symptomatic r.
    systemic r.
    vaccinoid r.
    Weil-Felix r.
    well-demarcated skin r.
    wheal and erythema r.
    wheal and flare r.
    whitegraft r.

reactivate

reactivation
    sunburn r.

reactive
    r. Hansen's disease
    r. metabolite
    r. molecules
    r. perforating collagenosis
    r. postinfectious synovitis
    r. proliferation

reactivity
    immediate skin r.

reading
    delayed patch test r.

reagin

reaginic hypersensitivity

Rea-Lo

rebound dermatitis

recalcitrance

recalcitrant
  r. acrodermatitis continua
  r. disease
  r. lesion
  r. palmoplantar eruptions
  r. pustular eruptions

recanalization

receptor
  r. antagonist
  cell membrane r.
  contact r.
  cutaneous r.
  end-organ r.
  Fc r.
  mannosyl-fucosyl r.
  r. molecule
  pain r.
  pressure r.
  sensory r.
  T-cell r. (TCR)
  tactile r.
  touch r.

recess

recession

recessive
  r. dystrophic epidermolysis
    bullosa
  r. inheritance type
  r. X-linked ichthyosis

recessus

recidivans
  leishmaniasis r.
  r. lesion
  r. type

recidive
  chancre r.
  r. cutaneous types

recirculation

Recklinghausen (von
  Recklinghausen)
    R's disease
    R's disease, type I
    R's disease, central, type II

Reclus disease

recombinant
  r. human granulocyte
    colony-stimulating factor
  r. human interleukin-4

recombination
  genetic r.

recrudescence
  r. supervene

recrudescent

rectal
  r. ulceration
  r. structures

rectocele

recurrens
  herpes simplex r.
  periadenitis mucosae
    necrotica r.

recurrent
  r. aphthous stomatitis
  r. cutaneous abscess
  r. erythema multiforme
    minor
  r. genital herpes simplex
    virus
  r. infection
  r. infundibulofolliculitis
  r. intraoral herpes simplex
    infection
  r. intraoral herpes simplex
    virus
  r. labial herpes simplex
    virus
  r. nevus
  r. palmar peeling
  r. palmoplantar hidradenitis
  r. ulcer
  r. urticaria

red
- r. albinism
- r. aniline
- r. ant
- "r. balls"
- r. bug
- r. bug bite
- r. dog
- r. eye
- r. granulation
- r. hair/blue eyes
- r. lunulae
- r. nodule
- r. papule
- r. papule and nodule
- r. pepper
- r. rash
- r. sweat
- r. top

"red man" syndrome

reddening
- r. of palm
- r. of soles of feet

reddish
- r. metachromasia
- r. purple periphery

reddishness

redundant plaques

reduplication

reduviid
- r. bite
- r. bug

Reduviidae

Reduvius
- *R. personatus*

redux
- chancre r.

Reed-Sternberg cells

reedy nail

reenameling

reepithelialization

reepithelialize

reflex
- erector spinae r.
- pilomotor r.
- r. sympathetic dystrophy (RSD)

refractile
- r. spherules

refractory
- r. disease
- r. hypoglycemia
- r. period
- r. wart

refringent
- r. parasites

Refsum
- R's disease
- R's syndrome

regimen
- continuous daily r.
- one-day-a-week r.

region
- intertriginous r.
- ringworm of genitocrural r.

regional
- r. enteritis
- r. granulomatous lymphadenitis
- r. internal carcinoma
- r. lymphadenopathy
- r. node metastasis
- r. predilection

Regranex

regressing atypical histiocytosis

regression
- spontaneous r.

regular borders

reinoculation

Reiter
- R's disease
- R's syndrome

rejection
    acute cellular r.
    allograft r.
    chronic allograft r.
    hyperacute r.
    primary r.

relapsing
    r. febrile nodular
        nonsuppurative
        panniculitis
    r. polychondritis

relaxation of the skin

relevant sting history

REM
    reticular erythematous
        mucinosis

remission
    pathologically confirmed
        complete r. (PCR)

remitting seronegative
    symmetrical synovitis

remodeling
    tissue r.

removal
    excisional r.

renal
    r. aplasia
    r. calculi
    r. cell carcinoma
    r. dialysis
    r. disease
    r. hamartomas

Rendu
    R.-Osler syndrome
    R.-Osler-Weber disease
    R.-Osler-Weber syndrome

Renova

Reovirus

repair
    tissue r.

repellent

repens
    dermatitis r.
    erythema gyratum r.

repetitive superficial freezes

repigmentation

Replens

replication
    mitogen-driven lymphocyte
        r.

RES
    reticuloendothelial system

reserpine

reservoir
    r. host
    r. of infection

residua

residual
    r. pigmentation
    r. rim

residue

residuum

resilience

resin
    podophyllum r.

resolution
    spontaneous r.

resorcin

resorcinol
    r. allergens
    r. monoacetate

respiratory
    r. atopy
    r. paralysis
    r. tree
    r. virus

response
    antibody-mediated immune
        r.
    anti-idiotype r.

response (*continued*)
  central cell regulating
    lymphoid r.
  delayed hypersensitivity r.
  irritant patch-test r.
  mitogen r.
  primary immune r.
  prompt r.
  secondary immune r.

resting
  r. phase
  r. stage

restrictive
  r. dermopathy

rete *pl.* retia
  dermal r.
  malpighian r.
  r. pegs
  r. ridges
  r. testis architecture

retention
  r. cyst

retial

reticular
  r. cells
  r. degeneration
  r. dermis
  r. erythema
  r. erythematous mucinosis
    (REM)
  r. lesion
  r. pigmentation
  r. pigmented anomaly of
    the flexures
  r. pigmented
    genodermatosis
  white r.

reticularis
  dermatopathia pigmentosa
    r.
  idiopathic livedo r.
  livido r.
  pars r.

reticulata
  folliculitis ulerythematosa r.

reticulate
  r. acropigmentation of
    Kitamura
  r. hyperpigmentation
  r. pigmentation

reticulated
  r. hyperkeratosis
  r. pigmentary dermatosis of
    the flexures
  r. pigmented anomaly
  r. papillomatosis
  r. papillomatosis of
    Gougerot-Carteaud
  r. pigmented poikiloderma

reticulation

reticulin fibers

reticuloendothelial
  r. cell
  r. system (RES)

reticuloendothelioma

reticuloendotheliosis

reticulogranuloma

reticulohistiocytic granuloma

reticulohistiocytoma

reticulohistiocytosis
  congenital self-healing r.
  r. cutanea hyperplastica
    benigna cum
    melanodermia
  multicentric r.
  self-healing r.

reticuloid
  actinic r.

reticulosis
  epidermotropic r.
  lipomelanotic r.
  medullary r.
  pagetoid r.

reticulum *pl.* reticula
  r.-cell sarcoma
  r. cutis

reticulum (*continued*)
    endoplasmic r.
    r. fibers
    r. unguis

retiform
    r. hemangioendothelioma
    r. network
    r. parapsoriasis
    r. subtype

Retin-A
    R. Micro gel

retinal
    r. arteriovenous aneurysm
    r. detachment
    r. hemorrhage
    r. pigmentary abnormality
    r. telangiectasia
    r. tumors
    r. vasculitis

retinitis
    r. pigmentosa

retinoblastoma

retinoic acid
    r. a. cream
    r. a. gel
    r. a. swabs

retinoids (*class of drugs*)
    r. therapy

retinopathy

retinyl
    r. esters
    r. palmitate

retraction

retroauricular skin

retroperitoneum

retrovirus group

revaccination

revulsion

Reye's syndrome

R-Gel

Rh imcompatibility

RH
    rheumatoid

rhabdomyoma

rhabdomyosarcoma (RD)

rhabdovirus

rhacoma

rhagadiform

rhagades
    r. of the lips

rheumatic nodule

rheumatica
    purpura r.
    scarlatina r.

rheumaticum
    erythema annulare r.

rheumatid

rheumatoid (RH)
    r. arthritis (RA)
    r. clawing
    r. disease
    r. episcleritis
    r. factor (RF)
    r. neutrophilic dermatosis
    r. nodule
    r. nodulosis
    r. scleritis
    r. vasculitis

rheumatologic disorders

rheumatology
    American College of R.
    (ACR)

Rheumatrex

rhinitis
    r. sicca

rhinocerebral infection

Rhinocladiella aquaspersa

rhinoconjunctivitis
    allergic r.

rhinoentomophthoromycosis

rhinopharyngitis

rhinophyma

rhinoscleroma
    r. bacillus

rhinoscleromatis
    Klebsiella r.

rhinosporidiosis

Rhinosporidium seeberi

Rhipicephalus
    R. sanguineus

Rhizoglyphus
    R. parasiticus

Rhizomucor
    R. pusillus

Rhizopus
    R. nigricans
    R. rhizopodoformis

rhizotomy

Rhodesian
    R. form
    R. trypanosomiasis

Rhodotorula rubra

rhus
    r. dermatitis
    r. toxicodendron
    r. toxin

Rhus
    R. diversiloba
    R. radicans
    R. toxicodendron
    R. toxicodendron antigen
    R. venenata
    R. venenata antigen
    R. vernix

rhyparia

rhytid

rhytidectomy

rhytidoplasty

Ribas-Torres disease

riboflavin deficiency

ribosomal RNA

ribosome

rice
    r. itch

Richner-Hanhart syndrome

Ricinus communis

ricinus
    Ixodes r.

rickets

Rickettsia
    R. akari
    R. australis
    R. conorii
    R. mooseri
    R. prowazekii
    R. rickettsii
    R. sibirica
    R. typhi
    R. vaccine, attenuated

rickettsia *pl.* rickettsiae

Rickettsiaceae

rickettsiae

rickettsial
    r. disease
    r. infection

Rickettsiales

rickettsialpox

rickettsicidal

Rickettsieae

rickettsii
    Rickettsia r.

rickettsiosis
    eastern tickborne r.
    Russian vesicular r.

rickettsiostatic

RID
    R. liquid
    R. mousse

ridge
    dermal r.
    rete r.
    skin r.

ridged wart

ridges
    interpapillary r.
    rete r.

ridging
    longitudinal r.

Rieger
    R's anomaly
    R's syndrome

Riehl
    R's melanoderma
    R's melanosis

rifabutin

rifampicin

rifampin and isoniazid

rigid plate

Riley
    R.-Day syndrome
    R.-Smith syndrome

Rilutek

ring
    incomplete r.
    irregular r.
    r. of hyperemia
    round r.
    r. ulcer

ringed
    r. creases
    r. hair

ringlike fibrosis

ringworm

ringworm (*continued*)
    black-dot r.
    crusted r.
    gray-patch r.
    honeycomb r.
    hypertrophic r.
    r. of the axillae
    r. of the beard
    r. of the body
    r. of the face
    r. of the foot
    r. of the body
    r. of the genitocrural region
    r. of the groin
    r. of the hand
    r. of the nails
    r. of the scalp
    Oriental r.
    scalp r.
    scaly r.
    Tokelau r.
    r. yaws

Rinse
    Nix Crème R.

risedronate

RIT

Ritter
    R's disease

river blindness

RNA
    ribonucleic acid

Ro and La antibody

road burn

Robaxin

Roberts' syndrome

Robicillin VK Oral

Robinson
    R. disease

Robitet Oral

Robles disease

Robomol

Rocky Mountain
    R. M. spotted fever
    R. M. spotted fever
      vaccine
    R. M. tick

rod
    gram-negative r.
    gram-positive r.

rod-shaped cytoplasmic
  granules

rodent
    r. carcinoma
    r. mite
    r. ulcer

rodenticide

rodonalgia

roentgen
    r. ray
    r. unit

roentgenograph

roentgenographic

roentgen
    r. ulcer
    r. units

RoEzIt skin moisturizer

Roferon-A

Rogaine

rolled
    r. edge
    r. shoulder lesion

Rollet
    R. chancre

Romaña's sign

Romberg
    R's sign
    R's syndrome

Rombo syndrome

root
    bitter r.
    mandrake r.
    nail r.
    r. of nail
    r. sheath

rope
    r. burn
    r. sign

rosacea
    acne r.
    corticosteroid r.
    r. fulminans
    granulomatous r.
    hypertrophic r.
    lupoid r.
    papular r.
    tuberculoid r.

rosaceaform dermatitis

rosacealike
    r. tuberculid
    r. tuberculid of
      Lewandowski

rosaceous lymphedema

Rosai
    R.-Dorfman disease
    R.-Dorfman syndrome

rose
    r. rash
    r. spot

rosea
    atypical pityriasis r.
    pityriasis r.

Rosenbach
    R. disease
    R. erysipeloid

Rosen's papular eruption

roseola
    epidemic r.
    r. fulminans
    idiopathic r.
    r. infantilis

roseola (*continued*)
 r. infantum
 syphilitic r.
 r. vaccinia

roseolalike
 r. facial dermatosis
 r. illness

roseolous

rosette
 EAC r.

rosin

Ross syndrome

Ro/SSA

rot
 Barcoo r.
 jungle r.

Roth
 Roth spot
 R.-Bernhardt disease

Rothmann-Makai syndrome

Rothmund
 R's syndrome
 R's type
 R.-Thomson syndrome

rough texture

roughness

rouleaux formation

round
 r. body
 r. fingerpad sign
 r. homogenous structures

roundish area

roundworm

Rous
 R.-associated virus (RAV)
 R. sarcoma
 R. sarcoma virus (RSV)
 R. sarcoma virus immune
  globulin intravenous
  (RSV-IGIV)

Rous (*continued*)
 R. tumor

routine monitoring

rove beetle

Rowasa

Rowell's syndrome

roxithromycin

Royl-Derm wound hydrogel
 dressing

RPC
 reactive perforating
  collagenosis

RPR
 rapid plasma reagin

RSV
 Rous sarcoma virus

RSV-IGIV
 Rous sarcoma virus
  immune globulin
  intravenous

rubber
 r. additive dermatitis
 r. band tourniquet
 r. man syndrome

rubbery

rubedo

rubefacient

rubefaction

rubella
 congenital r.
 r. HI test
 r. IgG ELISA test
 r. and mumps vaccines,
  combined
 r. vaccine virus
 r. virus
 r. virus vaccine, live

rubeola
 r. virus

rubeosis
 r. diabeticorum

ruber
 lichen r.

ruberous

rubescent

Rubinstein
 R.-Taybi syndrome
 R.-Taybi and Gardner
  syndrome

Rubivirus

rubor
 skin r.

ruborous

rubra
 miliaria r.
 pityriasis r.
 Rhodotorula r.
 stria r.

rubrous

rubrum
 eczema r.
 Trichophyton r.

ruby
 r. spots

ruddiness

rudiment
 hair r.

rudimentary
 r. cephalocele
 r. meningocele
 r. supernumerary digit

Rud's
 R. syndrome

rue

rufous
 r. albinism
 oculocutaneous albinism

ruga *pl.* rugae

rugose

rugous

rule
 r. of nines

Rumpel
 R.-Leede sign
 R.-Leede test

runaround

rupia
 r. escharotica

rupial
 r. blisters
 r. hyperkeratosis
 r. psoriasis
 r. syphilid

rupioid

rupioides
 psoriasis r.

rural cutaneous leishmaniasis

Russell bodies

Rutaceae (*family to which rue belongs*)

rutoside

S

SA
  salicylic acid

SAARD
  slow-acting antirheumatic drug

saber shin

Sabin-Feldman dye test

Sabouraud's agar

sacculations

sacral
  s. hypertrichosis
  s. zoster

sacrococcygeal
  s. lipoma

sacroiliitis
  psoriatic s.
  pyogenic s.

saddle
  s. nose
  s. nose deformity

saddleback
  s. caterpillar
  s. caterpillar sting

Saf-Clens wound cleanser

Safeguard

sagging

sailor's skin

Saint Anthony's fire

Saint Ignatius' itch

Saksenaea
  S. vasiformis

Salacid ointment

Sal-Acid plaster

Salagen oral

salicylate

salicylate (*continued*)
  choline s.
  s. toxicity

salicylic
  s. acid (SA)
  s. acid and lactic acid
  s. acid and propylene glycol
  s. acid collodion

Salicylic Acid
  S. A. acne treatment
  S. A. and Sulfur soap
  S. A. cleansing bar

salicylazosulfapyridine

salicylism

saline-solution compresses

salivary glands

salivation

salmon
  s. patch

Salmonella
  S. coinfection

salmonellal

Salmonelleae

salmonellosis

salpingitis
  reactive s.

salsalate

salt
  s.-split skin
  s.-split skin biopsy

saltwater
  s. boil
  s. marine dermatitis

Sanarelli-Shwartzman phenomenon

sand
  s. flea

sand (*continued*)
　　s. flea bite

sandal
　　keratodermic s.
　　s. strap dermatitis

sandfly
　　s. bite
　　s. inoculation

Sandoglobulin

sandpaper
　　s.-like texture
　　s. quality

sandworm disease

sanguine

sanguineous

sanguineus
　　nevus s.

sanguinopurulent
　　s. drainage

sanguinous
　　s. blisters

Santyl ointment

SAP
　　serum amyloid P

SAPHO syndrome
　　*s*ynovitis, *a*cne, *p*ustulosis,
　　　*h*yperostosis,
　　　*o*steomyelitis

saponification

saprophyte

saprophytic
　　s. floras
　　s. fungi
　　s. organism

Sarcodina
　　class S.

sarcodine

sarcoid

sarcoid (*continued*)
　　Boeck s.
　　s. of Boeck
　　Darier-Roussy s.
　　s. lesions
　　s. reactions
　　Spiegler-Fendt s.

sarcoidal granuloma

sarcoidosis
　　circinate type s.
　　cutaneous s.
　　large nodular type s.
　　s. of the skin, plaque form
　　small nodular type s.
　　subcutaneous s.
　　ulcerative s.

sarcoma *pl.* sarcomas,
　sarcomata
　　Abernethy s.
　　adipose s.
　　s. idiopathicum multiplex
　　　hemorrhagicum Kaposi
　　Kaposi s. (KS)
　　melanotic s.
　　multiple idiopathic
　　　hemorrhagic s.
　　pseudo-Kaposi s.
　　reticulum-cell sarcoma

sarcomatosis
　　s. cutis

sarcomatous
　　s. area
　　s. degeneration

Sarcopsylla

Sarcoptes scabiei

sarcoptic
　　s. acariasis
　　s. mange

Sarna
　　S. Anti-Itch foam
　　S. Anti-Itch lotion

Sastid Plain therapeutic
　　shampoo and acne wash

SAStid Soap

satellite
    s. brown macules
    s. cell necrosis
    s. lesion
    s. pigmentation
    s. pigmented spots

satellitosis

saucer-shaped ulcer

sauriderma

sauriasis

sauriosis

sauroderma

sausage
    s. appearance
    s. digit
    s. finger
    s.-shaped loops
    s. toe

"saw-toothed" configuration

sc
    subcutaneous

scab

scabby mouth

Scabene
    S. Lotion
    S. shampoo

scabetic

scabicidal

scabicides (*class of drugs*)

scabies
    Boeck s.
    crusted s.
    environmental s.
    hair follicle mite s.
    s. incognito
    nodular s.
    Norwegian s.
    s. preparation

scabietic
    s. mite

scabieticide

scabious

scabrities
    s. unguium

scald

scalded skin syndrome

scale
    branny s.
    carpet-tack s.
    lamellar s.
    lichen-type s.
    Lund-Browder burn s.
    micaceous s.
    ostraceous s.
    pityriasis-type s.
    psoriatic-type s.
    Sessing pressure ulcer
        assessment s.
    Shea pressure ulcer
        assessment s.
    silver-white s.
    silvery s.

scalene

scalenus anticus syndrome

scaliness

scaling
    s. base
    s. lesion
    s. nodule
    s. patches
    s. plaque
    s. skin-colored lesion

scalloped
    s. border
    s. pattern
    s. periphery

scalp
    s. alopecia
    dissecting cellulitis of s.
    dissection cellulites of s.

scalp (*continued*)
    s. dysesthesia
    s. electrodes
    gyrate s.
    s. hair follicle
    s. hair shafts
    s. hypothermia
    s. infection
    s. keloids
    s. louse
    s. margin
    s. melanoma
    s. of Ayres
    pilar tumor of s.
    s. pruritus
    ringworm of s.
    seborrheic dermatitis of the
      s.

scalpel

Scalpicin

scaly
    s. ringworm
    s. tetter

scan

scanning
    s. electron microscopy
    s. mode

Scanpor
    S. acrylate adhesive
    S. tape

scant spongiosis

scanty

scapus *pl.* scapi
    s. pili

scar
    atrophic white s.
    elevated hypertrophic s.
    s. formation
    hypertrophic s.
    ice-pick type s.
    keloidal s.
    keloidal type s.
    papular acne s.

scar (*continued*)
    papyraceous s.
    pitted s.
    postacne anetoderma-like
      s.
    radial s.
    s. sarcoid
    s. sarcoidosis
    shilling s.
    white s.

scarf nevus

scarification
    s. test

scarificator

scarifier
    Berkeley s.

scarify

scarlatina
    anginose s.
    s. hemorrhagica
    s. latens
    s. maligna
    s. rheumatica
    s. simplex

scarlatinella

scarlatiniform
    s. eruption
    erythema s.
    s. erythema
    s. reaction

scarlatinoid

scarlet
    s. fever
    s. red lipid stain

scarring
    s. alopecia
    s. basal cell cancer
    cigarette-paper s.
    keloidal s.
    patch test s.
    s. pemphigoid
    s. plaques

SCAT
  short-contact therapy
SCC
  squamous cell carcinoma
Schäfer
  S. syndrome
  S.-Branauer syndrome
Schamberg
  S's comedo extractor
  S's dermatitis
  S's dermatosis
  S's disease
  S's progressive pigmented
    purpuric dermatosis
  S's purpura
Schaumann's benign
  lymphogranulomatosis
schema
Schick test
Schilder's disease
Schimmelpenning
  S. syndrome
  S.-Feuerstein-Mims
    syndrome
Schinzel-Giedion syndrome
Schirmer's test
Schistosoma
  S. haematobium
  S. japonicum
  S. mansoni
  S. spindale
  S. spindale cercaria
schistosomacidal
schistosomacide
schistosomal dermatitis
Schistosomatium
schistosome
  s. cercarial dermatitis
  s. granuloma

schistosomiasis
  cutaneous .
  ectopic cutaneous s.
  visceral s.
schistosomicidal
schistosomicide
schizonychia
schizophrenia
schizotrichia
Schmidt syndrome
Schnitzler's syndrome
schoenleinii
  Trichophyton schoenleinii
Schönlein
  S's disease
  S's purpura
  S.-Henoch disease
  S.-Henoch purpura
  S.-Henoch syndrome
Schopf syndrome
Schridde cancer hair
Schüller
  S's disease
  S's syndrome
Schultz
  S's angina
  S's disease
  S's syndrome
Schultze
  S's acroparesthesia
  S.-type acroparesthesia
Schwann cells nuclei
schwannian
  s. cell
  s. tissue
schwannoma
  peripheral s.
  plexiform s.
Schweninger

Schweninger (*continued*)
    anetoderma of S.-Buzzi
    S.-Buzzi anetoderma
    S.-Buzzi type

SCID
    severe combined
      immunodeficiency
    severe combined
      immunodeficiency
      disorder

scirrhous
    s. carcinoma

scissura pilorum

SCLE
    subacute cutaneous lupus
      erythematosus

scleral
    s. pigmentation

scleredema
    s. adultorum
    s. adultorum Buschke
    Buschke's s.
    s. diutinum
    s. neonatorum

sclerema
    s. adiposum
    s. adultorum
    s. neonatorum

scleriasis

scleritis
    diffuse s.
    nodular s.
    nonrheumatoid s.
    posterior s.
    rheumatoid s.

scleroadipose

scleroatrophic syndrome of
  Huriez

scleroatrophy, sclerotylosis
    anetoderma s.
    atrophoderma s.
    lichen sclerosus s.

scleroatrophy (*continued*)
    striae s.

sclerodactylia
    s. annularis ainhumoides

sclerodactyly

scleroderma
    circumscribed s.
    diffuse s.
    environmental s.
    generalized s.
    linear s.
    localized s.
    pediatric s.
    s. septal panniculitis
    systemic s.

scleroderma-like
    s. eruption
    s. skin thickening

sclerodermatitis

sclerodermatomyositis

sclerodermatous
    s. changes
    s. condition
    s. plaques

sclerodermia progressiva

sclerodermiform basalioma

sclerodermoid change

scleroma

scleromyxedema

scleronychia

sclerose

sclerosed

sclerosing
    s. agent
    s. basal cell cancer
    s. cholangitis
    s. hemangioma
    s. lipogranuloma
    s. lymphangitis
    s. sweat duct carcinoma

sclerosis
   s. cutanea
   diffuse progressive systemic
     s.
   diffuse systemic s.
   drug-induced progressive
     symptom s.
   environment progressive
     symptom s.
   limited progressive
     systemic s.
   linear progressive systemic
     s.
   localized progressive
     systemic s.
   miliary s.
   multiple s.
   progressive symptom s.
     (PSS)
   progressive systemic s.
   systemic s.
   tuberous s.

sclerostenosis

sclerosus
   genital lichen s.
   lichen s.
   s. lichen

sclerotherapy

sclerothrix

sclerotic
   s. bands
   s. bodies
   s. densities
   s. plaque

Sclerotinia sclerotiorum

Sclerotiniaceae

sclerotrichia

sclerotylosis (*variant of*
   scleroatrophy)

sclerous

scoliosis

Scolopendra

Scolopendra (*continued*)
   S. heres
   S. heres bite
   S. subspinipes

scombroid

scopolamine

Scopulariopsis
   brevicaulis

scorbutic purpura

scorpion
   s. fish
   s. flower
   s. sting

Scorpionida

scorpionism

Scotch plaid pattern

Scotch Tape test

scotochromogen

scraping
   fungal s.

scratch
   s. marks
   s. test
   s. testing

scratches

scratching

screen
   skin s.
   solar s.
   s. test

Screening Patch Test Kit

scrofula

scrofuloderma
   s. gummosa
   papular s.
   pustular s.
   tuberculous s.
   ulcerative s.
   verrucous s.

scrofulosorum
  acne s.
  lichen s.

scrofulous
  s. nature

scrotal
  s. condylomata
  s. cyst
  s. epidermoid cyst
  s. erythema
  s. infundibular cyst
  s. rugae
  s. tongue

scrotalis
  lingua s.

scroti
  pruritus s.

scrub
  Exidine S.
  Techni-Care surgical s.
  s. typhus

scruff

scurf

scurvy
  s. fellow
  s. trick

Scutigera coleoptrata

scutula

scutular
  s. lesions

scutularis
  parakeratosis s.

scutulata
  ichthyosis s.
  porrigo s.

scutulum

scybala

Scytalidium
  S. dimidiatum
  S. hyalinum

sea
  s. anemone
  s. anemone sting
  s. chervil
  s. urchin
  s. urchin granuloma
  s. urchin sting

seabather's eruption

Searl ulcer

seasonal
  s. preponderance

seatworm infection

seaweed dermatitis

sebacea
  ichthyosis s.

sebaceous
  s. adenoma
  s. carcinoma
  s. cyst
  s. differentiation
  s. epithelioma
  s. gland
  s. gland carcinoma
  s. gland hyperplasia
  s. horn
  s. hyperplasia
  s. neoplasm
  s. oils
  s. trichofolliculoma
  s. tubercle
  s. tumor

sebaceus
  lupus s.
  nevus s.

sebaceum
  adenoma s.
  molluscum s.
  tuberculum s.

sebaceus
  nevus s.

Sebex
  S.-T shampoo

sebiferous

sebiparous

Sebizon lotion

sebolith

sebopsoriasis

seborrhea
  s. adiposa
  s. capitis
  s. cerea
  concrete s.
  s. congestiva
  s. corporis
  eczematoid s.
  s. faciei
  s. furfuracea
  s. generalis
  nasolabial s.
  s. nigra
  s. nigricans
  s. oleosa
  s. sicca
  s. squamosa neonatorum

seborrheal

seborrheic
  s. dermatitis
  s. dermatitis-like condition
  s. dermatitis-like eruption
  s. dermatitis of the scalp
  s. dermatosis
  s. eczema
  s. keratosis
  s. verruca
  s. verrucosis
  s. wart

seborrheica
  corona s.
  dermatitis s.

seborrhiasis

sebotropic

Sebucare

Sebulex
  S. shampoo

Sebulex (conintued)
  S. with conditioners

Sebulon shampoo

sebum
  cutaneous s.
  s. cutaneum
  s. overproduction
  s. preputiale
  s. secretion

Sebutone
  S. cream shampoo
  S. liquid shampoo

second
  s.-degree burn
  s. disease
  s. intention

secondary
  s. anetoderma
  s. clubbing
  s. cold urticaria
  s. crease
  s. cutaneous aspergillosis
  s. cutaneous lymphoma
  s. disease
  s. furunculosis
  s. hyperlipoproteinemia
  s. immune response
  s. infection
  s. lesion
  s. lues
  s. lymphedema
  s. lymphoma
  s. milia
  s. prurigo
  s. pyoderma
  s. Sjögren syndrome
  s. syphilid
  s. syphilis
  s. tufted hairs

second-line drug (SLD)

Secrétan's syndrome

secrete

secretion
  excessive s.

section
    tissue s.

seed
    s. corn
    s. wart

segmental
    s. anhidrosis
    s. colitis
    s. heterochromia
    s. hyalinizing vasculitis
    s. neurofibromatosis
    s. vitiligo

Seidlmayer syndrome

Seip-Lawrence syndrome

seizure

Seldane
    S.-D

selene
    s. unguium

selenium
    s. deficiency
    s. sulfate shampoo
    s. sulfide suspension

Selestoject
    "self" antigen

self-defense sprays

self-healing juvenile cutaneous
  mucinosis

self-induced

self-infection

self-inflicted trauma

self-limited
    s.-l. allergic reaction
    s.-l. course
    s.-l. infection

self-mutilation

sella turcica

Selsun
    S. Blue

Selsun (*continued*)
    S. Gold
    S. Gold for women

semelincident

semicircle

semicircular
    s. lipoatrophy

semiflexion

semi-impermeable membrane

seminal vesiculitis

semipermeable
    s. dressing
    s. filter

semisolid
    s. material

semisynthetic
    s. penicillin

semitranslucent nodule

Semprex
    S.-D

Senear
    S.-Usher disease
    S.-Usher syndrome

senile
    s. angioma
    s. atrophoderma
    s. cataracts
    s. ectasia
    s. fibroma
    s. freckle
    s. gangrene
    s. hemangioma
    s. keratoderma
    s. keratoma
    s. keratosis
    s. lentigo
    s. lentigines
    s. melanoderma
    s. pruritus
    s. purpura
    s. sebaceous adenoma

senile (*continued*)
    s. sebaceous hyperplasia
    s. skin
    s. wart

senilis
    alopecia s.
    keratosis s.
    lentigo s.
    pruritus s.
    purpura s.
    verruca s.
    verruca plana s.

sennetsu
    Ehrlichia s.

sensible perspiration

sensitiva
    trichosis s.

sensitivity
    acquired s.
    allergic s.
    animal dander s.
    antibiotic s.
    aspirin s.
    atopic s.
    photoallergic s.
    phototoxic s.
    salt s.

sensitization
    active s.
    autoerythrocyte s.
    s. dermatitis

sensitize

sensitizing
    s. dose
    s. injection
    s. substance

Sensorcaine
    S.-MPF

sensory
    s. dorsal root ganglion
    s. dorsal root ganglion cells
    s. ganglion
    s. nerve ganglion

sensory (*continued*)
    s. neuropathy
    s. peripheral neuropathy

sentinel cells

separation
    eschar s.

sepsis

Septa
    S. ointment
    S. topical

septal
    s. granulomas of epithelioid
      macrophages
    s. panniculitis

septate

septic
    s. dactylitis
    s. embolus
    s. staphylococcal emboli
    s. vasculitis

septicemia
    bacterial s.
    gonococcal s.
    streptococcal

septicemic hypotension

Septisol
    S. foam
    S. solution

Septra
    S. DS

Sequester

sequestra

sequestral

sequestration
    s. cyst
    s. dermoid

sequestrum

sera (*plural of* serum)

serial

serial (*continued*)
    s. dilutional intradermal
      skin test
    s. sections

seroconversion
    s. response

serodiagnosis

seroepidemiology

serologic
    s. data
    s. marker
    s. specificity
    s. test for syphilis (STS)

serology

seronegative
    s. arthropathy
    s. rheumatoid syndrome

seropositive

seroprevalence

seropurulent
    s. discharge

serosanguineous

serositis

serotaxis

serotoninergic

serotonin

serous
    s. discharge
    s. exudation

serovaccination

serovar

serotonin antagonist

serpentine hyperpigmentation

serpiginosa
    elastosis perforans s.
    zona s.

serpiginosum
    angioma s.
    s. angioma

serpiginosus
    lupus s.

serpiginous
    s. ecstatic arterioles
    s. patterns
    s. pustule
    s. ulcer

serpigo

Serratia marcescens

sertraline
    s. HCl
    s. hydrochloride

serum *pl.* serums, sera
    s. albumin
    s. alpha-fetoprotein levels
    s. ascorbic acid level
    s. bilirubin
    blister s.
    s. carcinoembryonic
      antigen
    s. catecholamines
    s. ceruloplasmin
    s. complement (C1-C9)
    s. complement level
    s. free testosterone
    s. hyaluronate
    s. iron
    s. porphyrins
    s. protein electrophoresis
    s. rash
    s. reaction
    s. sickness
    s. sickness reaction
    s. specimen
    s. tyrosine

serumal

serum-fast

sessile base

Sessing pressure ulcer
    assessment scale

seta *pl.* setae

setosa
    trichosis s.

severe
  s. acute allergic reaction
  s. allergic contact
    dermatitis
  s. combined
    immunodeficiency
    disorder (SCID)
  s. dissecting subcutaneous
    hematoma
  s. intracellular edema
  s. outbreaks
  s. scabietic infestation
  s. sunburn

sex
  s. hormone-binding
    globulin
  s.-linked
    agammaglobulinemia
  s.-linked recessive
    condition

sexual
  s. abuse
  s. climax
  s. impotence

sexually transmitted disease
  (STD)

Sézary
  S. cell
  S. erythroderma
  S. reticulosis
  S. syndrome

SGOT
  serum glutamic oxaloacetic
    transaminase

SGPT
  serum glutamic pyruvic
    transaminase

shadow cell

shaft
  hair s.
  naked hair s.

shagreen
  s. nodule

shagreen (*continued*)
  s. patch
  s. plaques
  s. skin

shallow
  s. shave biopsy
  s. ulcers

shampoo
  G-well S.
  Head and Shoulders s.
  Kwell s.
  P&S s.
  Scabene s.
  T/SAL s.
  Zincon s.

sharp
  s. borders
  s. dissection
  s. scissors excision

Sharp's syndrome

sharply
  s. circumscribed nodule
  s. circumscribed patch of
    alopecia
  s. circumscribed swelling
  s. circumscribed ulcer
  s. defined
  s. demarcated
  s. marginated

shave
  s. biopsy
  s. excision
  s. technique

Shaw scalpel

shawl
  s. distribution
  s. pattern

sheath
  s. cell
  cuticle of inner root s.
  fibrous s.
  inner root s.
  outer root s.

sheath (*continued*)
    outer root s.
    periarteriolar lymphoid s.
    root s.

shedding
    virus s.

sheep
    contagious ecthyma
      (pustular dermatitis) virus
      of s.

sheep-pox
    s.-p. virus

sheet
    keratinous s.
    Silk Skin s.

sheeting
    DermaSof s.
    New Beginnings topical gel
      s.

shell
    s. nail
    s. nail syndrome

shellac

Shelley
    S's method
    S's shoreline nails

shellfish

shelter foot

Shigella
    S. dysenteriae
    S. flexneri
    S. flexneri dysenteriae
    S. infection
    S. sonnei

Shigella-Salmonella
    medium

shigellosis

shilling scar

shimamushi disease

shin spot

shiner
    allergic s.

shingles

Shingles Relief Pak

shiny
    s. palms

SHML
    sinus histiocytosis with
      massive lymphadenopathy

shock
    anaphylactic s.

Shope
    S. fibroma
    S. fibroma virus
    S. papilloma
    S. papilloma virus

short
    s. dark hair
    s. duration
    s.-limbed dwarfism
    s. nanosecond pulse
    s. pulsed dye laser
    s. stature

shoulder
    s.-girdle syndrome
    s. pad sign

shrinking

shrunken
    s. appearing nucleus
    s. nuclei

Shulman's syndrome

Shwartzman
    S. phenomenon
    S. reaction

sialidosis

sialomucin

sib ship basal cell carcinoma

Sibine
    S. stimulea
    S. stimulea sting

sicca
cholera s.
keratoconjunctivitis s.
onychia s.
pityriasis s.
seborrhea s.
s. syndrome

siccalike syndrome

sickle
s. cell anemia
s. cell disease (SCD)
s.-shaped calcification

sickness
serum s.
spotted s.

side effect

sideroderma

siderophage

sign
cutaneous s.
Darier's s.
Dennie's s.
dimple s.
Elliot's s.
Gottron's s.
Leser-Trélat s.
Nikolsky's s.
Osler's s.
s. of Leser-Trelat
Pastia's s.
Romaña's s.
Raynaud's s.
Silex s.
Thomson's s.

signal transduction

signet ring lymphoma

Silex
S. sign

silica
s. granuloma

silicon
s. dioxide

silicone
s. gel sheeting
s. granuloma
s. sheeting
s. synovitis

silicosis

Silk Skin sheet

Siloskin dressing

Silvadene

silver
s. acupuncture needle
fused s. nitrate
molded s. nitrate
s. nitrate
s. nitrate crystals
s. oak
s. poisoning
s. sulfadiazine
toughened s. nitrate

silvery
s. scale
s. metallic hair
s.-white papules

Simmond
S's disease
S's syndrome

simple
s. drug
s. excision
s. elliptic excision
s. hypertrophy
s. lentigo
s. nevoid hypertrichosis
s. spongiosis

simplex
acne s.
angioma s.
dermatitis s.
disseminated herpes s.
EB s.
epidermolysis s.
epidermolysis bullosa s.
erythema s.

simplex (*continued*)
    herpes s.
    hidroacanthoma s.
    ichthyosis s.
    lentigo s.
    lichen chronicus s.
    lymphangioma superficium
        s.
    prurigo s.
    purpura s.
    scarlatina s.
    toxoplasmosis, other
        infections, rubella,
        cytomegalovirus infection,
        and herpes s. (TORCH)
    s. variant
    verruca s.

Simuliidae

Simulium

Sinequan

single
    s. hair matrix
    s. radial immunodiffusion
        (SRID)

sinopulmonary infection

sinus
    barber's hair s.
    barber's pilonidal s.
    coccygeal s.
    cutaneous s.
    dental s.
    s. histiocytosis
    s. orifice
    pilonidal s.
    sacrococcygeal s.
    s. tract
    s. unguis

Siphonaptera

Sister Mary Joseph's nodule

situ
    carcinoma in s.
    in s.
    malignant melanoma in s.

sixth
    s. disease
    s. venereal disease

size
    lesion s.

Sjögren
    S's disease
    S's syndrome (SS)
    S.-Larsson syndrome

SJS
    Stevens-Johnson syndrome

skeletal
    s. abnormality
    s. defects
    s. deformities

skin
    alligator s.
    s. atrophy
    s. biopsy
    blistering s.
    bronzed s.
    s. cancer
    citrine s.
    s.-colored
    collodion s.
    combination s.
    crocodile s.
    s. darkening
    deciduous s.
    diamond s.
    s. disease syndrome
    s. dissemination
    dry s.
    elastic s.
    s. elasticity
    s. eruption
    farmers' s.
    Favre-Rocouchot s.
    fish s.
    s. flap
    s. flexors
    s. flora
    s. folds
    s. fragility
    freeze-dried s.

skin (*continued*)
 glabrous s.
 glossy s.
 golfer s.
 golfer's s.
 s. graft
 granulomatous slack s.
 hanging s.
 hidden nail s.
 s. hyperextensibility
 hyperirritable s.
 India-rubber s.
 infantile acute hemorrhagic
   edema of the s.
 involvement of s.
 s. involvement
 islands of s.
 lax s.
 leopard s.
 s. lesion
 s. lipids
 loose s.
 s. lubrication
 s. lubrication therapy
 lymphocytic infiltration of
   the s.
 lyophilized s.
 s. manifestations
 marble s.
 s. metastases of
   melanoma/skin tumors
 s. metastases of tumors of
   internal organs
 s. microfilaria
 mixed tumor of s.
 monoclonal protein of s.
 nail s.
 parchment s.
 s. peel
 s. permeability barrier
 s. perpendicular
 piebald s.
 pig s.
 porcupine s.
 primary macular atrophy of
   s.
 primary neuroendocrine
   carcinoma of the s.

skin (*continued*)
 s. punch
 s. purpura
 s. rash
 s. reaction
 redundant s.
 s. rubor
 sailors' s.
 salt-split s.
 s. scrapings
 senile s.
 shagreen s.
 slack s.
 s. stones
 striate atrophy of s.
 s. tag
 s. tension line
 s. test
 s. testing
 thickened s.
 toad s.
 toasted s.
 s. trephine
 true s.
 s. tumor
 s. turgor
 tylotic s.
 s. type
 s. ulcer
 s. ulceration
 volar s.
 s. wheal
 s. window technique
 s. writing
 yellow s.

skinbound disease

skin-colored
 s.-c. lesion

skin disease
 exudative s. d.
 itching s. d.
 pustular s. d.

skin-puncture test

Skin-So-Soft

SkinTech medical tattooing
 device

Sklowsky symptom

sky-blue
  s.-b. moons
  s.-b. spot

slack skin

slackening

slapped
  "s. cheek" appearance
  "s. cheek" rash
  "s. face" appearance

slate blue discoloration

SLE
  systemic lupus
    erythematosus

Sleep-Eze 3 Oral

Sleepinal

SLE-like syndrome

slimy material

Slo-Niacin

slope shouldered lesion

slough

sloughed off

sloughing
  s. phagedena
  s. ulcer

slow-growing

slug caterpillar

slurry
  talc s.

slush
  carbon dioxide s.

small
  s. cell lymphoma
  s. cell lymphoma cutis
  s. intestinal atonia
  s. plaque parapsoriasis
  s. stature
  s. vessel vasculitis

smallpox
  fulminating s.
  hemorrhagic s.
  malignant s.
  modified s.
  s. vaccine
  s. vaccination
  s. virus
  West Indian s.

smear
  Tzanck s.

smegma

smegmalith

smegmatic

smoker
  s's keratosis
  s's patches

smooth
  s. beam
  s. leprosy
  s. lesion
  s. muscle bundle
  s. muscle cells
  s. muscle hamartoma
  s. shiny depressed scar
  s. skin-colored lesion
  s. stinger

smooth-bottomed

smooth-surfaced

"smudged"

snake
  Arizona coral s.
  s. bite
  copperhead s.
  coral s.
  cottonmouth s.
  eastern coral s.
  pit viper s.
  sea s.
  terrestrial s.
  Texas coral s.
  s. venom
  venomous s.
  water moccasin s.

snakebite

Sneddon
S's syndrome
S.-Wilkinson disease

snow
carbon dioxide s.

soak therapy

soap
Ayndet moisturizing s.
Baby Magic s.
Basis s.
Derma s.
Dermi-Vi s.

SOAP
Subjective, Objective,
Assessment, Plan (*format
for medical reports*)

social
s. nonsexual contact
s. wasp

soda
baking s.
bicarbonate of s.

sodden
s. appearance
s. epidermis
s. patch

sodium
s. antimony gluconate
solution
s. arsenite
s. bicarbonate
s. citrate and citric acid
s. cromoglycate
s. hypochlorite solution
s. hyposulfite
s. nitrate
s. nitroprusside
s. propionate
s. salt
s. silicate
s. stibogluconate
stibogluconate s.

sodium (*continued*)
s. succinate salt
s. sulfacetamide
s. tetradecyl sulfate
s. thiosulfate

sodoku

soft
s. chancre
s. corn
s. epidermal nevus
s. keratin
s. lesion
s. papilloma
s. sore
s. tick
s. tissue
s. tissue calcification
s. tissue hypertrophy
s. tissue mass
s. ulcer
s. wart

softened nails

Softform (Collagen Corporation)
implants

sola (*plural of* solum)

solar
s. cheilitis
s. dermatitis
s. eczema
s. elastosis
s. erythema
s. fever
s. keratosis
s. lentigo
s. purpura
s. urticaria

solare
erythema s.

solaris
s. urticaria
urticaria s.

Solatene

soldier

soldier (*continued*)
    s. ants
    s. patch

sole
    s. dyshidrosis

Solenoglypha

solenonychia

Solenopotes

Solenopsis
    S. geminata
    S. invecta
    S. invecta sting
    S. richteri
    S. richteri sting
    S. saevissima
    S. xyloni

Solganal

solid
    s. carbon dioxide
    s.-cystic basal cell carcinoma
    s. facial edema
    s. hidradenoma
    s. tumor
    s.-tumor marker

solitary
    s. angiokeratoma
    s. ash-leaf macules
    s. basal cell carcinoma
    s. benign cutaneous tumor
    s. clubbing
    s. cutaneous leiomyoma
    s. cutaneous neurofibroma
    s. cylindroma
    s. genital leiomyoma
    s. growth
    s. keratoacanthoma
    s. lytic changes
    s. macule
    s. mastocytoma
    s. nerve sheath tumor
    s. neurofibroma
    s. nodular lesion
    s. nonhereditary form

solitary (*continued*)
    s. palisaded encapsulated neuroma
    s. pigmented lesion
    s. pulmonary metastases
    s. reticulohistiocytoma
    s. simple lymphangioma
    s. skin lesion
    s. trichoepithelioma

soluble
    s. mediator substances
    s. protein antigens

Solu-Cortef

Solu-Medrol
    S. injection

solum *pl.* sola
    s. unguis

Solurex
    S. LA

solution
    aluminum acetate topical s.
    aluminum subacetate topical s.
    Burow's s.
    calcium hydroxide topical s.
    carbolfuchsin topical s.
    crystal violet s.
    Dakin's s.
    ferric subsulfate s.
    gentian violet topical s.
    methoxsalen topical s.
    methylrosaniline chloride s.
    Monsel's s.

solvent-based mascara

somatization

somatostatin

Sominex Oral

somnolence

soot wart

sorbic acid

sorbinil

sorbitol

Sorbsan alginate dressing

sordes

sore
　　bay s.
　　bed s.
　　canker s.
　　chrome s.
　　Cochin s.
　　cold s. (*coldsore*)
　　Delhi s.
　　desert s.
　　diphtheric desert s.
　　fever s.
　　fungating s.
　　Gallipoli s.
　　hard s.
　　mixed s.
　　s. mouth
　　Naga s.
　　Oriental s.
　　pressure s.
　　primary s.
　　septic s.
　　soft s.
　　summer s.
　　s. throat
　　tropical s.
　　Umballa s.
　　veldt s.
　　venereal s.
　　water s.

soreness

sorghum
　　s. grass

Soriatane

South African genetic porphyria

Southern blot test

sowda

spade finger

Spandex

Spanish
　　S. fly
　　S. fly sting
　　S. rapeseed oil

Spanlang-Tappeiner syndrome

sparganosis
　　application s.
　　ingestion s.

sparganum

spark-gap
　　s.-g. generator
　　s.-g. machine

sparse hair

sparsity of the hair

spastic
　　s. diplegia
　　s. paraplegia
　　s. quadriparesis

spatial coherence

special lesion

specialized germinative
　epithelium

specific
　　s. active immunity
　　s. alteration in immunologic
　　　reactivity
　　s. bactericide
　　s. disease
　　s. reaction
　　s. skin lesions in leukemia
　　s. Western blot serologic
　　　test

specificity

speck finger

speckled lentiginous nevus

Spectazole
　　S. topical

spectinomycin hydrochloride

spectrophotometer

spectroscopy

spectrum
    lichen planus s.

Sperling's disease

SPF
    sun protection factor

sphacelation

sphaceloderma

sphenoid
    s. dysplasia

spherical cells

spherocytosis
    hereditary s.

spheroid

spherule

sphingomyelinase D

sphygmomanometer cuff

spicule
    s. of cartilage

spider
    s. angioma
    antivenin, black widow s.
    arterial s.
    s. bite
    black widow s.
    brown recluse s.
    fiddle-back s.
    s. finger
    s. flower
    s. hemangioma
    s. mole
    s. nevus
    s. telangiectasia
    s. telangiectasis
    vascular s.
    s. venom
    violin-back s.

spider-burst

spidery splatters

Spiegler
    S's tumor
    S.-Fendt pseudolymphoma
    S.-Fendt sarcoid

spiloma

spiloplaxia

spilus
    nevus s.

spina
    s. bifida
    s. pedis

spinal
    s. cord tumor
    s. dysraphism

spindle
    s. cell
    s. cell carcinoma
    s. cell
        hemangioendothelioma
    s. cell lipoma
    s. cell nevus
    s. cell proliferation
    s. cell type

spine

spinocellular
    s. carcinoma

spinosa
    ichthyosis s.

spinosum
    stratum s.

spinothalamic tract

spinous
    s. fragments
    s. layer

spinulosa
    trichostasis s.

spinulosus
    lichen s.
    lichen planus seu s.

spiny keratoderma

spiradenitis

spiradenoma
eccrine s.

spiral
Herxheimer's s.

Spirillum
S. bacillus
S. minor
S. minus

Spirochaeta
S. pallida

spirochete
spiral s.

spirochetemia

spirochetes
commensal s.

spirochetosis

spiroma

Spirometra
S. mansonoides

spironolactone

Spiruroidea

Spitz nevus

Splendore-Hoeppli
phenomenon

splenectomy

splenomegaly

splinter hemorrhage

splintering

split
s. ends
s. papule

split-thickness graft

splitting nails

spondylitica
psoriasis s.

spondylitis
psoriatic s.

spondyloarthropathy (SpA)
seronegative s.

sponge
white s. nevus

spongiform
s. pustule
s. pustule of Kogoj

spongiosis
simple s.

spongiotic
s. dermatitis
s. epidermis
s. intraepidermal vesicles
s. vesicles

spontaneous
s. abortion
s. amputation
s. gangrene of newborn
s. hyphema
s. pseudoscar
s. remission
s. repigmentation
s. resolution

spoon
s. nails
s.-shaped nails

sporadic
s. condition
s. mosaic form
s. zoonosis

sporangium

Sporothrix schenckii

sporotrichoid
s. form
s. pattern

sporotrichosis
cutaneous s.
disseminated s.
fixed cutaneous s.
lymphangitic s.

sporotrichosis (*continued*)
    mucocutaneous s.
    visceral s.

sporotrichotic

sporotrichositic chancre

Sporotrichum
    S. schenckii

Sporozoa

sporozoa

sporozoan

Sporozoea

sporozoite

sporozoon

sporozoosis

sporulation

spot
    ash-leaf s.
    blue s.
    café au lait s.
    Campbell-De Morgan s.
    cayenne pepper s.
    cherry s.
    cold s.
    cotton-wool s.
    De Morgan's s.
    Forchheimer s.
    Fordyce's s.
    gift s.
    hot s.
    Koplik s.
    lance-ovate s.
    liver s.
    mongolian s.
    mulberry s.
    orange s.
    pain s.
    pink s.
    rose s.
    Roth's s.
    ruby s.
    sacral s.
    shin s.

spot (*continued*)
    sky-blue s.
    temperature s.
    s. test
    Trousseau s.
    typhoid s.
    warm s.
    s. weld

"spot-cell spot"

spotted
    s. fever
    Rocky Mountain s. fever
    s. sickness

spotted-fever tick

spotty
    s. coloration
    s. mucocutaneous
        pigmentation
    s. skin pigmentation

spreading phenomenon

Sprengel's deformity

sprue

spun-glass hair

SQ
    subcutaneous

squama, squame

squamate

squamatization

squame

squamosum
    eczema s.

squamous
    s. cell
    s. cell carcinoma (SCC)
    s. cell carcinoma in situ
    s. cell carcinoma of the lips
    s. cell carcinoma of the
        penis
    s. cell epithelioma
    s. cell layer
    s. cell lung cancer

squamous (*continued*)
    s. eddies
    s. epithelium
    s. metaplasia
    s. papules

square shouldered lesion

squash bug

squeeze effect

squirrel flea

SRF-A
    slow-reacting factor of
      anaphylaxis

SS
    Sjögren syndrome

SSA/Ro

SSD AF

SSD Cream

SSSS
    staphylococcal scalded skin
      syndrome

St. Anthony's fire

stabilizer

stable
    s. fly
    s. fly bite

stacking
    epidermal s.

stadium
    s. fluorescentiae

stage
    elicitation s.
    eruptive s.
    incubative s.
    induction s.
    s. of invasion
    patch s.
    plaque s.
    primary s.
    tumor s.

stain
    Alcian blue s.
    Brown-Brenn s.
    Giemsa s.
    s. eosinophilic
    Gram s.
    histopathologic s.
    Hotchkiss-McManus s.
    Levaditi's s.
    Masson s.
    silver s.
    Warthin-Starry silver s.
    Wright's s.

staining
    immunoperoxidase s.
    s. of growing teeth

stainless steel wire nail brace

stalk

staphylinid

Staphylinidae

staphylococcal
    s. abscess
    s. impetigo
    s. Lyell's syndrome
    s. scalded skin syndrome
      (SSSS)
    s. scarlatina

Staphylococcus
    S. albus
    S. aureus
    S. epidermidis

staphylococcus
    hemolytic s.

staphyloderma

staphylodermatitis

star
    venus s.

starch

starfish
    s. sting

starfishlike keratoses

starling mite

stasis
    dermatitis s.
    s. dermatitis
    s. eczema
    s. purpura
    s. ulcer
    s. vascular ulcer

state
    anaphylactic s.

static gangrene

Staticin topical

statistics
    National Center for Health
      S. (NCHS)

stature
    brittle hair, intellectual
      impairment, decreased
      fertility, short s. (BIDS)
    photosensitivity, ichthyosis,
      brittle hair, intellectual
      impairment, decreased
      fertility, and short s.
      (PIBIDS)

status dysraphicus

S-T cort

STD
    sexually transmitted
      disease

steatocystoma
    multiplex s.
    s. multiplex
    s. simplex

steatoma

steatomatosis

steatomery

steel-blue nodule

steely hair disease

steep sides

Stein-Leventhal syndrome

Steiner's method

stellate
    s. abscess
    s. bodies
    s. clefts
    s. hair
    s. pseudoscar

stem cell factor

Stemex

stenosis

stenotic auditory canals

Stenotrophomonas maltophilia

Sterapred oral

sterculia

stereopsis

sterigma

sterile
    s. abscess
    s. arthrosteitis
    s. eosinophilic pustulosis
    s. papules
    s. pustule
    s. saline
    s. technique

sterile normal saline solution

sterilize

sterilizer

Steri-Strip

sternoclavicular
    s. hyperostosis
    s. joint

sternocleidomastoid muscle

sternomastoid muscle

sternomanubrial junction

steroid
    s. acne

steroid (*continued*)
    class I s.
    s.-induced osteoporosis
    Psorcon topical s.
    s. sparing
    s.-sparing agent
    s. sulfatase
    s. sulfatase deficiency
    superpotent s.
    topical s.
    s. ulcer

steroidal agent

Stevens
    S.-Johnson disease
    S.-Johnson syndrome
    S.-Johnson-Fuchs syndrome

Stewart
    S.-Treves angiosarcoma
    S.-Treves syndrome

stibium

Sticker's disease

stickiness

stiff skin syndrome

stigmasterol

stigmata of pseudoxanthoma elasticum

stillbirth

Still's disease

stimulation

stimuli

sting
    Africanized honeybee s.
    ant s.
    Apis mellifera s.
    arthropod s.
    ash-gray blister beetle s.
    bark scorpion s.
    bee s.
    blister beetle s.
    blue bottle s.
    Bombus s.

sting (*continued*)
    box jellyfish s.
    brown moth larvae s.
    brown-tail moth s.
    bumblebee s.
    caterpillar s.
    catfish s.
    Centruroides exilicauda s.
    Centruroides sculpturatus s.
    Centruroides vittatus s.
    Chironex fleckeri s.
    coelenterate s.
    common striped scorpion s.
    Dolichorespula s.
    Epicauta fabricii s.
    Epicauta vittata s.
    Euproctis chrysorrhoea s.
    European blister beetle s.
    fire ant s.
    fire coral s.
    gypsy moth larva s.
    honeybee s.
    hornet s.
    Hymenoptera s.
    insect s.
    io moth larva s.
    jellyfish s.
    Lymantria dispar s.
    Lytta vesicata s.
    marine animal s.
    Megabombus s.
    Megalopyge opercularis s.
    millipede s.
    Paederus gemellus s.
    Paederus limnophilus s.
    Paravespula s.
    Polistes s.
    Portuguese man-of-war s.
    puss caterpillar s.
    Pyrobombus s.
    red imported fire ant s.
    saddle back caterpillar s.
    scorpion s.
    sea anemone s.
    sea cucumber s.
    sea urchin s.
    Sibine stimulea s.
    Solenopsis invecta s.

sting (*continued*)
    Solenopsis richteri s.
    Spanish fly s.
    starfish s.
    sting ray s.
    striped blister beetle s.
    Vespula s.
    wasp s.
    yellow jacket s.

stinger
    barbed s.
    imbedded s.
    smooth s.

stinging
    s. caterpillar

stingray
    s. injury

stink bug

stint placement

stippled

STIR
    short tau inversion recovery

stockinette dressing

stocking
    s.-glove distribution
    s. nevus

Stockman nodule

Stokes Gard Outdoor cream

stomatitis *pl.* stomatitides
    angular s.
    s. angularis
    s. aphthosa herpetica
    aphthous s.
    s. candidomycetica
    drug-induced s.
    s. medicamentosa
    s. nicotina
    nicotine s.

Stomoxys bite

stone
    skin s.

stonefish

stone-hard concretions

stone
    skin s's

storage disease

storiform

strabismus

strata (*plural of* stratum)

stratification

stratified
    s. filaments
    s. formations
    s. squamous epithelial wall
    s. squamous epithelium
    s. squamous mucosa

stratum *pl.* strata
    s. basale
    s. basale epidermidis
    s. corneum
    s. corneum epidermidis
    s. corneum unguis
    s. cylindricum
    s. cylindricum epidermidis
    s. germinativum
    s. germinativum
      epidermidis (Malpighii)
    s. germinativum unguis
    s. granulosum
    s. granulosum epidermidis
    s. lucidum
    s. lucidum epidermidis
    malpighian s.
    s. malpighii
    s. membranosum telae
      subcutaneae
    s. membranosum telae
      subcutaneae abdominis
    s. mucosum
    s. papillare corii
    s. papillare cutis
    s. papillare dermidis
    s. reticulare corii
    s. reticulare cutis

stratum (*continued*)
    s. reticulare dermidis
    s. spinosum
    s. spinosum epidermidis
    s. subcutaneum

straw
    s. itch

strawberry
    s. angioma
    s. birthmark
    s. hemangioma
    s. mark
    s. nevus
    s. tongue

streak

streaking
    linear s.

stream
    hair s.

strength
    Clocort Maximum S.
    Cortaid Maximum S.

streptobacillary fever

streptobacilli

Streptobacillus
    S. moniliformis

streptococcal
    Gram A beta-hemolytic s.
        skin infection
    s.-induced impetigo
    s. pharyngitis

streptococci
    microaerophilic beta-
        hemolytic s.

Streptococcus
    S. agalactiae
    S. anginosus
    S. faecalis
    S. infection
    S. iniae
    penicillin-resistant *S.
        pneumoniae* (PRSP)

Streptococcus (*continued*)
    S. pneumoniae
    S. pyogenes
    S. viridans

streptoderma

streptodermatitis

streptogenous impetigo

Streptomyces
    S. somaliensis

streptomycin sulfate

streptozocin

streptozotocin

stretch marks

stretchability

stria *pl.* striae
    s. alba
    s. albicans
    s. albicantes
    s. atrophicae
    s. cutis distensae
    s. distensae
    s. gravidarum
    elastotic s.
    s. rubra
    Wickham's s.

strialike

striata
    dermatitis pratensis s.
    melanonychia s.

striatal

striate
    s. atrophy of skin
    s. keratoderma

striated
    s. beaded lines
    s. muscles
    s. xanthomas

striatum
    atrophoderma s.

striatus
    lichen s.

stridor

striped
    s. appearance
    s. blister beetle
    s. blister beetle sting

stroma

stromal
    s. invasion
    s. spindle cell

Strongyloides stercoralis

strongyloidiasis
    cutaneous s.
    systemic s.

strophulosus
    lichen s.

strophulus
    s. adultorum
    s. candidus
    s. infantum
    s. intertinctus
    s. pruriginosus

structural
    s. outline
    s. units

structure
    hairlike s.
    pilosebaceous s.

Strümpell-Westphal
    pseudosclerosis

STS
    serologic test for syphilis

stucco keratosis

stunted growth

stupe

Sturge
    S. disease
    S. syndrome
    S.-Weber disease

Sturge (*continued*)
    S.-Weber
        encephalotrigeminal
        angiomatosis
    S.-Weber syndrome

stye

stylet

styptic solution

styptics

Styrax

SU
    solar urticaria

subacuta
    prurigo simplex s.

subacute
    s. bacterial endocarditis
    s. cutaneous lupus
        erythematosus (SCLE)
    s. dermatitis
    s. lupus erythematosus
    s. prurigo

subarachnoid space

subbasal lamina

subchondral
    s. cyst

subclavian
    s. atherosclerosis
    s. vein occlusion

subclinical
    s. genital herpes
    s. outbreak

subconjunctival hemorrhage

subcorneal
    s. blister
    s. pustular dermatitis
    s. pustular dermatosis
    s. vesicopustule
    s. vesiculation

subcutanea
    lipogranulomatosis s.

subcutanea (*continued*)
  urticaria s.

subcutaneous (sc, SQ)
  s. calcification
  s. capillaries
  s. fat
  s. fat cells
  s. fat necrosis
  s. fat necrosis of the
    newborn
  s. fungal infection
  s. granuloma annulare
  s. granulomatous nodule
  s. hemorrhage
  s. injection
  s. leiomyosarcoma
  s. morphea
  s. mycosis
  s. myiasis
  s. necrotizing infection
  s. neurofibroma
  s. nodule
  s. phycomycosis
  s. plexiform neurofibromas
  s. rheumatoid nodule
  s. sclerosis
  s. swelling
  s. T-cell lymphoma
  s. tissue
  s. vessels

subcuticular

subcutis

subdermic

subendothelial hyaline deposit

subependymal nodules

subepidermal
  s. abscess
  s. blister
  s. bulla
  s. calcified nodule
  s. fibrotic plaque
  s. nodular fibrosis
  s. papillae
  s. space

subepidermal (*continued*)
  s. vesicle formation
  s. vesicular dermatosis
  s. vesiculation
  s. zone

subepidermic

subepithelia

subepithelial

subepithelium

subfascial muscle

subinfection

subintegumental

subitum
  exanthema s.

subjective symptoms

sublamina
  s. densa
  s. densa deposits

subluxation

submammary
  s. folds
  s. region

submental region

submucosal
  s. plaque

submucous fibrosis

suboptimal absorption

subpapillary
  s. layer
  s. plexus
  s. vessels

subpapular

subperiosteal hemorrhage

substance
  onychogenic s.
  s. P

subtegumental

subtropical

subtype

subungual
  s. abscess
  s. exostosis
  s. hematoma
  s. hemorrhage
  s. hyperkeratosis
  s. isoproterenol
    hydrochloride
  s. keratin
  s. keratosis
  s. hyperkeratosis
  s. hyperpigmentation
  s. melanoma
  s. papules
  s. splinter hemorrhages
  s. squamous cell carcinoma
  s. traumatic hematoma
  s. wart

subungualis
  hyperkeratosis s.

succinic semialdehyde
  dehydrogenase deficiency

succulence

Sucquet
  S.-Hoyer anastomosis
  S.-Hoyer canal

sucralfate

sucrose

sudamen

Sudamina

sudaminal

sudation

sudden death

Sudeck's syndrome

sudogram

sudomotor

sudor

sudor (*continued*)
  s. sanguineus
  s. urinosus

sudoral

sudoresis

sudoriferous
  s. hemangioma
  nevus s.

sudorific

sudorikeratosis

sudoriparous
  s. abscess
  s. angioma

sudorometer

sudorrhea

suffodiens
  folliculitis abscedens et s.
  folliculitis et perifolliculitis
    abscedens et s.
  perifolliculitis abscedens et
    s.
  perifolliculitis capitis
    abscedens et s.

suggillation

suid herpesvirus

sulcatum
  keratoderma plantare s.
  keratolysis plantare s.
  keratoma plantare s.

sulciform

sulconazole
  s. nitrate

Sulcosyn Topical

sulcus *pl.* sulci
  s. cutis
  s. matrices unguis
  s. of matrix of nail
  s. of skin

Sulfacet-R topical

sulfadiazine
    s. cream
    silver s.
    s., sulfamethazine, and
      sulfamerazine

sulfadoxine and pyrimethamine

Sulfamethoprim

sulfamethoxazole
    s./trimethoprim

Sulfamylon topical

sulfapyridine

sulfasalazine

sulfated acid
    mucopolysaccharide
    chondroitin sulfate

Sulfatrim
    S. DS

sulfisoxazole
    erythromycin and s.
    s. and phenazopyridine

sulfites

sulfonamide

sulfone

sulfonylurea
    s. antidiabetic medication
    s. diuretics

sulfhydrates

sulfhydryl

sulfisoxazole

sulfonamide
    s. hypersensitivity reaction

sulfone therapy

Sulfoxyl
    S. Regular lotion

sulfur
    s. flakes
    s. granules
    s. mustard gas

sulfur (*continued*)
    precipitated s.
    s. and salicylic acid
    s. and sodium
      sulfacetamide
    sublimed s.

Sulfur Soap bar

sulfureum
    Trichophyton tonsurans var.
      s.

sulfuryl fluoride

Sulzberger
    S.-Bloch syndrome
    S.-Garbe disease
    S.-Garbe syndrome

sumac, sumach
    poison s.
    swamp s.

summer
    s. acne
    s. eruption
    s. itch
    s. prurigo
    s. rash
    s. sore

Sumycin Oral

sun
    s. and chemical
      combination damage
    s. exposure
    s. precautions
    s. protection factor
    (SPF)

sunburn
    s. reactivation

sunburnlike
    s. rash
    s. reaction

sun-exposed surfaces

sun-induced
    s.-i. DNA damage
    s.-i. skin cancer

sunscreen
    chemical s.
    physical s.

sunscreening action

superabsorbent gel

superantigen

superficial
    s. angioma
    s. bacterial infection
    s. basal cell carcinoma
    s. basal cell epithelioma
    s. blood vessels
    s. burn
    s. capillaries
    s. channels
    s. corium
    s. dermis
    s. exfoliation
    s. fascia
    s. follicular pyoderma
    s. fungous infection
    s. granulomatous pyoderma
    s. hemangioma
    s. infection
    s. inflammatory dermatosis
    s. inflammatory process
    s. liquid nitrogen
        application
    s. lymphatic malformation
    s. malignant melanoma
    s. molting
    s. multicentric basal cell
        carcinoma
    s. papillary adenomatosis
    s. papular lesion
    s. perivascular lymphocytic
        infiltrate
    s. punctate keratitis
    s. pustular folliculitis
    s. pustular perifolliculitis
    s. pyoderma
    s. shave biopsy
    s. spreading melanoma
        (SSM)
    s. thrombophlebitis
    s. ulceration

superficial (*continued*)
    s. vascular plexus
    s. varicosities
    s. vein thrombosis
    s. venules
    s. wounds

superficialis
    lupus s.

superfluous hair

superinduce

superinfection

superior
    s. auricular fold
    s. cosmesis
    s. vena cava

supernatant

supernumerary
    s. breasts
    s. digits
    s. nipple
    s. ribs
    s. structures

superpigmentation

support hose

supportive therapy

suppository
    Anucort-HC s.
    Anuprep HC s.
    Anusol-HC s.
    Truphylline s.

suppuration

suppurativa
    s. folliculitis
    genital hidradenitis s.
    s. hidradenitis

suppurative/granulomatous
    bacterial infection

suppression

suppressive therapy

suppressor cell

suppuration
s. of the bubo

suppurativa
genital hidradenitis s.
hidradenitis s.

suppurative
s. dermatitis
s. synovitis

suprabasal
s. bullae
s. cleft lacuna
s. clefting

suprabasalar
s. acantholysis

suprabasilar

supraorbital ridges

suprapapillary plate

suprarenal insufficiency

suprasternal notch

supraventricular tachycardia

Sure-Closure skin stretching
system

surface
s. active agents
dorsal s.
s. epidermis
extensor s.
flexor s.
s. irritation

surfactant

surfer's nodule

surgery
acne s.
laser s.
Mohs' micrographic s.
wire-brush s.

surgical
s. ablation

surgical (*continued*)
s. cutting current
s. drainage
s. erysipelas
s. excision
s. extirpation
s. margin
s. scarring
s. therapy
s. treatment

surrounding macular erythema

sursanure

suspension

sutilains

Sutton
S's disease
S's major aphthous ulcer
S's nevus
S's ulcer
S.-Rendu-Osler-Weber
syndrome

suture (*material*)
Ethilon s.
Vicryl s.

suture (*technique*)
s. puncture site

swamp
s. fever
s. fever virus
s. itch

swan-neck deformity

swarming

sweat
s. bee
bloody s.
blue s.
fetid s.
s. gland
s. gland carcinoma
s. gland epithelium
s. gland nevus
green s.

sweat (*continued*)
  insensitive s.
  phosphorescent s.
  red s.

sweating
  excessive s.

sweat-inhibiting property

sweat-retention syndrome

sweaty feet syndrome

Sweet
  S.-like reaction
  S's syndrome

swelling
  boggy s.
  joint s.
  nodules, eosinophilia, rheumatism, dermatitis, and s. (NERDS)

Swift's disease

swimmer's
  s. dermatitis
  s. itch

swimming pool granuloma

swine
  s. vesicular disease

swinepox
  s. virus

Swiss
  S. cheese appearance
  S.-type thymic dysplasia

sycoma

sycosiform
  s. fungous infection
  s. tinea barbae

sycosiforme
  ulerythema s.

sycosis
  bacillogenic s.
  s. barbae
  coccogenic s.

sycosis (*continued*)
  s. contagiosa
  s. framboesia
  s. framboesiformis
  herpetic s.
  hyphomycotic s.
  lupoid s.
  s. lupoides
  nonparasitic s.
  s. nuchae
  s. nuchae necrotisans
  parasitic s.
  s. staphylogenes
  tinea s.
  s. vulgaris

symbiotic
  s. organism

symblepharon

Symmers
  S. disease

Symmetrel

symmetrica
  erythrokeratodermia progressive s.
  keratodermia s.

symmetrical
  s. dermatosis
  s. dyschromatosis
  s. gangrene
  s. pallor
  s. peripheral gangrene
  s. polyarthritis-like rheumatoid arthritis
  s. sympathetic punctate leukonychia
  s. vermiform facial atrophy of childhood
  s. vesicular hand dermatitis

sympathectomy

sympathetic
  s. denervation
  s. trunk

symptom

symptom (*continued*)
    classic allergy s.
    frequency of allergy s.
    gastrointestinal s.
    severity of allergy s.
    Sklowsky s.
    Wartenberg s.

symptomatic
    s. erythema
    s. fever
    s. lymphedema
    s. porphyria
    s. pruritus
    s. pulmonary disease
    s. reaction
    s. relief
    s. therapy
    s. treatment
    s. ulcer
    s. visceral involvement

symptomatica
    alopecia s.
    livedo reticularis s.
    purpura s.

Synacort

Synalar
    S.-HP topical
    S. topical

synanthem

synchronous behavior

synchrony

syncope

syndactylia

syndactyly

syndet
    synthetic detergent

syndroma mucocutaneo-
    oculare Fuchs

syndrome
    acquired immune
      deficiency s. (AIDS)

syndrome (*continued*)
    acquired
      immunodeficiency s.
      (AIDS)
    Albright's s.
    Albright-McCune-Sternberg
      s.
    Alezzandrini's s.
    angioedema-urticaria-
      eosinophilia s.
    angry back s.
    ataxia-telangiectasia s.
    atypical mole s.
    autoerythrocyte
      sensitization s.
    BADS s.
    Bäfverstedt's s.
    Bart's s.
    basal cell nevus s.
    Bazex' s.
    blue rubber bleb nevus s.
    Bourneville-Pringle s.
    brittle nail s.
    brown spot s.
    Brunsting's s.
    Buschke-Ollendorff s.
    bypass arthritis-dermatitis s.
    calcinosis cutis, Raynaud
      phenomenon, esophageal
      motility disorder,
      sclerodactyly,
      telangiectasia s.
    Canada-Cronkhite s.
    CHILD s.
    craniocarpotarsal syndrome
    CREST s.
    Cronkhite-Canada s.
    CRST s.
    Danlos s.
    Degos' s.
    dysplastic nevus s.
    ectrodactyly-ectodermal
      dysplasia-clefting s.
    EEC s.
    Ehlers-Danlos s.
    erythrocyte
      autosensitization s.
    Favre-Racouchot s.

syndrome (*continued*)
  Felty's s.
  Feuerstein-Mims s.
  Fèvre-Languepin s.
  Fiessinger-Leroy-Reiter s.
  Forsius-Eriksson s.
  Gardner-Diamond s.
  Gianotti-Crosti s.
  Goltz' s.
  Goltz-Gorlin s.
  Gorlin's s.
  Gorlin-Goltz s.
  Gougerot-Blum s.
  Gougerot-Carteaud s.
  Graham Little s.
  Grönblad-Strandberg s.
  hand-foot-and-mouth s.
  Hartnup s.
  Henoch-Schönlein s.
  hereditary flat adenoma s.
  Hermansky-Pudlak s.
  Howel-Evans' s.
  intestinal
    polyposis–cutaneous
    pigmentation s.
  Jadassohn-Lewandowski s.
  Kasabach-Merritt s.
  keratitis-ichthyosis-deafness
    (KID) s.
  Klippel-Trénaunay s.
  Klippel-Trénaunay-Weber s.
  LEOPARD s.
  linear sebaceous nevus s.
  Löfgren's s.
  Louis-Bar's s.
  Lyell's s.
  Mauriac s.
  Melkersson's s.
  Melkersson-Rosenthal s.
  multiple lentigines s.
  Nelson's s.
  Netherton's s.
  nevoid basal cell carcinoma
    s.
  nevoid basalioma s.
  nonstaphylococcal scalded
    skin s.
  s. of immediate reactions

syndrome (*continued*)
  painful bruising s.
  Profichet's s.
  Riley-Smith s.
  Rothmann-Makai s.
  Rothmund-Thomson s.
  Rud's s.
  Schäfer's s.
  Schönlein-Henoch s.
  Senear-Usher s.
  Senter s.
  Sézary s.
  Sjögren s.
  Sjögren-Larsson s.
  Sneddon's s.
  spun glass hair s.
  staphylococcal scalded skin
    s.
  Stevens-Johnson s.
  Sulzberger-Garbe s.
  sweat retention s.
  Sweet's s.
  Touraine-Solente-Golé s.
  uncombable hair s.
  unilateral nevoid
    telangiectasia s.
  Unna-Thost s.
  Vohwinkel's s.
  Waterhouse-Friderichsen s.
  Weber-Christian s.
  Weber-Cockayne s.
  Weil's s.
  Weill-Marchesani s.
  Werner's s.
  Woringer-Kolopp s.
  yellow nail s.
  Zinsser-Cole-Engman s.

syndromic

synechia

Synemol
  S. topical

synergism

synergistic
  s. gangrene
  s. role

synergistic (*continued*)
  s. toxicity

syngeneic
  s./autologous GVHD
  s. graft

syngenesioplasty

syngenesiotransplantation

syngenic

syngraft

synophridia

synophrys

synostosis

synovial
  s. cyst
  s. hemangioma
  s. lipoma

synovitis
  nodular s.
  pigmented villonodular s.
    (PVNS)
  proliferative s.
  reactive postinfectious s.
  villonodular s.

synthesis
  genes directing s.
  protein s.
  vitamin D s.

synthetic
  s. chemicals
  s. detergent (syndet)
  s. phase
  s. resin dermatitis
  s. retinoid therapy

syphilid
  acneform s.
  acuminate papular s.
  annular s.
  bullous s.
  corymbose s.
  ecthymatous s.
  erythematous s.

syphilid (*continued*)
  flat papular s.
  follicular s.
  frambesiform s.
  gummatous s.
  impetiginous s.
  lenticular s.
  lichenoid s.
  macular s.
  maculopapular s.
  miliary papular s.
  nodular s.
  nummular s.
  palmar s.
  papular s.
  papulosquamous s.
  pemphigoid s.
  pigmentary s.
  plantar s.
  pustular s.
  rupial s.
  secondary s.
  tertiary s.
  varioliform s.

syphilide

syphilis
  Captia test for s.
  s. chancre
  congenital s.
  s. connata
  cutaneous s.
  s. d'emblée
  early latent s.
  endemic s.
  gumma of tertiary s.
  s. hereditaria tarda
  inflammatory late
    congenital s.
  late s.
  late benign s.
  late latent s.
  late osseous s.
  latent s.
  nonvenereal s.
  primary s.
  quaternary s.
  relapsing secondary s.

syphilis (*continued*)
    secondary s.
    serologic test for s. (STS)
    tertiary s.

syphilitic
    s. alopecia
    s. chancre
    s. dactylitis
    s. fever
    s. gumma
    s. leukoderma
    s. roseola
    s. rupia
    s. ulcer

syphilitica
    acne s.
    alopecia s.

syphiliticum
    tuberculum s.

syphiliticus
    lichen s.

syphiloderm

syphilologist

syphilology

syphiloma of Fournier

syphilomatous

syphilophobia

syringoacanthoma

syringoadenoma
    s. papilliferum

syringocarcinoma

syringocystadenoma
    s. papilliferum

syringocystoma

syringoma
    chondroid s.
    disseminated s.

syringomyelia

syringosquamous metaplasia

system
    antibody assay s.
    CD designation s.
    dermal s.
    dermoid s.
    feedback control s.
    humoral and cell-mediated
      immune s.
    integumentary s.
    keratinizing s.
    malpighian s.
    melanocyte s.
    mononuclear phagocyte s.
      (MPS)
    pigmentary s.

systematized
    s. nevus
    s. type

systemic
    s. amyloidosis
    s. anaphylaxis
    s. argyria
    s. candidiasis
    s. chemotherapy
    s. corticosteroid
    s. disease
    s. floxins
    s. fungal infection
    s. granulomatous disease
    s. lupus erythematosus
      (SLE)
    s. mast cell disease
    s. mastocytosis
    s. mycobacterial infection
    s. plaques
    s. PUVA
    s. reaction
    s. retinoids
    s. retinoid therapy
    s. sarcoidosis
    s. scleroderma
    s. sclerosis
    s. steroidal agent
    s. steroid
    s. therapy
    s. toxicity
    s. vasculitis

T

T
  T cell
  T Gamma/Delta cells
  T helper cell (Th)
  T helper cell type 2 (Th2)
  T lymphocyte
  T piece
  T zone
  T zone complexion

Tabanidae

tabes dorsalis

tabetic

Tablet
  Kenacort T.

TAC
  triamcinolone cream

Tac-3

tache
  t. bleuâtre
  t. cérébrale
  t. méningéale
  t. noire
  t's noire sclérotiques
  t. spinale

tachetic

tachyphylaxis

tacrolimus (Topical FK506)

tactile cell of Merkel-Ranvier

TAD
  transient acantholytic
    dermatosis

Taenia solium

Taenzer
  T. disease

tag
  auricular t.
  cutaneous t.
  sentinel t.
  skin t.

Tagamet
  T. HB

Takahara's disease

Takayasu
  T's arteritis
  T's disease
  T's syndrome

TAL
  triamcinolone lotion

talc

talcum powder

talon
  t. noir

tamoxifen

tan

tangentiality

Tangier disease

tannate

tanner's ulcer

tannin

tanning
  t. bed
  delayed t.
  immediate t.
  t. lamps

TAO
  triamcinolone
    ointment

tape
  Cath-Secure t.
  ColorZone t.
  Cordran t.
  Dermicel t.
  Micropore t.
  Scanpor t.

TAR syndrome

tar
- t. acne
- birch t.
- coal t.
- t. cream
- juniper t.
- t. keratosis
- t. melanosis
- t. oil
- ointment of t.
- pine t.
- t. shampoo

tarantula
- American t.
- black t.
- European t.

tarda
- porphyria cutanea t. (PCT)
- syphilis hereditaria t.

Tardieu petechia

tardus
- nevus t.

target
- antigenic t.
- t. lesion

targetoid
- t. hemosiderotic hemangioma
- t. lesion
- t. purpuric lesion

Targretin

tartrate

tartrazine

tattoo
- amalgam t.
- eyeline t.
- oral t.

tattooing
- accidental t.
- t. effect
- intentional t.

taut
- t. skin

tautologic

Tavist
- T.-1

taxonomy

Tay's syndrome

Taylor's disease

tazarotene

Tazicef

Tazidime

Tazorac

TCA
- trichloroacetic acid

T cell (*noun*)

T-cell (*adjective*)
- T-c. activation
- T-c. antigen receptor
- T-c. erythroderma
- T-c. factors
- T-c. growth factor
- T-c. helper function
- T-c. immunoblastic lymphoma
- T-c. immunodeficiencies
- T-c. independent antigens
- T-c. infiltrate
- T-c. interaction
- T-c. lymphoma
- T-c. mediated delayed type hypersensitivity dermatitis
- T-c. phenotype
- T-c. proliferation
- T-c. pseudolymphoma
- T-c. receptor CD3
- T-c. receptor clonal rearrangement
- T-c. receptor gene
- T-c. receptor gene rearrangement
- T-c. suppressor function

TCR
- T-cell (antigen) receptor

T/Derm
    Neutrogena T.

te sudor abest

teardrop-shaped vesicle

tearlessness

Techni-Care surgical scrub

technique
    aseptic t.
    Blenderm patch t.
    ELISA t.
    Mohs' t.
    Mohs' fresh-tissue t.
    t. of Shelley
    periodic acid–Schiff t.
    shave t.
    skin window t.

Tegaderm semipermeable
  dressing

Tegison

Tegrin
    Advanced Formula T.
    T. for Psoriasis cream
    T.-HC
    T.-LT shampoo/conditioner
    T. Medicated gel shampoo
    T. Medicated Extra
      Conditioning

tegument

tela *pl.* telae
    t. subcutanea
    t. subcutanea abdominis
    t. submucosa

Telachlor Oral

Teladar

telangiectases (*plural of*
  telangiectasis)

telangiectasia
    ataxia t.
    calcinosis cutis, Raynaud
      phenomenon, esophageal
      motility disorder,
      sclerodactyly, t. (CREST)

telangiectasia (*continued*)
    cephalo-oculocutaneous t.
    dermatomal superficial t.
    essential t.
    generalized t.
    hemorrhagic t.
    hereditary hemorrhagic t.
    t. macularis eruptive
      perstans (TMEP)
    nevoid t.
    periungual t.
    primary t.
    secondary t.
    spider t.
    threadlike t.
    unilateral dermatomal
      superficial t.
    unilateral nevoid t.
    t. verrucosa
    oculocutaneous t's

telangiectasis *pl.* telangiectases
    hereditary hemorrhagic t.
    linear t's
    multiple hereditary
      hemorrhagic t.
    spider t.
    stellate t.
    tortuous t.

telangiectatic
    t. erythema
    t. lipoma
    t. wart

telangiectatica
    livedo t.

telangiectaticum
    granuloma t.

telangiectodes
    elephantiasis t.
    purpura annularis t.

telar

Teldrin oral

teleological

teleology

teletactor

Teline Oral

telogen
 t. effluvium
 t. effluvium diffuse hair loss
 t. follicle
 t. hair
 t. phase

telomere
 t. length monitoring

Temaril

Temovate
 T. ointment
 T. topical

temperature-dependent dermatosis

temperature-sensitive
 t.-s. oculocutaneous albinism

template

Templeton's skin tags

temporal
 t. arteritis
 t. artery biopsy
 t. balding
 t. canthus
 t. coherence
 t. scalp

temporomandibular pain

temporo-occipital fringe

temporoparietal hairline

TEN
 toxic-epidermal necrolysis

tendinosum
 xanthoma t.

tendinous xanthoma

tendon
 Achilles t.
 t. xanthoma

teniposide

Tenormin

tenosynovectomy

tenosynovitis
 de Quervain t.
 stenosing t.

tenotomy scissors

TENS
 transcutaneous electrical nerve stimulation

tensile strength

tension vesicles of bullae

tentacles

tentorium
 t. cerebelli
 t. of cerebellum

teratogen

teratogenesis

teratogenetic effect

teratogenicity

teratogenous

teratogeny

teratoma
 benign cystic t.
 cystic t.
 mature t.

terbinafine
 t. hydrochloride

terbutaline
 t. sulfate

terebrans

terfenadine
 t. and pseudoephedrine

terminal
 t. arteriole
 t. follicle
 t. hair

terminal (*continued*)
    t. hematuria
    t. hemorrhagic diathesis
    t. ileitis
    t. phalangeal tufts
    t. phalanges

terpene

Terra-Cortril
    T. Ophthalmic suspension

Terramycin
    T. IM injection
    T. ophthalmic ointment
    T. oral
    T. with Polymyxin B
        ophthalmic ointment

terrestrial snake

Terry
    T.-like nails
    T's nail

tertiary
    t. lues
    t. syphilid
    t. syphilis

test
    ACADERM patch t.
    adhesion t.
    alkali patch t.
    antibiotic sensitivity t.
    bacterial agglutination t.
    basophil degranulation t.
    Candida skin t.
    coccidioidin skin t.
    Casoni intradermal t.
    Casoni skin t.
    chrome patch t.
    closed patch t.
    complement fixation t.
    CSD skin t.
    cutaneous t.
    diagnostic t.
    Draize t.
    Draize Repeat Insult patch
        t.
    epicutaneous t.

test (*continued*)
    false-negative patch t.
    false-positive patch t.
    false-positive syphilis t.
    Frei t.
    Hanger t.
    immunofluorescence t.
    insulin skin t.
    intradermal skin t.
    Ito-Reenstierna t.
    Jadassohn-Bloch t.
    Keller ultraviolet t.
    Kolmer t.
    Kveim t.
    leishmanin t.
    lepromin t.
    Mecholyl skin t.
    midpoint skin t.
    Mitsuda t.
    negative patch t.
    nontreponemal t.
    nontreponemal antigen t.
    occlusive patch t.
    open patch t.
    patch t.
    photo-patch t.
    PPL skin t.
    predictive patch t.
    prick t.
    prick-prick t.
    prick puncture t.
    Rose t.
    scarification t.
    Scotch Tape t.
    scratch t.
    skin t.
    skin-puncture t.
    T.R.U.E. T.
    T.R.U.E. allergy patch t.
    tuberculin skin t.
    Tzanck t.

testicular
    t. cancer
    t. hypoplasia

testing
    epidermal t.
    mouse foot pad t.

test (*continued*)
    patch t.
    prick t.
    scratch t.
    skin t.

Testoderm patch

testosterone

tetanus
    t. prophylaxis

tetracaine
    t. hydrochloride
    t. with dextrose

Tetracap oral

tetracycline (TCN, TET)
    t. resistance

tetrad
    acne t.

Tetralan oral

Tetram oral

tetter
    branny t.
    brawny t.
    crusted t.
    dry t.
    honeycomb t.
    humid t.
    milk t.
    moist t.
    scaly t.
    wet t.

Texier's disease

texture

textus

T/Gel

TGM
    transglutaminase

Th
    T helper cell

thalassemia
    t. major

thalidomide

thallium poisoning

Thallophyta

Thaumetopoea processionea

thawing fluids

thecal cell tumor

thelerethism

thelium *pl.* thelia

thenar eminence

theophylline

thèque

therapeutic
    t. agents
    t. modality

Theraplex Z

therapy
    antibacterial t.
    antifungal t.
    antipruritic t.
    arsenic t.
    beam t.
    constant t.
    dressing t.
    grenz ray t.
    hormone t.
    hyperbaric oxygen t.
    intermittent t.
    light t.
    medical t.
    photodynamic t.
    PUVA (psoralens and ultraviolet A) t.
    radiation t.
    skin lubrication t.
    soak t.
    surgical t.
    symptomatic t.
    systemic antibacterial t.
    systemic antifungal t.
    topical t.
    topical antibacterial t.
    topical antifungal t.

thermal
- t. anhidrosis
- t. barrier
- t. burn
- t. damage
- t. elastosis
- t. flushing
- t. injury

Thermazene

thermocouple

thermodynamics

thermogenic

thermographic

thermography

thermolysis

thermometer

thermoregulation

thermoregulatory system

Theroxide wash

thesaurismosis

thesaurosis

THH
- targetoid hemosiderotic hemangioma

thiabendazole

thiamine deficiency

thiazide
- t. diuretic

Thibierge-Weissenbach syndrome

thick
- t. and sticky mucus
- t. tongue

thickened
- t. granular layer
- t. scapula
- t. nails
- t. skin

thickener

thickening
- disciform t.
- t. of nails
- scleroderma-like skin t.

thickness

Thibierge-Weissenbach syndrome

thimerosal

thin
- t. brittle fingernails
- t. platinum tips

thinning

thin-walled vessel

thiocarbamide

thioflavine

thioglycolate
- ammonium t.
- calcium t.

thioguanine

thiol

thioridazine

thiourea
- t. compound

third
- t. degree burn
- t. disease

thiuram

Thompson
- T's dermatoplasty
- T's syndrome

Thomson
- T's disease
- T's poikiloderma congenitale
- T's scattering
- T's sign

Thor-lo

thoracic
t. nerves
t. sympathetic ganglion
t. zoster

thoracocentesis

Thorazine

thorns

threadlike telangiectasia

three-day measles

threshold
erythema t.
low t.

thrix
t. annulata

throat culture

thromboangiitis
t. cutaneointestinalis
disseminata
t. obliterans

thrombocythemia

thrombocytopenia
autoimmune t. (AITP)
autoimmune neonatal t.
drug-induced t.
familial t.
immune t.
isoimmune neonatal t.
sepsis-induced t.

thrombocytopenic
t. hemangiomatosis
t. purpura

thromboembolia

thromboembolism

thrombosis

thrombotic
t. gangrene
t. occlusion
t. phase
t. thrombocytopenic
purpura (TTP)

thrush
oral t.

Thuja

thuja

thumb sucking

Thygeson's disease

thylacitis

thymectomy

thymic
t. cyst
t. dysplasia
t. hypoplasia
t. medulla

thymion

thymol

thymoma

thymopentin

thymus

thyroglossal
t. cyst
t. duct cyst

thyroid
t. acropachy
t. adenocarcinoma
t. carcinoma
t. follicles
t. goiter

thyroiditis
Hashimoto t.

thyroiditis, Addison disease,
Sjögren syndrome,
sarcoidosis syndrome (TASS
syndrome)

thyrotoxicosis

tic douloureux

tick
t. bite
t. bite alopecia

tick (*continued*)
    t. bite pyrexia
    black-legged t.
    California black-legged t.
    deer t.
    dog t.
    t. fever
    hard t.
    Ixodes dammini t.
    Ixodes pacificus t.
    Ixodes ricinus wood t.
    ixodid t.
    Lone Star t.
    Pacific t.
    t. paralysis
    t. pyrexia
    Rocky Mountain t.
    seed t.
    soft t.
    spotted-fever t.
    western black-legged t.
    wood t.

tickborne
    t. disease
    t. encephalitis (Central
        European subtype)
    t. encephalitis (Eastern
        subtype)
    t. encephalitis virus
    t. relapsing fever
    t. spirochete
    t. virus

ticklishness

ticlopidine
    t. HCl

Tietze's syndrome

tigertail appearance

TILS
    tumor-infiltrating
        lymphocyte

tin ethyl etiopurpurin

Tinactin powder

TinBen

TinCoBen

tinctorial change

tincture
    compound benzoin t.
    Fungoid t.
    t. of benzoin
    t. of cantharidin
    t. of cinchona

tinea
    t. amiantacea
    asbestoslike t.
    t. axillaris
    t. barbae
    t. barbae profunda
    black-dot t. capitis
    t. capitis
    t. capitis profunda
    t. ciliorum
    t. circinata
    t. circinata tropical
    t. colli
    t. corporis
    t. cruris
    t. decalvans
    t. dermatitis
    t. faciale
    t. faciei
    t. favosa
    t. flava
    t. furfuracea
    t. glabrosa
    t. imbricata
    t. incognito
    t. inguinalis
    t. kerion
    t. manus
    t. manuum
    t. nigra
    t. nodosa
    t. pedis
    t. pedis et manus
    t. profunda
    t. sycosis
    t. tarsi
    t. tonsurans
    t. trichophytica

tinea (*continued*)
    t. tropicalis
    t. unguium
    t. versicolor

tinted
    Oxy-5 T.

Tinver
    T. lotion

Ti-Screen

Tisit

tissue
    t. ablation
    t. breakdown
    t. culture
    cyst-bearing t.
    t. damage
    dartoic t.
    dartoid t.
    t. debris
    distensible t.
    t. expander
    granulation t.
    t. hydration
    necrotic t.
    t. repair
    scar t.
    t. section
    soft t.
    t.-sparing technique
    subcutaneous t.
    subcutaneous fatty t.

titanium
    t. oxide
    t. hydrochloride

TMEP
    telangiectasia macularis
        eruptive perstans

TMP
    trimethyl psoralen

TMP-SMX
    trimethoprim-
        sulfamethoxazole

TNF

TNF (*continued*)
    tumor necrosis factor

TNMB system
    involvement of the skin (T),
        the lymph node (N), the
        viscera (M), and the
        peripheral blood (B)

TNM
    tumor, node, metastasis

toadskin
    "toasted skin" syndrome

tobacco smoke tar

tobramycin
    t. and dexamethasone

toe
    black t.
    hammer t.
    Hong Kong t.
    t. itch
    mallet t.
    sausage t.
    tennis t.
    t. tips

toenail
    t. disorder
    t. dysplasia
    ingrowing t.
    ingrown t.

toeweb

Togaviridae

togavirus

Tokelau ringworm

tolazoline HCl

tolnaftate
    t. powder
    t. solution

toluene
    t. sulfonamide

toluidine blue O

tomato

tomato (*continued*)
    t. tumor

tongue
    black hairy t.
    t. blade
    burning t.
    t. carcinoma
    coated t.
    fissured t.
    furrowed t.
    geographic t.
    glossy t.
    hobnail t.
    painful t.
    raspberry t.
    red strawberry t.
    scrotal t.
    strawberry t.
    thick t.
    white strawberry t.

tonic pupils

tonofibril

tonofilament
    t./desmosome attachment

tonsillar pillars

tonsillitis

tonsurans
    tinea t.

top
    red t.

tophus *pl.* tophi
    synovial membrane t.
    t. syphiliticus

topical
    Aclovate t.
    Actinex t.
    Akne-Mycin t.
    Ala-Quin t.
    t. aluminum chloride
    t. androgen
    t. anesthetic
    t. anthralin
    t. antibacterial therapy

topical (*continued*)
    t. anticandidal imidazole
      cream
    t. antifungal therapy
    t. antipruritic
    Aquacare t.
    Aquaphor Antibiotic t.
    A/T/S t.
    Baciguent t.
    BactoShield t.
    Bactroban t.
    t. BCNU
    Benadryl t.
    Caldesene t.
    Carmol t.
    Carmol HC t.
    Cloderm t.
    Cordran t.
    Cordran SP t.
    Corque t.
    t. corticoids
    t. corticosteroid
    Cortin t.
    Cruex t.
    Cutivate t.
    Cyclocort t.
    t. cytotoxic therapy
    Debrisan t.
    t. decongestant
    Del-Mycin t.
    Dermacomb t.
    Derma-Smoothe/FS t.
    Desitin t.
    DesOwen t.
    Dyna-Hex t.
    Efudex t.
    Elase t.
    Elase-Chloromycetin t.
    Elocon t.
    Emgel t.
    EMLA t.
    Erycette t.
    EryDerm t.
    Erygel t.
    Erymax t.
    erythromycin t.
    E-Solve-2 t.
    ETS-2% t.

topical (*continued*)
        Eurax t.
        Exelderm t.
        Florone t.
        Florone E t.
        Fluonex t.
        Fluonid t.
        Fluoroplex t.
        Flurosyn t.
        t. formaldehyde
        FS Shampoo t.
        Furacin t.
        t. FK 506
        Garamycin t.
        G-myticin t.
        Halog t.
        Halog-E t.
        Halotex t.
        t. hemostatic agent
        Hibiclens t.
        Hibistat t.
        t. hydrocortisone cream
        Hysone t.
        Lamisil t.
        Lanaphilic t.
        Lanvisone t.
        Lida-Mantle HC t.
        Lidex t.
        Lidex-E t.
        Maxiflor t.
        Meclan t.
        Merlenate t.
        t. methoxsalen
        Micatin t.
        t. minoxidil
        t. moisturizer
        Monistat-Derm t.
        Mycifradin Sulfate t.
        Mycitracin t.
        Mycogen II t.
        Mycolog-II t.
        Myconel t.
        Mycostatin t.
        Mytrex F t.
        Naftin t.
        Neo-Cortef t.
        Neomixin t.
        NGT t.

topical (*continued*)
        Nilstat t.
        t. nitrogen mustard
        t. nitroglycerin
        Nizoral t.
        Novacet t.
        Nutraplus t.
        Nystex t.
        Nyst-Olone II t.
        Oxistat t.
        Oxsoralen t.
        Pedi-Cort V t.
        Pedi-Pro t.
        Polysporin t.
        Pontocaine t.
        Psorcon t.
        t. PUVA
        Quinsana Plus t.
        Racet t.
        Retin-A t.
        t. retinoids
        Spectazole t.
        Staticin t.
        t. steroid
        t. sucralfate
        Sulcosyn t.
        Sulfacet-R t.
        t. sucralfate suspension
        Sulfamylon t.
        Synalar t.
        Synalar-HP t.
        Synemol t.
        Temovate t.
        t. therapy
        Travase t.
        Tridesilon t.
        Triple Antibiotic t.
        Tri-Statin II t.
        T-Stat t.
        UAD t.
        Ultra Mide t.
        Ultravate t.
        Undoguent t.
        Ureacin-20 t.
        Ureacin-40 t.
        Vioform t.
        Vitec t.
        Vytone t.

topical (*continued*)
    Zovirax t.

Topicort
    T.-LP

TORCH

toxoplasmosis, other infections,
    rubella, cytomegalovirus
    infection, and herpes simplex
            TORCH serology
            TORCH syndrome

torpid
    t. papule

torque

torti
    pili t.

torticollis
    dermatogenic t.

tortuous
    t. bulge
    t. capillaries
    t. channels
    t. line
    t. telangiectasis

Torula capsulatum

torulosis

torulus *pl.* toruli
    toruli tactiles

torus
    t. palatinus
    pilus t.

Totacillin
    T.-N

total
    t. hemolytic complement
        level
    t. surgical excision

totalis
    alopecia t.
    alopecia capitis t.

toto
    in t.

Touraine
    T. centrofacial lentigo
    T. syndrome (III)

Touraine-Solente-Golé
    syndrome

tourniquet

Touton giant cell

toxic
    t. alopecia
    t. degenerative eczema
    t. epidermal necrolysis
        (TEN)
    t. erythema
    t. hydroxylamine
        metabolites
    t. metabolites
    t. morbilliform erythema
    t. oil syndrome (TOS)
    t.-producing strains
    t. psychoses
    t. pustuloderma
    t. shock syndrome
    t. shock–like syndrome
        (TSLS)
    t. shock syndrome (TSS)
    t. systemic reaction

toxica
    alopecia t.

toxicity

Toxicodendron
    T. diversilobum
    T. radicans
    T. verniciferum

toxicodendron
    t. dermatitis
    Rhus t.

toxicoderma

toxicodermatitis

toxicodermatosis

toxicopathic

toxicosis

toxicum
  erythema t.

toxin
  botulinal t.
  botulinum t.
  botulinus t.
  t. neutralization assays
  t.-producing organism

toxinic

toxinogenic

toxinogenicity

toxinology

toxinosis

toxins

toxipathic

toxipathy

Toxocara

toxocariasis

toxoid

toxonosis

Toxoplasma
  T. gondii

toxoplasmosis
  epidermotropic cutaneous
    t.

TPI test

trabecular carcinoma

tracer

tracheobronchitis

tracheobronchomegaly

trachoma

trachomatis
  Chlamydia t.

trachyonychia

tract
  burrowing sinus t.

tract (*continued*)
  chronic fistulous t.
  chronic suppuration t.
  epithelial-lined sinus t.
  follicular t.

traction
  t. alopecia
  t. atrophy

tragacanth

tragi of the ears

tragomaschalia

trailing scale

transaminase

transcobalamin
  t. II (TCII)

transcriptase
  t. inhibitor

transcription factors

Transderm ScMp patch

transdermic

transduction
  signal t.

transection

transepidermal
  t. neutrophil migration

transfection

transferrin

transformant

transformation
  blast t.
  malignant t.

transient
  t. acantholytic dermatosis
    (TAD)
  t. acantholytic dyskeratosis
  t. bullous dermolysis of the
    newborn
  t. erythroporphyria of
    infancy

transient (*continued*)
  t. facial papules
  t. facial pustules
  t. hyperbilirubinemia
  t. hypercoagulable state
  t. neonatal pustular
    melanosis
  t. paresis

transitory
  t. benign plaques

translucent
  t. papule

transmembrane
  t. tyrosine kinase KIT
    receptor

transmission
  airborne t.
  bedbug disease t.

transmitter

transovarial

transsphenoidal microsurgical
  excision

transpiration

Trans-Plantar transdermal patch

transplantation
  t. antigen

transthyretin

transudation

transvaginal sonography

Trans-Ver-Sal transdermal patch

transverse
  t. depression
  t. fracture
  t. grooves
  t. palmar creases

transversion mutation

trauma *pl.* traumas, traumata
  inadvertent t.

traumatic

traumatic (*continued*)
  t. alopecia
  t. anserine folliculosis
  t. asphyxia
  t. avulsion
  t. calcinosis
  t. dermatitis
  t. distortion
  t. fat necrosis
  t. herpes
  t. imbedding
  t. lesion
  t. myiasis
  t. neuroma
  t. purpura

traumatically induced
  inflammatory disease

traumatization

Travase topical

Treacher Collins
  T. C. syndrome
  T. C.–Franceschetti
    syndrome

treatment
  Castellani t.
  duration of t.
  energetic t.
  Gennerich t.
  Goeckerman t.
  light t.
  nonpharmacologic
    measure of t.
  oatmeal t.
  preventive t.
  prolonged t.
  prophylactic t.
  slush t.

trefoil dermatitis

Trematoda

trematode

trematodiasis

tremelloid

tremellose

trench
- t. fever
- t. foot
- t. hand
- t. mouth

Trental

trephine
- skin t.

Treponema
- *T.* antibody
- *T. carateum*
- *T. endemicum*
- *T. pallidum*
- *T. pallidum* hemagglutination
- *T. pallidum* immobilization reaction
- *T. pallidum* immobilization test
- *T. pertenue*

treponema-immobilizing antibody

treponemal disease

treponemata

treponematosis
- endemic t.
- nonsyphilitic t.
- nonvenereal t.

treponeme
- commensal oral t.

tretinoin
- t. crème
- t. gel
- t. in a polyolprepolymer
- t. lotion
- t. solution

triacetin

triacylglycerol

triad
- follicular occlusion t.
- Gougerot t.
- Hutchinson t.

triad (*continued*)
- t. of skin lesions
- retention t.

triamcinolone
- t. acetonide
- t. cream (TAC)
- t. diacetate
- t. hexacetonide
- t. lotion (TAL)
- nystatin and t.
- t. ointment (TAO)

triangular
- t. cross-sectional appearance
- t. lunulae
- t. mouth
- t. nicking

triangularis
- alopecia t.

Triatoma
- *T. gerstaeckeri*
- *T. gerstaeckeri* bite
- *T. protracta*
- *T. sanguisuga*
- *T. sanguisuga* bite

triatoma

trichatrophia

trichatrophy

trichauxis

trichiasis

trichilemmal
- t. carcinoma
- t. cyst

trichilemmoma
- desmoplastic t.

Trichina
- *T. spiralis*

trichina

Trichinella
- *T. spiralis*

trichinelliasis

trichinellosis

trichiniasis

trichinosis

trichitis

trichiura
    Trichuris t.

trichoepithelioma

trichomegaly

trichlorfon spray

Tri-Chlor

trichloroacetic acid

trichloroethylene

trichoadenoma

trichobezoar

trichoblastoma

trichoclasia

trichoclasis

trichocryptomania

trichocryptosis

trichocryptotillomania

Trichoderma viride

trichodiscoma

trichodystrophy

trichoepithelioma
    acquired t.
    desmoplastic t.
    t. formation
    hereditary multiple t.
    multiple t.
    t. papillosum multiplex

trichofolliculoma
    sebaceous t.

trichogen

trichogenous

trichoglossia

trichographism

trichohyalin

trichokinesis

trichokleptomania

tricholemmoma

tricholith

trichologia

trichology

trichoma

trichomatose

trichomatosis

trichomatous

trichomatrioma

trichomegaly

Trichomonas
    T. vaginalis
    T. vulvovaginitis

Trichomonas vaginitis

trichomoniasis

trichomycetosis

trichomycosis
    t. axillaris
    t. axillaris nodosa
    t. axillaris nodularis
    t. chromatica
    t. favosa
    t. nigra
    t. nodosa
    t. nodularis
    t. palmellina
    t. pustulosa
    t. rubra

trichonocardiosis
    t. axillaris

trichonodosis

trichonosis

trichonosus
    t. versicolor

trichopathic

trichopathophobia

trichopathy

trichophagy

trichophobia

trichophytia
t. barbae profunda
t. profunda capitis

trichophytic
t. granuloma

trichophytica
acne t.

trichophyticus
lichen t.

trichophytid

trichophytin

Trichophyton, Trichophytum
T. beigelii
T. concentricum
T. crateriforme
T. cutaneum
T. epilans
T. equinum
T. gypseum
T. megninii
T. mentagrophytes
T. purpureum
T. rubrum
T. schoenleinii
T. simii
T. soudanense
T. sulfureum
T. tonsurans
T. verrucosum
T. violaceum

trichophytosis
t. barbae
t. capitis
t. corporis
t. cruris
t. unguium

trichopoliodystrophy

trichopoliosis

trichoptilosis

trichorhinophalangeal
syndrome

trichorrhea

trichorrhexis
t. invaginata
t. nodosa
t. nodosa-like fracture

trichorrhexomania

trichoschisia

trichoschisis

trichoscopy

trichosiderin

trichosis
t. carunculae
t. sensitiva
t. setosa

Trichosporon, Trichosporum
T. beigelii

trichosporonosis

trichosporosis

trichostasis spinulosa

trichothiodystrophy
t. syndrome

trichotillomania

trichotoxin

trichotrophy

trichrome
t. vitiligo

Trichuris trichiura

triclocarban

triclosan

Tridesilon
T. topical

trifluorothymidine

trifluridine

trigeminal
    t. cranial nerve
    t. nerve
    t. trophic lesions

trigger finger

triglycerides

triiodomethane

Tri-Kort

trilaminar

Trilisate

Trilog

Trilone

trimeprazine tartrate

trimethadione

trimethoprim
    t. and polymyxin b
    t.-sulfamethoxazole
      (TMP-SMX)

trimethyl psoralen (TMP)

trioxsalen

triparanol

tripelennamine
    t. citrate
    t. HCl

Triple Antibiotic topical

Triple paste

triple
    t.-jawed pedicellaria
    t. palms

Tripneustes

Trisoject

trisomy
    t. 21,22
    t. 20 syndrome

Trisoralen
    T. Oral

Tri-Statin II topical

Tritin
    Dr Scholl's Maximum
      Strength T.

troche
    clotrimazole t.
    Mycelex t.

Trombicula
    T. akamushi
    T. deliensis
    T. irritans

trombiculiasis

trombiculid
    t. mite
    t. red mite

Trombiculidae

trombidiasis

Trombidiidae

trombidiosis

trophic ulcer

trophodermatoneurosis

trophoneurosis

trophoneurotic leprosy

trophozoite

tropica
    acrodermatitis
      vesiculosa t.
    Leishmania t.
    leishmaniasis t.
    phagedena t.
    pyosis t.

tropical
    t. acne
    t. anhidrotic asthenia
    t. boil
    t. bubo
    t. disease

tropical (*continued*)
 t. dyschromic lichenoid
  disorder
 t. eczema
 t. lichen
 t. measles
 t. milieu
 t. phagedena
 t. phagedenic ulcer
 t. rate mite
 t. sloughing phagedena
 t. sore
 t. swelling
 t. typhus
 t. ulcer

tropicalis
 acne t.
 Blomia t.
 Candida t.
 tinea t.

tropicum
 granuloma inguinale t.
 papilloma inguinale t.
 ulcus t.

tropicus
 lichen t.

Trousseau
 T's sign
 T's spot
 T's syndrome

T.R.U.E.
 T. allergy patch test
 T. test

true
 t. fungi
 t. progeria
 t. skin

trumpet nail

trumpeter's wart

truncal lesion

trypanid

Trypanosoma
 T. brucei

Trypanosoma (*continued*)
 T. cruzi
 T. gambiense
 T. protracta
 T. rhodesiense

trypanosome
 t. chancre

trypanosomiasis
 African t.
 American t.

trypanosomicidal

trypanosomid

Trypanozoon

trypsin

trypsin, balsam peru, and castor
 oil

tryptase

tryptophan dysmetabolism

TS
 temperature sensitive

T/SAL Shampoo

TSEB
 total skin electron beam

tsetse
 t. fly
 t. fly bite

TSH
 thyroid-stimulating
  hormone

TSLS
 toxic shock–like syndrome

TSS
 toxic shock syndrome

T-Stat topical

tsutsugamushi
 t. disease
 t. fever

TTP

TTP (*continued*)
   thrombotic
      thrombocytopenic
      purpura

tubba

tuber *pl.* tubers, tubera

tubercle
   anatomical t.
   t. bacilli
   butcher's t.
   dissection t.
   naked t.
   necrogenic t.
   postmortem t.
   prosector's t.
   sebaceous t.

tubercula (*plural of* tuberculum)

tubercula dolorosa

tubercular

tuberculate, tuberculated

tuberculation

tuberculatum
   erythema t.

tuberculid
   bacillary-barren t's
   micronodular t.
   micropapular t.
   nodular t.
   papular t.
   papulonecrotic t.
   rosacealike t.

tuberculin
   t. skin test

tuberculin-type hypersensitivity

tuberculitis

tuberculization

tuberculocidal

tuberculoderma

tuberculoid

tuberculoid (*continued*)
   t. granuloma
   t. leprosy
   t. macules
   t. rosacea

tuberculosis (TB)
   t. abscess
   acute miliary t.
   t. colliquativa
   t. colliquativa cutis
   cutaneous t.
   t. cutis
   t. cutis colliquativa
   t. cutis follicularis
      disseminata
   t. cutis indurata
   t. cutis indurativa
   t. cutis lichenoid
   t. cutis lichenoides
   t. cutis luposa
   t. cutis miliaris
   t. cutis miliaris disseminata
   t. cutis orificialis
   t. cutis papulonecrotica
   t. cutis verrucosa
   dermal t.
   t. fistulosa subcutanea
   t. fungosa cutis
   t. gumma
   t. indurativa
   t. lichenoides
   t. miliaris cutis
   t. miliaris disseminata
   t. miliaris ulcerosa cutis et
      mucosae
   miliary t.
   multidrug-resistant t. (MDR-
      TB)
   Mycobacterium t. (MTB)
   orificial t.
   papulonecrotic t.
   t. papulonecrotica
   t. primaria cutis
   primary t.
   primary inoculation t.
   t. of skin
   t. ulcer
   t. ulcerosa

tuberculosis (*continued*)
   t. verrucosa cutis
   warty t.

tuberculostat

tuberculostatic

tuberculosus
   lupus t.

tuberculous
   t. abscess
   t. arteritis
   t. chancre
   t. dactylitis
   t. lymphadenitis
   t. synovitis
   t. wart

tuberculum *pl.* tubercula
   t. sebaceum
   t. syphiliticum

tuberoeruptive xanthomas

tuberosa
   urticaria t.

tuberosis

tuberositas *pl.* tuberositates

tuberosum
   xanthoma t.

tuberous
   t. sclerosis
   t. xanthoma
   t. xanthomata

TubiFast bandage

tubiferous

tubocurarine

Tucks
   T. Take-Alongs cleansing pads
   T. Clear gel

tuft
   hair t.

tularemia

tularemic chancre

tumbu fly

tumefacient

tumefaction

tumentia

tumescent

tumid
   t. lepromas
   t. lupus erythematosus
   t. process

tumor
   Abrikosov (Abrikossoff) t.
   adenomatoid t.
   adipose t.
   adnexal t.
   amyloid t.
   angiomatoid t.
   t. antigen
   Bednar t.
   benign t.
   blood t.
   Brooke's t.
   t. burden
   Buschke-Löwenstein t.
   carcinoid t.
   t. cell line
   connective t.
   cutaneous t.
   dermal duct t.
   dermoid t.
   desmoid t.
   epithelial t.
   t. extirpation
   fatty t.
   fibrohistiocytic t.
   glomus t.
   granular cell t.
   Gubler's t.
   haarscheibe t.
   innocent t.
   Koenen's t.
   malignant t.
   malignant mixed müllerian t. (MMMT)

tumor (*continued*)
    melanotic neuroectodermal
      t. of infancy
    Merkel cell t.
    mixed t.
    mixed t. of skin
    mucoepidermoid t.
    t. necrosis
    t., node, metastasis (TNM)
    t. of follicular infundibulum
    oil t.
    papillary t.
    pilar t. of scalp
    Pinkus t.
    potato t. of neck
    premalignant t.
    premalignant fibroepithelial
      t.
    proliferating trichilemmal t.
    sebaceous t.
    t. suppressor gene
    tomato t.
    turban t.
    villous t.
    wing-beating t.

tumoral calcinosis

tumoricidal activity

tumoriform

tumorigenesis

tumorigenic

tumorous
    t. development
    t. lesion
    t. swelling

Tunga
    T. penetrans
    T. penetrans bite

tungiasis

tunica
    t. dartos
    t. propria corii

tunnel

turban tumor

turbid fluid

turgescence

turgid

turgidization

turgometer

turgor
    t. vitalis

Turner
    T's familial syndrome
    T's male syndrome
    T's phenotype with normal
      karyotype
    T's syndrome
    T's syndrome in females
      with normal X
      chromosome
    T.-Kieser syndrome

turpentine

twenty-nail
    t.-n. dystrophy
    t.-n. dystrophy of childhood

twin transfusion syndrome

twinning

twisted
    t. hair

two feet-one hand syndrome

tyloma

tylosis *pl.* tyloses
    t. ciliaris
    t. linguae
    t. palmaris et plantaris

tylotic hand and foot eczema

tyloticum
    eczema t.

Tyndall effect

type
    t. 1 NF

type (*continued*)
    t. 2 5-alpha-reductase
      inhibitor
    t. 2 helper T cell
    t. 2 isoenzyme
    t. 3 (mixed) NF
    t. 4 (variant) NF
    t. 6 NF
    t. A acanthosis nigricans
    t. A lymphomatoid
      papulosis
    t. B acanthosis nigricans
    t. C acanthosis nigricans
    t. 1-24 cornification
    t. 1 cytokines
    t. 2 cytokines (IL-10)
    t. 3 hyperlipoproteinemia
    epidermolysis bullosa,
      dermal t.
    epidermolysis bullosa,
      epidermal t.
    epidermolysis bullosa,
      junctional t.
    t. I bovine collagen
    t. I collagen
    t. I disease
    t. IA oculocutaneous
      albinism
    t. IB oculocutaneous
      albinism
    t. II neuraminidase
      deficiency
    t. II ocular albinism
    t. II oculocutaneous
      albinism
    t. II pachyonychia congenital
    t. III collagen
    t. IV collagen
    t. V collagen
    t. VII collagen gene COL7A1
    t. I-MP oculocutaneous
      albinism
    t. I hypersensitivity
    t. I ocular albinism
    t. I oculocutaneous
      albinism
    t. I-TS oculocutaneous
      albinism

type (*continued*)
    t. IV delayed
      hypersensitivity reaction
    t. IV delayed-type
      sensitization
    t. V disease
    keratosis palmaris et
      plantaris of the Meleda t.
    skin t.
    t. V collagenase
    t. VI collagen
    t. VII collagen
    t. VIII collagen
    t. XI collagen
    t. XIV collagen

typhoid

typhus
    African tick t.
    endemic t.
    epidemic t.
    European t.
    exanthematous t.
    flea-borne t.
    Indian t.
    louse-born t.
    mite t.
    murine t.
    Queensland tick t.
    prison fever t.
    recrudescent t.
    scrub t.
    tick t.
    topical t.
    t. vaccine

typical
    t. infantile strawberry
      hemangioma
    t. nevi

Tyroglyphus
    T. longior
    T. siro

Tyrophagus
    T. longior
    T. putrescentiae
    T. siro

tyrosinase
    t.-negative oculocutaneous
     albinism
    t.-positive albino
    t.-positive oculocutaneous
     albinism
    t.-related oculocutaneous
     albinism
    t.-related protein 1
     (TRP-1)

tyrosine metabolism

tyrosinemia
    neonatal t.
    type I, II t.

Tyson
    T's crypts
    T's glands

Tzanck
    T. cell
    T. preparation
    T. smear
    T. test

U

U1 RNP antibody

UAD topical

ubiquitous
  u. autoantigen
  u. molds

U-Cort

UCTD
  undifferentiated connective
    tissue disease

Udder Butter lubricant/emollient

ulcer
  acute decubitus u.
  Aden u.
  amebic u.
  amputating u.
  anesthetic u.
  aphthous genital u.
  aphthous oral u.
  atonic u.
  burrowing phagedenic u.
  Buruli u.
  chancroid u.
  chancroidal genital u.
  chiclero u.
  chrome u.
  chronic u.
  chronic undermining
    burrowing u.
  cockscomb u.
  cold u.
  constitutional u.
  corneal u.
  corrosive u.
  crateriform u.
  creeping u.
  cutaneous u.
  decubital u.
  decubitus u.
  deep punched-out u.
  diabetic u.
  diabetic foot u.
  diphtheritic u.
  frambesia u.

ulcer (*continued*)
  genital aphthous u.
  gravitational u.
  gummatous u.
  hard u.
  healed u.
  herpetic u.
  hypertensive ischemic u.
  indolent u.
  inflamed u.
  inflammatory u.
  ischemic u.
  Jacob's u.
  u. lesion
  Lipschütz u.
  lupoid u.
  Malabar u.
  Marjolin's u.
  Meleney's u.
  Meleney's chronic
    undermining u.
  nasopharyngeal u.
  necrotic u.
  neurotrophic u.
  in noma u.
  oral aphthous u.
  Oriental u.
  penetrating u. of foot
  perambulating u.
  phagedenic u.
  phlegmonous u.
  plantar u.
  pressure u.
  pudendal u.
  recurrent u.
  ring u.
  rodent u.
  serpiginous u.
  serpiginous syphilitic u.
  sickle cell u.
  skin u.
  sloughing u.
  soft u.
  stasis vascular u.
  steroid u.
  symptomatic u.

ulcer (*continued*)
    syphilitic u.
    tanner's u.
    trophic u.
    tropical u.
    tropical phagedenic u.
    undermining u.
    undermining burrowing u.
    varicose u.
    vascular u.
    venereal u.
    venous stasis u.
    Zambesi u.

ulcera (*plural of* ulcus)

ulcerans
    Mycobacterium u.

ulcerate

ulcerated
    u. hypopigmented area

ulcerating
    u. granuloma of pudendum

ulceration
    gangrenous u.
    gastric u.
    gummatous u.
    intertrigo with u.
    ischemic u.
    mucous membrane u.
    nasal mucosal u.
    oral u.
    u. of oral mucosa
    ragged u.
    rectal u.

ulcerative
    u. colitis
    u. dermatosis
    u. form
    u. gingivitis
    u. lesion
    u. lichen planus
    u. pharyngitis
    u. proctocolitis
    u. stomatitis

ulceroglandular

ulceronecrotic
    u. Mucha-Habermann
      disease
    u. skin lesions

ulcerous

ulcero-vegetating plaque

ulcus *pl.* ulcera
    u. ambulans
    u. ambustiforme
    arteriosclerotic u. cruris
    u. cruris mixtum
    u. cruris postthromboticum
    u. cruris venosum
    u. durum
    u. hypostaticum
    u. interdigitale
    u. migrans
    u. molle
    u. molle cutis
    u. rodens
    u. scorbuticum
    u. syphiliticum
    u. terebrans
    u. tropicum
    u. venereum
    u. vulvae acutum

ulerythema
    u. acneiforme
    u. centrifugum
    u. ophryogenes
    u. sycosiforme

ulerythematosa
    atrophodermia u.

Ullrich-Turner syndrome

ulnar bands

ulodermatitis

ulotrichous

Ultra
    Grisactin U.
    U. Mide topical
    U. Tears solution

ultracentrifugation

ultramicronized
  u. form
  u. particles

ultrapulsed laser resurfacing

ultrasonography

ultrasound
  A-mode u.
  Doppler u.

ultrastructural features

Ultravate
  U. topical

ultraviolet (UV)
  u. actinotherapy
  u. A (UVA)
  u. B (UVB)
  u. B-range (UVB)
  u. C (UVC)
  u. irradiation
  u. lamp
  u. light
  u. light exposure
  u. radiation
  u. spectrum
  u. treatment

ultraviolet-induced erythema

Umbelliferae

umbilical artery
  catheterization

umbilicated

umbilication

Uncinaria

uncinariasis

uncinariatic

uncombable hair syndrome

unction

unctuosa
  cutis u.

unctuous

undecylenic
  u. acid
  u. acid and derivatives

undercover cosmetic

underdeveloped nails

underdevelopment

undermining ulcer

underpants-pattern erythema

undersurface

Underwood disease

undifferentiated
  u. cell
  u. connective tissue disease
    (UCTD)

Undoguent topical

undressable hair

undulate

unencapsulated

ungual
  u. digital dystrophy
  u. melanocytic band

unguent

unguenta (*plural of*
  unguentum)

unguenti (*genitive of*
  unguentum)

unguentum *pl.* unguenta

ungues
  u. hippocratici

unguinal

unguis *pl.* ungues
  u. incarnates
  u. incarnatus
  leukopathia u.
  lunula u.
  pterygium u.
  vallum u.

unguium
    achromia u.
    atrophia u.
    canities u.
    defluvium u.
    dystrophia u.
    fragilitas u.
    gryposis u.
    scabrities u.
    tinea u.
    trichophytosis u.

ungula

unicameral cyst

unidirectional current

uniform
    u. basaloid cells
    u. border
    u. pits
    u. spindle cells

unilateral
    u. cerebral atrophy
    u. clubbing
    u. degenerative retinitis
    u. dermatomal superficial
      telangiectasia
    u. eczema
    u. glaucoma
    u. hemangiomatosis
    u. hemidysplasia
    u. hemidysplasia
      cornification disorder
    u. laterothoracic
      exanthem
    u. macular degeneration
    u. nevoid telangiectasia
    u. palmar hyperhidrosis
    u. uveitis

unilocular cyst

uninflamed

uniocular

Unipen
    U. injection
    U. oral

unit
    dermal microvascular u.
    epidermal-melanin u.
    follicular melanin u.
    pilosebaceous u.
    skin test u.

unius
    nevus u. lateris

universal
    u. acquired melanosis
    u. angiomatosis
    u. erythroderma
    u. redness
    u. vitiligo

universale
    angiokeratoma corporis
      diffusum u.
    melasma u.

universalis
    alopecia u.
    calcinosis u.
    hypertrichosis u.
    psoriasis u.

unmyelinated
    u. C fibers
    u. nerve endings

Unna
    U's boot
    U's cell
    U's comedo extractor
    U's dermatosis
    U's disease
    U's mark
    U's nevus
    U's syndrome
    U.-Thost disease
    U.-Thost keratoderma
    keratosis palmaris et
      plantaris of U.-Thost
    U.-Thost syndrome

unsaturated polyester resins

unusual
    u. lupus erythematosus–like
      syndrome
    u. opportunistic infection

upcurved punch

upper
    u. costochondral junction
    u. dermal collagen sclerotic
    u. dermal infiltrate
    u. dermal infiltrate of
        mononuclear cells
    u. dermal vessels
    u. dermal vessels
        telangiectatic
    u. dermis
    u. epidermal intercellular
        IgA staining
    u. stratum malpighii
    u. thoracic sympathectomy

upward proliferation

uranitis plasmacellularis

Urbach
    U.-Oppenheim disease
    U.-Wiethe disease
    U.-Wiethe syndrome

urban cutaneous
    leishmaniasis

urea
    u. and hydrocortisone
    u. cream
    u. mixture
    u. preparation

Ureacin
    U.-10 topical lotion
    U.-20 topical cream

Ureaphil Injection

Ureaplasma urealyticum

uredo

uremia

uremic
    u. pruritus

urethral
    u. meatus
    u. orifice
    u. stricture

urethritis
    chlamydial u.
    gonorrheal u.
    nongonococcal u.

urhidrosis
    u. crystallina

uric acid crystals

uridrosis
    u. crystallina

urinalysis

urinary
    u. electrophoresis
    u. gas chromatography
    u. porphyrin
    u. uroporphyrins

urine

urinidrosis

uritis

urogenital system

Uroplus DS

Uroplus SS

uroporphyrin
    u. type I
    u. type III

uroporphyrinogen
    u. decarboxylase
    u. III synthase

ursodeoxycholic acid

Urtica
    U. dioica

urticans
    purpura u.

urticant

urticaria
    u. acuta
    acute u.
    acute allergic u.
    allergic u.
    aquagenic u.

urticaria (*continued*)
    u. bullosa
    bullous u.
    cholinergic u.
    chronic u.
    u. chronica
    cold u.
    cold-induced u.
    u. conferta
    congelation u.
    contact u.
    cystic u.
    u. dermagraphism
    endemic u.
    u. endemica
    u. epidemica
    u. factitia
    factitious u.
    febrile u.
    u. febrilis
    giant u.
    u. gigantea
    heat u.
    hemorrhagic u.
    u. hemorrhagica
    heredofamilial u.
    idiopathic u.
    idiopathic cold u.
    immunological contact u.
    irritant contact u.
    light u.
    u. maculosa
    u. mechanica
    u. medicamentosa
    Milton u.
    u. multiformis endemica
    papular u.
    u. papulosa
    u. papulosa chronica
    u. papulosa infantum
    u. perstans
    u. photogenica
    physical u.
    u. pigmentosa
    pressure u.
    recurrent u.
    solar u.
    solaris u.

urticaria (*continued*)
    u. solaris
    u. subcutanea
    subcutaneous u.
    u. tuberosa
    u. vesiculosa
    vibratory u.

urticarial
    u. dermatographia
    u. dermatographism
    u. erythema multiforme
    u. fever
    u. patch
    u. plaque
    u. vasculitis

urticariogenic substance

urticarioides
    acarodermatitis u.

urticarious

urticata
    acne u.

urticate

urtication

urticatus
    lichen u.

urushiol

ustilaginism

Ustilago

uta

uteri
    ichthyosis u.

uterine
    u. bleeding
    u. carcinoma
    u. fibroma
    u. leiomyoma
    u. sarcoma

Uticort

UV
    ultraviolet

UV (*continued*)
UV light-cured acrylate
lacquer

UVA
long-wavelength ultraviolet
light
ultraviolet A
UVA I
UVA II

UVB
midrange-wavelength
ultraviolet light
ultraviolet B
ultraviolet B-range
ultraviolet light

UVB (*continued*)
UVB phototherapy
UVB therapy

UVC
ultraviolet C

uveitis
anterior u.

uveoparotid fever

uviofast

uvioresistant

uviosensitive

UVL
ultraviolet light

V

V
  V area
  V gene
  V chain

vaccina

vaccinal

vaccinate

vaccination

vaccinator

vaccinatum
  eczema v.

vaccine
  V. Adverse Events Reporting
    System (VAERS)
  AIDS v.
  v. antigen
  aqueous v.
  autogenous v.
  bacterial v.
  chickenpox v.
  foot-and-mouth disease
    virus v.
  heterogenous v.
  measles, mumps, and
    rubella v. (MMR)
  measles virus v.
  MMR v.
  polyvalent v.
  smallpox v.
  Staphylococcus v.
  Staphylococcus aureus v.
  varicella v.
  variola v.

vaccinia
  v. gangrenosa
  generalized v.
  v. immune globulin
  v. infection
  v. necrosum
  progressive v.
  variola v.

vaccinia (*continued*)
  v. virus
  v. virus-induced
    dermatoses

vaccinial

vacciniform

vacciniforme
  hydroa v.

vaccinist

vaccinization

vaccinogen

vaccinogenous

vaccinoid
  v. reaction

vaccinostyle

vaccinum

vacuolar
  v. alteration
  v. changes
  v. interface dermatitis
  v. interface reaction pattern

vacuolated
  v. cytoplasm
  v. epithelium
  v. histiocytes
  v. leukocytes
  v. Paget's cell
  v. prickle cell

vacuolating virus

vacuolation

vacuole

vacuolization
  basket-weave v.
  v. of the basal cells

vacutome

vacuum tube

VAERS
  Vaccine Adverse Events
    Reporting System

vagabond's disease

Vagi-Gard
  V. Advanced Sensitive
    Formula
  V. vaginal cream

vaginal
  v. bioadhesive moisturizer
  v. mucosa
  v. pruritus

vaginal
  Monistat V.

vaginalis
  Trichomonas v.

vaginitis
  Gardnerella v.
  granular v.

vaginosis

vagrant's disease

valacyclovir
  v. HCl

valerate
  betamethasone v.

Valisone

Valium
  V. injection
  V. oral

vallecula *pl.* valleculae
  v. unguis

vallecular

vallum *pl.* valla
  v. unguis

Valnac

valproate sodium

Valrelease Oral

Valsalva maneuver

Valtrex

valvular disease

vancomycin
  v. hydrochloride
  v. red-man syndrome
  v.-resistant strain

vancomycin-resistant
  enterococci (VRE)

van der Waals forces

vanilla
  v. pods

vanillin

vanillism

Van Lohuizen's syndrome

Vanoxide

Vanoxide-HC

vaporization

variabilis
  Dermacentor v.
  erythrokeratodermia v.
  erythrokeratodermia
    figurata v.

variable
  v. region
  v. vascular spaces

variant
  dystrophic v.
  generalized morphea v.
  junctional v.
  linear scleroderma v.
  Miller-Fisher v.
  morphea v.
  v. neurofibromatosis
  simplex v.
  ulcerative v.

varicella
  congenital v.
  v. disease
  v. gangrenosa
  v. infection

varicella (*continued*)
  v. pneumonia
  pustular v.
  v. pustulosa
  v. vaccine
  v. virus vaccine live
  v. zoster
  v. zoster virus

varicellation

varicella-zoster (VZ)
  v.-z. immune globulin
  v.-z. immunoglobulin
    (VZIG)
  v.-z. infection
  v.-z. virus (VZV)

varicelliform
  v. lesion
  Kaposi v. eruption

varicelloid

varicellosus
  herpes zoster v.

varices
  v. of the tongue

varicocele

varicolored lesion

varicose
  v. eczema
  v. glands
  v. ulcer
  v. veins

varicosis

varicosity
  venous v.

varicosum
  lymphangioma capillare v.

variegata
  parakeratosis v.
  parapsoriasis v.

variegate porphyria (VP)

variegated

variegatum
  Hyalomma v.

variola
  v. benigna
  v. crystallina
  v. hemorrhagica
  v. inserta
  v. major
  v. maligna
  v. miliaris
  v. minor
  v. mitigata
  v. pemphigosa
  v. siliquosa
  v. sine eruptione
  v. vaccine
  v. vaccinia
  v. vera
  v. verrucosa
  v. virus

variolar

variolate

variolation

variolic

varioliform
  v. scarring
  v. scars
  v. syphilid

varioliformis
  acne v.
  parapsoriasis v.
  parapsoriasis acuta et v.

variolization

varioloid

variolous

variolovaccine

Varivax

varix

vascular
  v. alopecia
  v. damage

vascular (*continued*)
v. disturbance
v. endothelial cell
v. endothelium
v. hamartoma
v. hemophilia
v. leakage
v. leiomyoma
v. malformation birthmark
v. neoplasia
v. nevus
v. occlusion
v. proliferation
v. proliferative lesion
v. sclerosis
v. spider
v. stigmata
v. thrombosis
v. tree
v. tumor
v. type
v. ulcer

vasculare
poikiloderma v. atrophicans
poikiloderma atrophicans v.

vascularis
nevus v.

vascularity

vascularization

vasculitic lesion

vasculitis *pl.* vasculitides
v. allergic
allergic v.
v. allergica profunda
cutaneous v.
cutaneous necrotizing v.
granulomatous v.
Henoch-Schönlein v.
v. hyperergica cutis
hypersensitivity v.
hypocomplementemic v.
hypocomplementemic
urticarial v.
leukocytoclastic v. (LCV)
v.-like reaction

vasculitis (*continued*)
livedo v.
livedoid v.
lymphomatoid v.
necrotizing v.
nodular v.
nodular granulomatous v.
v. nodularis Montgomery
v. of arterioles
v. racemosa
septic v.
systemic v.
urticarial v.

vasculopathy

vasculosus
nevus v.

Vaseline
V. gauze
V. Intensive Care
moisturizer
V. petroleum jelly

vasoactive
v. amines
v. endogenous
substance

vasoconstriction
v. bioassay
hypoxic v.

vasodilatation

vasodilating drugs

vasomotor
v. disorder
v. lability
v. nerve

vasoreactive material

vasospasm
cold-induced v.

Vater-Pacini corpuscle

vaulted palate

V-Cillin K Oral

VDRL

VDRL (*continued*)
Venereal Disease Research
Laboratory
VDRL test

vection

vector
biological v.
mechanical v.
v. of plague
recombinant v.

vectorial

vecuronium

Veetids Oral

vegetans
dermatitis v.
keratosis v.
pemphigus v.
pyoderma v.

vegetative bacteriophage

veiled cell

vein
broken v.
saphenous v.

Velban

Velcro closure

veldt sore

vellus
v. hair
v. hair cyst
v. olivae

Veltane tablet

velvety palms

venectomy

venenata
acne v.
cheilitis v.
dermatitis v.
Rhus v.

venenatum

venenatum (*continued*)
erythema v.

venerea, venereum
granuloma v.
lymphogranuloma v. (LGV,
LVG)
lymphopathia v.
papilloma v.
ulcus v.

venereal
v. bubo
v. disease
v. lymphogranuloma
v. sore
v. ulcer
v. virus
v. wart

Venereal Disease Research
Laboratory (VDRL)

Venetian red

venlafaxine
v. HCl

Venoglobulin
V.-I
V.-S

venography

venom
bee v.
v. extract
flea v.
v. hemolysis
Hymenoptera v.
v. immunotherapy
snake v.
spider v.
v. testing

venom-bathed nematocyst

venom-bearing spine

venomous
v. fish
v. lizard
v. snake

venosus
   nevus v.

venous
   v. congestion
   v. dermatitis
   v. disease
   v. duplex
   v. ectasia
   v. gangrene
   v. insufficiency
   v. lake
   v. ligation
   v. malformation
   v. reconstruction
   v. rheography
   v. stasis disease
   v. stasis ulcer
   v. stripping
   v. thrombosis
   v. ulcer
   v. ulceration
   v. varicosities

ventral

ventricosus
   dermatitis pediculoides v.
   Pediculoides v.
   Pyemotes v.

venular lesion

venulitis
   cutaneous necrotizing v.

Venus
   collar of V.
   crown of V.
   necklace of V.

ver du cayor

vera
   cutis v.
   polycythemia v.
   variola v.

verapamil

vergeture

Vergogel Gel

vermicular
   v. atrophoderma

vermicularis
   atrophoderma v.
   Enterobius v.
   Oxyuris v.

vermiculatum
   atrophoderma v.

vermiform mite

vermilion
   v. border
   v. mucous membrane
   v. surface

vermilionectomy

Vermox

vernacular

Verneuil
   hidradenitis axillaris of V.
   V. neuroma

verniciferum
   Toxicodendron v.

vernix
   Rhus v.

Verocay body

verruca *pl.* verrucae
   v. acuminata
   v. digitata
   v. filiformis
   v. glabra
   v. mollusciformis
   v. necrogenica
   v. peruana
   v. peruviana
   v. plana
   v. plana juvenilis
   v. plana senilis
   v. planta
   v. plantaris
   seborrheic v.
   v. seborrheica
   v. seborrheica senilis
   v. senilis

verruca (*continued*)
  v. simplex
  v. tuberculosa
  v. vulgaris

verruciform
  v. scales
  v. xanthoma

verruciformis
  acrodermatitis v.
  acrokeratosis v.
  epidermodysplasia v.

verrucoid plaques

verrucosa
  v. cutis
  dermatitis v.
  elephantiasis nostra v.
  pachyderma v.
  Phialophora v.
  telangiectasia v.
  tuberculosis cutis v.
  variola v.

verrucose

verrucosis
  v. generalisata
  lymphostatic v.

verrucosum
  eczema v.
  erysipelas v.
  molluscum v.

verrucosus
  lichen planus v.
  lichen ruber v.
  lupus v.
  nervus v.

verrucous
  v. angiokeratoma
  v. carcinoma
  v. dyscrasia
  v. epidermal hyperplasia
  v. epidermal nevus
  v. epidermophytosis
  v. excrescence
  v. hemangioma

verrucous (*continued*)
  v. lupus erythematosus
  v. melanoma
  v. nevus
  v. papule
  v. plaque
  v. scrofuloderma
  v. streak
  v. tumor
  v. vascular malformation
  v. vegetative lesion
  v. white plaques
  v. xanthoma

verruga
  v. peruana

versicolor
  Aspergillus v.
  pityriasis v.
  tinea v.
  trichonosus v.

vertebrate
  v. protein

vertex
  v. region

vertical
  v. diaphysis
  v. growth phase
  v. transmission

vertigo

vesica

vesicae
  pachyderma v.

vesicant

vesicate

vesication

vesicatory

vesicle
  v. formation
  tense v.

vesicobullous
  v. eruption
  v. lesion

vesicopustular
    v. eruption

vesicopustule

vesicular
    v. bullous pemphigoid
    v. dermatophytid
    v. dermatitis
    v. eruption
    v. exanthema
    v. exanthema of swine virus
    v. eczema of palms and
        soles
    v. form
    v. lesions
    v. nucleus
    v. ringworm
    v. palmoplantar eczema
    v. stomatitis
    v. stomatitis virus
    v. viral infection

vesiculate

vesiculated

vesiculation
    creeping v.
    intraepidermal v.
    subepidermal v.

vesiculiform

vesiculobullous
    v. disease
    v. hand eczema

vesiculopapular

vesiculopustular

vesiculosa
    urticaria v.

vesiculose

vesiculosis

vesiculosum
    eczema v.
    hydroa v.

vesiculotomy

vesiculous

Vesiculovirus

vespid
    Hymenopterous v.
    v. venom

Vespula
    V. crabro
    V. sting

vessel
    dilated superficial blood v.
    v. lumina

vestibular
    v. bands
    v. cyst
    v. papilla
    v. system

vestibuloauditory symptoms

vestimenti
    pediculosis v.

vestimentorum
    pediculosis corporis vel v.

vibesate

vibex *pl.* vibices

Vibramycin
    V. injection
    V. oral

Vibra-Tabs

vibratory
    v. angioedema
    v. stimuli
    v. urticaria

Vibrio
    V. vulnificus

vibrio

vibrissa

Vicryl suture

Vidal's disease

vidarabine

Vierra sign

Vigilon dressing

vigorous hydration

villi

villoma

villonodular
  v. synovitis

villous
  v. atrophy
  v. fold
  v. frond
  v. tumor

villus

vimentin

vinblastine
  v. sulfate

Vinca alkaloid

Vincent
  V's angina
  V's disease
  V's infection
  V's white mycetoma

vincristine

Vinson's syndrome

vinyl
  v. chloride
  v. chloride exposure
  v. dental trays
  v. monomers

Vioform
  V. topical

violaceous
  v. color
  v. erythema
  v. halo
  v. hue
  v. macule
  v. plaque
  v. zone

Violaceum

violet
  v.-blue erythema
  crystal v.
  gentian v.
  hexamethyl v.
  methyl v.

violin-back
  v.-b. spider
  v.-b. spider bite

Vira-A
  V. injection
  V. Ophthalmic

viral
  v. antigens
  v. blister
  v. culture
  v. enzyme thymidine kinase
  v. exanthema
  v. genome
  v. particle
  v. vesicle
  v. wart

viremia

viricidal

viricide

viridans hemolysis

virilism

virilization

virion
  live and dead v.

viroid

virologist

virology
  v. laboratory

Viroptic Ophthalmic

virucidal

virucide

virulent
  v. bacteriophage

viruliferous

virus
African tick v.
AIDS-related v. (ARV)
bacterial v.
chickenpox v.
v. colonies
contagious pustular
  stomatitis v.
enteric cytopathogenic
  human orphan (ECHO) v.
  *(former name for
  echovirus)*
measles v.

viscera (*plural of* viscus)

visceral
v. disease virus
v. dissemination
v. fat
v. involvement
v. leishmaniasis
v. neoplasm
v. sporotrichosis
v. syphilis
v. tuberculosis

viscerocutaneous
loxoscelism

viscerotropic
v. leishmaniasis

viscid
v. fluid
v. necrotic material

viscous Xylocaine

viscus *pl.* viscera

Vistaril

vitamin
v. A
v. A deficiency
v. A hypervitaminosis
v. B complex
v. B deficiency
v. B_1 deficiency
v. B_2 deficiency

vitamin (*continued*)
v. B_6
v. B_{12} deficiency
v. D
v. D cutaneous
  photosynthesis
v. D deficiency
v. D excess
v. D_2
v. E
v. E deficiency
v. K
v. K deficiency
v. K–dependent clotting
  factors II, VII, IX, X

Vitec topical

vitiligines (*plural of* vitiligo)

vitiliginous skin

vitiligo *pl.* vitiligines
acral v.
acrofacial v.
v. capitis
Cazenave v.
Celsus v.
circumscribed v.
facial v.
generalized v.
localized v.
perinevic v.
segmental v.

vitiligoidea

vivo
in v.

VKHS
Vogt-Koyanagi-Harada
  syndrome

VLDL
very-low-density lipoprotein

Vogt
V.-Koyanagi syndrome
V.-Koyanagi-Harada
  syndrome

Vohwinkel

Vohwinkel (*continued*)
  V's keratoderma
  mutilating keratoderma of
    V.
  V's syndrome

Voigt line

volar
  v. skin

volatile
  v. gases
  v. odor

volcanic border

volume-reducing surgery

von
  v. Gierke glycogen storage
    disease
  v. Hippel-Lindau disease
  v. Hippel-Lindau syndrome
  v. Recklinghausen's disease
  v. Recklinghausen's
    neurofibromatosis
  v. Willebrand factor
    multimers
  v. Zumbusch's disease
  v. Zumbusch's psoriasis
  v. Zumbusch's pustular
    psoriasis

Vorner variant of Unna-Thost
  keratoderma

vortex *pl.* vortices
  v. coccygeus
  v. pilorum

VP
  variegate porphyria

V-shaped pattern

vulgaris
  acne v.
  apple jelly papule of lupus
    v.
  Faba v.
  ichthyosis v.
  impetigo v.

vulgaris (*continued*)
  lupus v.
  pemphigus v.
  Proteus v.
  sycosis v.
  Thermoactinomyces v.
  verruca v.
  xerosis v.

vulva *pl.* vulvae
  kraurosis v.
  leukoplakia v.
  pruritus v.

vulvar
  v. intraepithelial neoplasia
  v. lesion
  v. lichen sclerosus
  v. melanosis
  v. muscle
  v. vestibulitis syndrome
  v. wart

vulvitis
  atrophic v.
  chronic atrophic v.
  v. chronica plasmacellularis
  follicular v.
  leukoplakic v.
  v. plasma cell
  pseudoleukoplakic v.

vulvodynia

vulvovaginal
  v. area
  v. candidiasis (VVC)

vulvovaginitis

Vumon injection

VVC
  vulvovaginal candidiasis

VX
  verruciform xanthoma

Vytone topical

VZ
  varicella-zoster

VZIG

W

Waardenburg
  W's syndrome
  W.-Shah syndrome

Waldenström
  W's benign
    hypergammaglobulinemic
    purpura
  W's
    hypergammaglobulinemic
    purpura
  hypergammaglobulinemia
    of W.
  W's macroglobulinemia
  W's purpura
  W's syndrome

wall
  bacterial cell w.
  nail w.
  shaggy thick w.

Wallace's line

Walsh pressure ring

wandering
  w. erysipelas
  w. rash

Wangiella dermatitidis

waning
  waxing and w.

warehouseman's itch

warfarin
  w.-induced necrosis
  w. sodium

warm water immersion foot

wart
  acuminate w.
  anatomical w.
  asbestos w.
  common w,
  digitate w.
  filiform w.
  flat w.

wart (*continued*)
  fugitive w.
  genital w.
  infectious w.
  juvenile w.
  moist w.
  mosaic w.
  mucocutaneous w.
  myrmecia w.
  necrogenic w.
  paronychial w.
  periungual w.
  peruvian w.
  pitch w.
  plane w.
  plantar w.
  pointed w.
  postmortem w.
  prosector's w.
  seborrheic w.
  seed w.
  senile w.
  soft w.
  soot w.
  subungual w.
  telangiectatic w.
  tuberculous w.
  venereal w.
  viral w.
  vulvar w.

wartlike excrescence

water
  hamamelis w.
  lime w.

Warthin
  W.-Starry silver stain
  W.-Starry-staining bacillus

wartpox

warty
  w. dyskeratoma
  w. excrescence
  w. exophytic mass
  w. horn

warty (*continued*)
    w. keratotic plaques
    w. tuberculosis

wash
    Benzac AC W.
    SAStid Plain Therapeutic
      Shampoo and Acne W.
    Theroxide W.

washerman's mark

washerwoman's itch

wasp
    w. sting
    w. venom immune globulin

Wassermann
    W. antibody
    W. reaction
    W. test

wasting
    w. disease
    w. syndrome

watchglass nails

water
    w. bugs
    w. canker
    w. fleas
    w.-free facial foundation
    w.-impermeable,
      non–silicone-based
      occlusive dressing
    w. itch
    w. moccasin
    w. sore

water-based
    w.-b. facial foundation
    w.-b. formulation
    w.-b. mascara
    w.-b. paints

water-free facial foundation

Waterhouse-Friderichsen
    syndrome

water impermeable,
    non–silicone-based occlusive
    dressing

watermelon stomach

waterpox

waveform

wavelength

wax depilatory

waxing and waning

waxy
    w. fibrillar tissue
    w. finger
    w. skin

weal

weaverfish

web formation

webbed
    w. neck
    w. pattern

Weber
    W.-Christian disease
    W.-Christian panniculitis
    W.-Christian syndrome
    W.-Cockayne disease
    W.-Cockayne syndrome

wedge
    w. biopsy
    w. excision
    w.-shaped

weep

weeping
    w. dermatitis
    w. eczema
    w. lesion

weepy lesion

Wegener
    W's granulomatosis
    W.-Klinger syndrome

Weibel-Palade bodies

weight loss

weight-bearing joints

Weil
    W's disease
    W.-Felix reaction
    W.-Felix test

weld
    spot w.

well-circumscribed
    w.-c. dermal nodule
    w.-c. mantle

well-defined
    w.-d. border

well-demarcated skin reaction

well-differentiated
    w.-d. squamous cell
        carcinoma
    w.-d. superficial lesion
    w.-d. tubular structure

well-formed palisaded lesion

Wells' syndrome

welt
    indurated w.

wen

Werlhof
    W's disease
    W's purpura

Werner
    W's gene
    W's syndrome

Werther
    W's disease
    W's nevus

West
    W. African fever
    W. Indian smallpox
    W. Nile fever
    W. Nile virus

Westcort

Westergren sedimentation rate

Western Blot test

western
    w. black-legged tick
    w. poison oak

Westphal's
    W's disease
    W's pseudosclerosis
    W.-Strümpell disease
    W.-Strümpell
        pseudosclerosis

wet
    w. cutaneous leishmaniasis
    w. compress
    w. dressing
    w. flush
    w. gangrene
    w. pellagra
    w. smear

whale finger

wheal
    w. and flare
    skin w.

wheal-and-erythema reaction

wheal-and-flare reaction

whelp

Whipple
    W's bacillus
    W's disease

whisker hair

Whistling face syndrome

white
    w. clot syndrome
    w. dermatographia
    w. dermographism
    w. finger
    w. frontal forelock
    w. gangrene
    w. graft
    w. hair
    w. lesion
    w. line
    w. line response
    w. melanin

white (*continued*)
  w. nails
  w. petrolatum
  w. piedra
  w. scalp hair
  w. scar
  w. sclerae dominant
  w. sponge nevus
  w. spot disease
  w. strawberry tongue
  w. superficial
    onychomycosis

White disease

white-faced hornet

whitegraft reaction

whitehead

whitepox

Whitfield's Ointment

whitlow
  herpes w.
  herpetic w.
  melanotic w.
  thecal w.

Whitmore
  W's disease
  W's fever
  W's melioidosis

WHO
  World Health Organization
    WHO Class IV
    WHO criteria

whorl
  digital w.

whorled
  w. nevoid hypermelanosis

Wickham's striae

wide
  w. excision
  w. local excision
  w. mouth
  w. spectrum

widespread
  w. distribution
  w. dysplastic process
  w. erythema
  w. papular skin lesions
  w. uncontrolled infection

widow's peak

wildfire rash

Wilks disease

Willan's disease

Wilms' tumor

Wilson
  W. disease
  W's lichen
  W's syndrome

Winchester's syndrome

windburn

windmill-vane hand syndrome

Winiwarter-Buerger disease

Winkler's disease

winter
  w. eczema
  w. itch

Winterbottom's sign

wire-loop lesion

Wiskott-Aldrich syndrome

wit

witch hazel

witkop

Witkop-Von Sallman disease

Wohlfahrtia vigil

womanish proportions

Wood
  W's glass
  W's lamp
  W's light
  W's light examination

wood
  w. preservatives
  w. tick

wood-grain
  w.-g. appearance
  w.-g.-pattern scales

woolly hair

woolly-hair
  w.-h. nevus

woolsorter's disease

Woringer-Kolopp disease

World Health Organization
  (WHO)

wormlike

Woronoff ring

wound
  w. contraction
  w. edge ischemia
  w. healing
  w. myiasis
  puncture w.

wrap
  elastic w.

Wright
  W's stain
  W's syndrome

wrinkle

wrinkling

writing
  skin w.

wryneck deformity

WS
  Waardenburg
    syndrome

Wuchereria
  W. bancrofti

wuchereriasis

Wyburn-Mason syndrome

Wycillin injection

Wynn method

xanchromatic

xanthelasma
    generalized s.
    x. palpebrarum

xanthelasmatosis

xanthelasmoidea

xanthism

xanthochroia

xanthochromatic

xanthochromia
    x. striata palmaris

xanthochromic

xanthochroous

xanthoderma

xanthoerythrodermia
    x. perstans

xanthogranuloma
    juvenile x.
    necrobiotic x.

xanthogranulomatosis

xanthogranulomatous

xanthoma *pl.* xanthomata
    diabetic x.
    x. diabeticorum
    diffuse plane x.
    disseminated x.
    x. dissemination
    x. disseminatum
    eruptive x.
    x. eruptivum
    fibrous x.
    generalized plane x.
    hypercholesteremic x.
    hyperlipemic x.
    juvenile x.
    x. multiplex
    normocholesteremic x.
    palmar x.

xanthoma (*continued*)
    x. palpebrarum
    palpebrarum x.
    x. pigmentosum
    x. pigmentosum tardivum
    planar x.
    plane x.
    x. planum
    x. striata palmaris
    x. striatum palmare
    x. tendinosum
    tendinous x.
    tendon x.
    tuberoeruptive x.
    x. tuberosum
    x. tuberosum multiplex
    tuberous x.
    verrucous x.
    verruciform x.

xanthomatosis
    biliary
        hypercholesterolemic x.
    cerebrotendinous x.

xanthomatous
    x. biliary cirrhosis
    x. tumor

Xanthomonas maltophilia

xanthopathy

xanthopsydracia

xanthosis
    x. cutis
    x. diabeticorum

xanthous

X chromosome

XD
    xanthoma
        disseminatum

xenogeneic
    x. graft

xenogenic

xenogenous

xenograft

Xenopsylla
 X. cheopis
 X. cheopis bite

Xerac AC

xerasia

xerochilia

xeroderma (*variant* xerodermia)
 follicular x.
 Kaposi x., x. of Kaposi
 x. pigmentosa
 x. pigmentosum

xerodermatic

xerodermia *variant of*
 xeroderma)

xerodermoid
 pigmented x.

xeronosus

xerophthalmia

xerosis
 x. conjunctiva
 conjunctival x.
 x. corneae
 corneal x.
 x. cutis
 s. generalisata
 x. vulgaris

xerostomia

xerotes

xerotic
 x. eczema

xerotica
 balanitis x. obliterans

xerotripsis

X-linked
 X-l. cutis laxa
 X-l. dominant
 X-l. dominant disorder
 X-l. dominant trait
 X-l. dominant
  chondrodysplasia
  punctata
 X-l. EDS-EDS type V
 X-l. hypogammagl-
  obulinemia
 X-l. ichthyosis
 X-l. lymphoproliferative
  syndrome
 X-l. mucopolysaccharidosis
  II
 X-l. recessive
 X-l. recessive disorder
 X-l. recessive ichthyosis
 X-l. recessive inheritance

XOAN
 X-linked (Nettleship) ocular
  albinism

XO genotype

x-radiation

x-ray
 x-r. chronic dermatitis
 x-r. dermatitis
 x-r. epilation
 x-r. ulcer

X-seb T

Xylocaine
 X. Viscous solution
 X. with Epinephrine

Xylohypha bantiana

xylol

XYY syndrome

Y

yabapox

YAG
  yttrium-aluminum-garnet
    YAG laser

Yatapoxvirus

yaw
  mother y.

yaws
  Bosch y.
  bush y.
  crab y.
  early y.
  foot y.
  forest y.
  guinea corn y.
  late y.
  mother y.
  ringworm y.
  tertiary y.

yeast
  y. extract
  y. form
  y. infection

Yeast-Gard
  Y.-G. Medicated Disposable
    Douche Premix solution
  Y.-G. Medicated Douche
  Y.-G. vaginal suppositories

yeastlike fungi

yellow
  y. albinism
  y. azo-benzene dye
  y. disease
  y. dye tartrazine
  y. fever
  y. hornet
  y. jacket
  y. jacket sting
  y. jaundice
  y. lesion
  y. mutant albinism
  y. nail
  y. nail syndrome
  y. oculocutaneous
    albinism
  y. pus
  y. skin

yellows

Yersinia
  Y. enterocolitica
  Y. pestis
  Y. pestis bite

Yersinieae

yperite

yttrium

Z

Zaditor

zafirlukast

Zahorsky's disease

zalcitabine

Zambesi ulcer

Zaufal's sign

ZDV
    zidovudine

Zeasorb-AF
    Z. Powder

Zefazone

Zeis' gland

zeisian stye

zeism

zeismus

Zerit (d4T)

Zetar
    Z. shampoo
    Z. Emulsion bath oil

Zetran injection

zidovudine (ZDV)

Zimmer Pulsavac wound
   debridement system

Zimmerman-Laband syndrome

Zinacef infection

zinc
    z. absorption
    z. acetate
    z. bacitracin
    z. caprylate
    z. carbonate
    z. chloride
    z. deficiency
    z. gelatin
    medicinal z. peroxide

zinc (*continued*)
    z. oxide
    z. oxide, cod liver oil, and
      talc
    z. shampoo
    z. stearate
    z. sulfate
    z. undecylenate
    white z.

zinciferous

Zincon
    Z. shampoo

Zinsser-Cole-Engman syndrome

ZIP
    zoster immune plasma

zirconium
    z. granuloma
    z. lactate
    z. salt preparations

zit

Zithromax

Zn
    zinc

ZNP Bar

zoacanthosis

Zolicef

zona
    z. coronae
    z. dermatica
    z. epithelioserosa
    z. facialis
    z. ignea
    z. ophthalmica
    z. serpiginosa

zonal type reaction

Zonalon
    Z. cream

zonary

zonate

zone
 grenz z.
 Head's z's
 z's of hyperalgesia
 z. of hyperemia
 hyperesthetic z.
 keratogenous z.
 z. of leukoderma
 papillary z.
 T z.
 vascular z.

zonesthesia

zoning

zoodermic

zoografting

Zoon
 Z's balanitis
 balanitis of Z.
 Z's balanitis
  plasmacellularis
 Z's disease
 Z's erythroplasia

zoonosis

zoonotic
 z. cutaneous leishmaniasis
 z. infection
 z. potential

zoophilic

zooplasty

zootoxin

ZORprin

zoster
 acute herpes z.
 z.-associated pain
 z. encephalomyelitis
 z. gangrenosus
 z. generalisatus

zoster (*continued*)
 z. hemorrhagicus
 herpes z. (HZ)
 z. immune globulin
 z. immune plasma (ZIP)
 z. mucosae
 ophthalmic z.
 z. ophthalmicus
 z. sine eruptione
 z. sine herpetic
 z. varicellosus

zosteriform
 z. distribution
 z. pattern

zosteroid

Zostrix
 Z. cream
 Z.-HP

Zosyn

Zovirax
 Z. injection
 Z. oral
 Z. topical

Z-plasty procedure

Zumbusch
 Z's disease
 generalized pustular
  psoriasis of von Z.
 Z's psoriasis

zygoma

Zygomycetes

zygomycosis

zygospore

zymosan

zymotic papilloma

Zyplast collagen

Drugs Used in Dermatology

Following are names of generic and R brand name drugs used in dermatology, as shown in the *Saunders Pharmaceutical Xref Book.* The drugs are categorized by their "indications"—also called "designated use," "approved use," or "therapeutic action"—which group drugs used for a similar purpose. The indications shown here are broad categories of therapeutic action. Individual drugs may be placed in subcategories or have specifically targeted diseases beyond the scope of this listing. For complete information about the drugs listed in this appendix, including each drug's availability, specific indications, forms of administration, and dosages, please consult the current edition of *Saunders Pharmaceutical Word Book.*

Acne Products, Systemic
Accutane
Achromycin V
cyproterone acetate
Diane-35 (CAN)
Dynacin
E-Base
E-Mycin
Ery-Tab
ERYC
erythromycin
erythromycin estolate
Estrostep 21
Gen-Cyproterone (CAN)
Ilosone
isotretinoin
Minocin
minocycline HCl
Not-Tet
Ortho Tri-Cyclen
Panmycin
PCE
PMS-Minocycline (CAN)
Rhoxal-minocycline (CAN)
Robimycin
Robite:
Sumycin
Sumycin '250'; Sumycin '500'
Teline; Teline-500
Tetracap
tetracycline HCl
Tetralan
Tetralan '250'; Tetralan-500
Vectrin
Acne Products, Topical
A/T/S
adapalene

Acne Products (*continued*)
Akne-mycin
Altinac
Atrisone
Avita
azelaic acid
Azetex
Benzac AC 2½; Benzac W 2½;
    Benzac 5; Benzac AC 5; Benzac W 5;
    Benzac 10; Benzac AC 10; Benzac
    W 10
Benzac AC Wash 2½; Benzac AC Wash
    5; Benzac W Wash 5; Benzac AC Wash
    10; Benzac W Wash 10
Benzaclin
5 Benzagel; 10 Benzagel
Benzagel Wash
Benzamycin
Benzashave
Benzox-10
benzoyl peroxide
Brevoxyl
Brevoxyl Cleansing
Brevoxyl Creamy Wash
C/T/S
Cleocin T
Clinda-Derm
clindamycin
clindamycin phosphate
Clindets
Dalacin T (CAN)
Del Aqua-5; Del Aqua-10
Del-Mycin
Desquam-E; Desquam-E 5; Desquam-E
    10
Desquam-X 5 Wash; Desquam-X 10
    Wash

481

Acne Products (*continued*)
Desquam-X 5; Desquam-X 10
Differin
Emgel
Erycette
EryDerm 2%
Erygel
Erymax
Erythra-Derm
erythromycin
Finevin
Hyacne
Klaron
Meclan
meclocycline sulfosalicylate
Novacet
Panoxyl
Panoxyl AQ 2½; Panoxyl 5; Panoxyl AQ 5; Panoxyl 10; Panoxyl AQ 10
Percxin A 5; Peroxin A 10
Persa-Gel; Persa-Gel W 5%; Persa-Gel W 10%
PROPApH Foaming Face Wash
pyrithione zinc
Rejuva-A (CAN)
Renova
Retin-A
Retin-A Micro
salicylic acid (SA)
Septi-Soft
Septisol
Staticin
Sulfacet-R
sulfacetarnide sodium
Sulfoxyl Regular; Sulfoxyl Strong
sulfur, precipitated
sulfur, sublimed
T-Stat
tazarotene
Tazorac
tetracycline HCl
Theramycin Z
Topicycline
tretinoin
Triaz
triclosan
Vanocin
Vanoxide-HC
Vitinoin (CAN)

Antibiotics, Topical
A/T/S
AK-Neo-Dex
Akne-mycin

Antibiotics (*continued*)
AK-Tracin
Ala-Quin
Atridox
bacitracin
bacitracin zinc
Bactroban
Bactroban Nasal
Benzaclin
Benzamycin
C/T/S
Castellani Paint Modified
chloramphenicol
chloramphenicol palmitate
chlorhexidine gluconate
chlortetracycline HCl
Cleocin T
Clinda-Derm
clindamycin phosphate
Clindets
clicquinol
Corque
Cortisporin
Cytolex
Dalacin T (CAN)
Del-Mycin
doxycycline hyclate
Elase-Chloromycetin
Emgel
Erycette
EryDerm 2%
Erygel
Erymax
Erythra-Derm
erythromycin
1+1-F Creme
fuchsin, basic
Fucidin (CAN)
Furacin
fusidate sodium
fusidic acid
G-myticin
Garamycin
gentamicin sulfate
Klaron
Locilex
mafenide
mafenide acetate
MetroCream
MetroGel; MetroLotion
mupirocin
mupirocin calcium
Myco-Bictic II

Antibiotics (*continued*)

Neo-Cortef
Neo-Dexair
Neo-Dexameth
NeoDecadron
neomycin sulfate
Neosporin G.U. Imigant
nitrofurazone
Noritate
Novacet
oxytetracycline HCl
Pedi-Cort V Creme
pexiganan acetate
polymyxin B sulfate
Protegrin
Sebizon
Silvadene
silver sulfadiazine (SSD)
SSD; SSD AF
Staticin
Storz-N-D
Sulfacet-R
sulfacetamide sodium
Sulfamylon
T-Stat
tetracycline HCl
Theramycin Z
Thermazene
Topicycline
Vanocin

Antifungals, Topical

Ala-Quin
amphotericin B
amphotericin B deoxycholate
amphotericin B lipid complex (ABLC)
Bensal HP
benzoic acid
betamethasone dipropionate &
   clotrimazole
butenafine HCl
Castellani Paint Modified
ciclopirox
ciclopirox olamine
clioquinol
clotrimazole (CLT)
clotrimazole & betamethasone
   dipropionate
Corque
econazole nitrate
Exelderm
Exsel
1+1-F Creme
fuchsin, basic

Antifungals (*continued*)

Fungizone
Fungoid
Fungoid-HC
gentian violet
haloprogin
Halotex
ketoconazole
Lamisil DermGel
Loprox
Lotrimin
Lotrisone
Mentax
miconazole nitrate
Monistat-Derm
Mycelex
Myco-Biotic II
Myco-Triacet II
Mycogen II
Mycolog-II
Myconel
Mycostatin
Mytrex
N.G.T.
naftifine HCl
Naftin
Nilstat
Nizoral
nystatin
Nystex
oxiconazole nitrate
Oxistat
Oxizole (CAN)
Pedi-Cott V Creme
Pedi-Dri
Penlac
resorcinol
selenium sulfide
Selsun
Spectazole
sulconazole nitrate
terbinafine HCl
tolnaftate
Tri-Statin II
undecylenic acid

Anti-hyperhidrotics

aluminum chloride
aluminum chlorohydrate
aluminum sulfate
Drysol
formaldehyde solution
Formalyde-10
Lazer Formalyde

Anti-inflammatory Agents

Aclovate
Acticort 100
Aeroseb-Dex
Aeroseb-HC
Ala-Cort
Ala-Quin
alclometasone dipropionate
Alphatrex
amcinonide
Aristocort
Aristocort A
Aristocort Intralesional
Aristospan Intralesional
Beta-Val
betamethasone benzoate
betamethasone dipropionate
betamethasone dipropionate &
   clotrimazole
betamethasone dipropionate, augmented
betamethasone sodium phosphate
betamethasone valerate
Betatrex
Capex
Carmol HC
Celestoderm-V; Celestoderm-V/2 (CAN)
Celestone Soluspan
Cetacort
clobetasol propionate
clocortolone pivalate
Cloderm
clotrimazole & betamethasone
   dipropionate
Cordran
Cordran SP
Cormax
Corque
Cort-Dome
Cortate (CAN)
cortisone acetate
Cortisporin
Cortone Acetate
Cutivate
Cyclocort
Dalalone
Dalalone L.A.
Decadron-LA
Decadron Phosphate
Decaject
Decaject-L.A.
Delta-Tritex
depMedalone 40; depMedalone 80
Depo-Medrol

Anti-inflammatory Agents (continued)

Depoject
Depopred-40; Depopred-80
Derma-Smoothe/FS
Dermacort
Dermatop
desonide
DesOwen
Desoxi (CAN)
desoximetasone
dexamethasone
dexamethasone acetate
dexamethasone sodium phosphate
Dexasone
Dexasone L.A.
Dexone
Dexone LA
diclofenac potassium
diflorasone diacetate
dimethyl sulfoxide (DMSO)
Diprolene
Diprolene AF
Diprosone
Duralone-40; Duralone-80
Elocom (CAN)
Elocon
Enzone
Epifoam
1+1-F Creme
Finevin
Florone
Florone E
fluocinolone acetonide
fluocinonide
Fluonex
Fluonid
flurandrenolide
Flurosyn
Flutex
fluticasone propionate
FS Shampoo
Fungoid HC
1% HC
halcinonide
halobetasol propionate
Halog
Halog-E
Hexadrol Phosphate
Hi-Cor 1.0; Hi-Cor 2.5
Hycort
Hydeltra-T.B.A.
HydroTex
Hydrocort

Anti-inflammatory Agents (*continued*)

hydrocortisone (HC)
hydrocortisone acetate (HCA)
hydrocortisone buteprate
hydrocortisone butyrate
hydrocortisone probutate
hydrocortisone valerate
Hydrocortisone Iodoquinol 1%
Hydrocortone Acetate
Hytone
Hytone 1%
Kemsol (CAN)
Kenaject-40
Kenalog
Kenalog-H
Kenalog-10; Kenalog-40
Kenonel
Kutapressin
LactiCare-HC
Lida-Mantle-HC
Lidex
Lidex-E
liver derivative complex
Locoid
Lotrisone
Luxiq
Lyderm (CAN)
M-Prednisol-40; M-Prednisol-80
Mantadil
Maxiflor
Maxivate
Medralone 40; Medralone 80
methylprednisolore acetate
mometasone furcate
Myco-Biotic II
Myco-Triacet II
Mycogen II
Mycolog-II
Myconel
Mytrex
N.G.T.
Nasonex
Neo-Cortef
NeoDecadron
Nutracort
Olux
orgotein
OxSODrol
Pandel
Pedi-Cort V Creme
Penecort
Pramosone
prednicarbate

Anti-inflammatory Agents (*continued*)

Prednisol TBA
prednisolone tebutate
Protopic
Psorcon E
S-T Cort
Solurex
Solurex LA
Synacort
Synalar
Synalar-HP
Synemol
Tac-3
tacrolimus
Teladar
Temovate
Temovate Emollient
Texacort
Topicort
Topicort LP
Tri-Kort
Tri-Statin II
Triacet
Triam-A
triamcinolone acetonide
triamcinolone diacetate
triamcinolone hexacetonide
Triamonide 40
Triderm
Tridesilon
Trilog
U-Cort
Ultravate
Valisone
Valisone Reduced Strength
Vanoxide-HC
ViaFoam
Vytone
Westcort
Zemaphyte
Zone-A Forte

Antiseptics

alcohol
benzalkonium chloride (BAC)
Castellani Paint Modified
chlorhexidine gluconate
chlorobutanol
chloroxylenol
Erygel
gentian violet
hexachlorophene
hexylresorcinol
ichthammol

Antiseptics (*continued*)
iodine
isopropyl alcohol
Lugol
Ovide
phenol
pHisoHex
potassium iodide
povidone-iodine
Septi-Soft
Septisol
Strong Iodine
thimerosal
Tinver
triclosan
Versiclear
Xerac AC

Corticosteroids, Systemic
A-Hydrocort
A-Methapred
ACTH
ACTH-80
Actbar
Adlone
Alti-Dexamethasone (CAN)
Amcort
Apo-Prednisone (CAN)
Aristocort
Aristocort Forte
Aristospan Intra-articular
Articulose-50
Articulose L.A.
Atolone
Betaject (CAN)
betamethasone
betamethasone acetate
betamethasone sodium phosphate
Cel-U-Jec
Celestone
Celestone Phosphate
Celestone Soluspan
Cortef
corticotropin
cortisone acetate
Cortone Acetate
Dalalone
Dalalone D.P.
Dalalone L.A.
Decadron
Decadron-LA
Decadron Phosphate
Decadron with Xylocaine
Decaject

Corticosteroids (*continued*)
Decaject-L.A.
Delta-Cortef
Deltasone
depMedalone 40; depMedalone 80
Depo-Medrol
Depoject
Depopred-40; Depopred-80
Dexameth
dexamethasone
dexamethasone acetate
dexamethasone sodium phosphate
Dexasone
Dexasone L.A.
Dexone
Dexone LA
Duralone-40; Duralone-80
Florinef Acetate
fludrocortisone acetate
H.P. Acthar Gel
Hexadrol
Hexadrol Phosphate
Hydeltra-T.B.A.
Hydeltrasol
hydrocortisone (HC)
hydrocortisone acetate (HCA)
hydrocortisone sodium phosphate
hydrocortisone sodium succinate
Hydrocortone
Hydrocortone Acetate
Hydrocortone Phosphate
Key-Fred 25; Key-Pred 50
Kenacort
Kenaject-40
Kenalog-10; Kenalog-40
Key-Pred-SP
Liquid Pred
M-Prednisol-40; M-Prednisol-80
Medralone 40; Medralone 80
Medrol
methylprednisolone
methylprednisolone acetate
methylprednisolone sodium phosphate
methylprednisolone sodium succinate
Meticorten
Orapred
Orasone
Panasol-S
Pediapred
PMS-Dexamethasone (CAN)
Predalone 50
Predcor-50
Prednicen-M

Corticosteroids (*continued*)
Prednisol TBA
prednisolone
prednisolone acetate
prednisolone sodium phosphate
prednisolone tebutate
prednisone
Prelone
Solu-Cortef
Solu-Medrol
Solurex
Solurex LA
Sterapred; Sterapred DS
Tac-3
Tac-40
Tri-Kort
Triam Forte
Triam-A
triamcinolone
triamcinolone acetonide
triamcinolone diacetate
triamcinolone hexacetonide
Triamolone 40
Triamonide 40
Trilog
Trilone
Tristoject

Depigmenting Agents
Alustra
Glyquin
hydroquinone
Lustra; Lustra-AF
Melanex
Melpaque HP
Melquin HP
Nuquin HP
Solaquin Forte
Viquin Forte

Dermatitis Herpetiformis Agents
dapsone

Emollients and Protectants
Accuzyme
allantoin
aloe
aluminum acetate
Alustra
ammonium lactate (lactic acid netralized
  with ammonium hydroxide)
ascorbic acid (L-ascorbic acid; vitamin C)
bismuth subnitrate
Carmol HC
cocoa butter
cod liver oil

Emollients and Protectants (*continued*)
colloidal oatmeal
Cosmederm-7 (CAN)
Derma-Smoothe/FS
dimethicone
glycerin
glycolic acid
Glyquin
Gordon's Urea 40%
Lac-Hydrin
lactic acid
Lactinol
Lactinol-E
lanolin
Lustra; Lustra-AF
mineral oil
Panafil
Panafil White
Papain Urea Chlorophyllin
Papain Urea Debriding
Peruvian balsam
petrolatum
propylene glycol
shark liver oil
silicone
urea
vitamin A
vitamin A palmitate
vitamin E
zinc oxide

Hair and Scalp Agents
Ala-Scalp
betamethasone valerate
Capitrol
chloroxine
coal tar
Drithocreme; Drithocreme HP 1%;
  Dritho-Scalp
eflomithine HCl
finasteride
ketoconazole
Luxiq
minoxidil
Nizoral
Ohix
phenol
povidone-iodine
Propecia
pyrithione zinc
Sal-Oil-T
salicylic acid (SA)
sulfur, precipitated
Vaniqa

Keratolytic Agents
Alustra
Bensal HP
Castellani Paint Modified
Emersal
Finevin
glycolic acid
Glyquin
Lustra; Lustra-AF
Mono-Chlor
monochloroacetic acid
resorcinol
salicylic acid (SA)
silver nitrate
Tinver
Tri-Chlor
trichloroacetic acid
Versiclear

Pholodamaged Skin Agents
Actinex
Altinac
5-aminolevulinic acid HCl (5-ALA HCl)
Avita
diclofenac potassium
Levulan Kerastick
masoprocol
Rejuva-A (CAN)
Renova
Retin-A
Retin-A Micro
Solage
Solaraze
tretinoin
Vitinoin (CAN)

Psoriasis Agents, Systemic
acitretin
Amevive
calcitriol (1,25-hydroxycholecalciferol;
　1,25-hydroxyvitamin D_3)
etretinate
Folex PFS
methotrexate (MTX)
methotrexate sodium
methoxsalen (8-methoxsalen)
Oxsoralen-Ultra
P-53
Rheumatrex
Rocaltrol
Soriatane
Tegison
Trexall

Psoriasis Agents, Topical
Anthra-Derm

Psoriasis Agents (*continued*)
anthralin
calcipotriene
coal tar
Dovonex
Drithocreme; Drithocreme HP 1%;
　Dritho-Scalp
Lasan
Lasan HP-1
maxacalcitol
mercury, ammoniated
methenamine sulfosalicylate
methoxsalen (8-methoxsalen)
MG217 Dual Treatment
Miconal
Prezios
Sal-Oil-T
salicylic acid (SA)
Unguentum Bossi
Zetar Emulsion

Rosacea Agents
MetroCream
MetroGel; MetroLotion
metronidazole
Noritate

Vitiligo Agents
Benoquin
methoxsalen (8-methoxsalen)
monobenzone
8-MOP
Oxsoralen
trioxsalen
Trisoralen

Wart and Corn Removers
Bichloracetic Acid
cantharidin
Condylox
dichloroacetic acid
DuoPlant
Gordofilm
Paplex Ultra
Podocon-25
podofilox
Podofin
podophyllum
podophyllum resin
salicylic acid (SA)
Verr-Canth
Verrex
Wartec[CAN]

Dermatological Preparations, Other
aminobenzoate potassium
Dermprotective Factor (DPF)

Dermatological (*continued*)
Glylorin
monolaurin
Potaba

SERPACWA (Skin Exposure Reduction
Paste Against Chemical Warfare Agents)
TopiCare